EIGHTH EDITION

Physical Education, Exercise and Sport Science

IN A CHANGING SOCIETY

William H. Freeman, PhD
Campbell University
Buies Creek, North Carolina

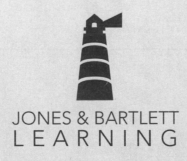

JONES & BARTLETT
LEARNING

World Headquarters
Jones & Bartlett Learning
5 Wall Street
Burlington, MA 01803
978-443-5000
info@jblearning.com
www.jblearning.com

Jones & Bartlett Learning books and products are available through most bookstores and online booksellers. To contact Jones & Bartlett Learning directly, call 800-832-0034, fax 978-443-8000, or visit our website, www.jblearning.com.

Production Credits

Executive Publisher: William Brottmiller
Publisher: Cathy L. Esperti
Acquisitions Editor: Ryan Angel
Senior Managing Editor: Maro Gartside
Editorial Assistant: Kayla Dos Santos
Associate Director of Production:
  Julie Champagne Bolduc
Production Assistant: Alyssa Lawrence
Senior Marketing Manager: Andrea DeFronzo

VP, Manufacturing and Inventory Control:
  Therese Connell
Composition: Laserwords Private Limited, Chennai, India
Cover Design: Michael O'Donnell
Photo Research and Permissions Coordinator:
  Amy Rathburn
Cover Image: © Photodisc/Thinkstock
Printing and Binding: Edwards Brothers Malloy
Cover Printing: Edwards Brothers Malloy

To order this product, use ISBN: 978-1-284-03408-0

Library of Congress Cataloging-in-Publication Data
Freeman, William Hardin, 1943- author.
  Physical education, exercise, and sport science in a changing society / by William H. Freeman. – Eighth edition.
    p. ; cm.
  Includes bibliographical references and index.
  ISBN 978-1-4496-9104-2 – ISBN 1-4496-9104-8
  I. Title.
  [DNLM: 1. Physical Education and Training–history. 2. Exercise. 3. Kinesiology, Applied. 4. Sports–history.
QT 11.1]
  GV211
  613.7'1–dc23
                                              2013023520

6048

Printed in the United States of America
17 16 15 14 13   10 9 8 7 6 5 4 3 2 1

For Ronald W. Hyatt
Professor, barbecue aficionado, and friend

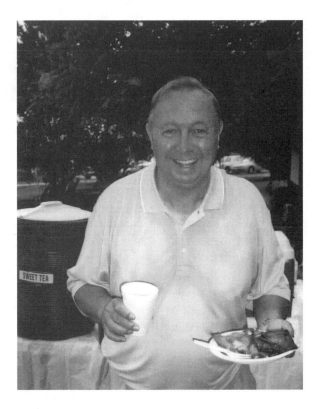

This *Eighth Edition* examines the disciplines and interests in the broad field of exercise science, including physical education, kinesiology, and sport as it is today. Although the book has gradually changed from the earlier editions, the foundational and philosophical concepts that underlie its structure remain the same.

This edition continues to expand its scope to the widening interests of the field, though it still heavily emphasizes the traditional focal field of physical education and sport. Our field is presented as a broad field that now includes three career areas: the professional (teaching), the discipline (scholarly), and the rapidly growing new professions (applied careers, such as sport management). Those three emphases are facets of the same broad interests and should not be antagonistic competitors. The core interest in physical activity draws us together, whatever our more specific professional or disciplinary interests may be.

Part 1 serves as an introduction by defining the field of exercise science and sport, and then overviews the disciplines that study the field's cultural, social, and scientific foundations. Part 2 surveys our cultural heritage, first with a broad overview of the history of exercise science and sport, and then by discussing in Part 3 the philosophical heritage and its application in the field, with a strong focus on ethical concerns. Part 4 examines career development and job options in the field, looking at the traditional field of teaching and coaching, the expanding career options outside the schools, and the new world of the technological workplace, along with an overview of the traits that lead to success in the field. Part 5 examines exercise science and sport in today's world, with chapters on comparative international programs, current issues, and our future directions.

Though their relative share of space in the text has changed, history and philosophy are presented as comprising the cornerstone of the study of exercise science and sport as a profession and as a discipline. I take this view because I believe that we can more easily find our directions for the future when we know our past in thought, word, and deed. The area of ethics and ethical problems is still treated as of critical importance, just as it was in the first edition three decades ago. Indeed, it is increasingly critical in a world that seems at times to have lost its direction. The function of the primary research disciplines is described in detail, but the depth of coverage is deliberately limited because most of those disciplines are studied in complete separate courses. This text emphasizes material that is rarely presented in other required courses.

The essential treatment of the concepts and issues presented is for the beginning student rather than for the upper-level student. The primary goal is to discuss the material in a clear and simplified manner, but the reader is encouraged to pursue the subjects to more scholarly levels. The reading lists that follow each chapter are suggested as a means of expanding your exposure to the work of specialists in those areas. The lists serve as a starting point for the interested student. They are *not* meant to be "approved" readings; they will give diverse and (at times) conflicting ideas that you should learn to examine critically.

Acknowledgments

I want to express my sincere appreciation to the people who had a formative influence on the existence of this book. Professor F. W. Clonts of Wake Forest University taught the broad view of the scope of history, combined with his requirement of clear, precise prose. Professor Betty F. McCue of the University of Oregon was an invaluable, supportive advisor and critic. Professor Bill Bowerman of Oregon, the 1972 United States Olympic Track Coach, provided critical experiences, an association of lasting value and meaning, and an example of commitment to the broad view of the university, of education, and of the development of the whole person.

My good friend, the late Professor Ron Hyatt of the University of North Carolina, shared many discussions on life and the progress of our field over barbecue and sweet tea. Jan Mintiens, Jenifer Haas, and Debora Ellis provided help and significant encouragement for the earlier editions. Jan Mintiens provided significant assistance during the editing process of this edition.

Professor Donna Woolard of Campbell University has been a significant sounding board for several revisions. The interest and confusion of my students at Campbell University for 20 years were also significant contributors.

I want to thank the reviewers of this manuscript for their helpful suggestions. I am most appreciative of the many teachers and students who have used the previous editions of this text. As always, comments from readers and teachers are welcomed.

PART 1

Defining Our Field

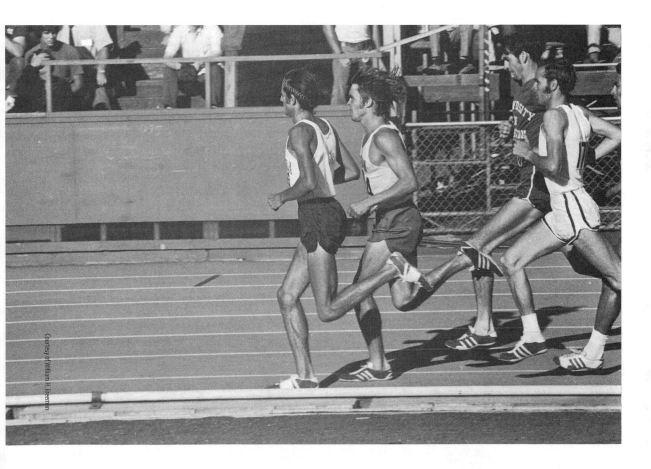

Courtesy of William H. Freeman

What Is Our Field?

"Our Field": A Term to Represent a Broad Range of Interests

Our field uses physical activity, primarily in the play and sport settings, to produce holistic improvements in a person's physical, mental, and emotional qualities. It treats each person as a unity, a whole being, rather than as having separate physical and mental qualities that bear no relation to and have no effect on each other. Our field is, in reality, a broad field of interests. Its core concern is the improvement of human movement. More specifically, it deals with the relationship between human movement and other areas of education—the relationship of the body's physical development to its mind and soul as they are being developed. This focus on the effect of physical development on other areas of human growth and development contributes to the uniquely broad scope of our field. No other single field is concerned with the total development of the human.

Many names are used to describe our field. From physical education to exercise science, from fitness to sport science, human performance, kinesiology, and many other titles, we find that our field is difficult to describe to others because we have no universally accepted single identifier. For that reason, in this text I will often simply use "our field" to represent the host of areas in which we work and study.

A survey in 1989 found more than 100 different titles used by college departments in our field, while another survey in 2010 found an increase in the number of terms used in departmental titles.[1] That is one reason many introductory textbooks, including this one, use multiple terms in their titles. While some of the terms represent narrower areas of study, most of them have large overlapping areas of concern.

The reason for this confusing state of affairs is discussed in this chapter. It identifies what people in our field study, how our field's component interests came to be, and the shades of difference from one title to another. As you will learn, this confusion of titles is not recent, even though some of the titles are relatively new. Even in the formative years of American physical education in the late 1800s many different titles were used for programs that had essentially the same focus.

Our field today has its sometimes unclear focus as a result of changes that began half a century ago in the core field of physical education. First, look at the changing motivations for human movement, and then the changing terms for human movement and the changing approaches to human movement.

Changing Motivations for Human Movement

Our field is interested in people's motivation for movement. Why do we exercise? Why do we take part in sport? From prehistoric times to today, we find changing motivations for human movement.

Survival Skills

Survival was the basic aim of education in primitive society—for both the individual and the group. The education of young males was primarily accomplished by physical means that were strongly oriented toward physical strength and cunning. Good hunting and fighting skills were necessary if early men were to feed themselves and their families and provide protection from outside forces.

Primitive education was concerned with learning in two areas: survival skills and conformity conduct.[2] Survival skills included the ability to defend oneself and others; the ability to provide food, clothing, and shelter; and the skills necessary to survive as an individual in the world.

Conformity Conduct

Conformity conduct was designed to ensure the survival of the group by putting the skills of the individual at the service of the group. People had to be able to work with others to meet the needs of the group, or the group would not survive. If the group did not survive, then humans might eventually become extinct.

Fitness and Heath

As society advanced and basic survival was no longer the greatest concern, people gradually realized that movement and physical activity affected their health and fitness. That awareness appeared in early large cultures, but we are most aware of it in the ancient Greeks, with their concept of "a sound mind in a sound body."

As we move toward modern times, the growing awareness of the impact of movement and fitness on health affected developing theories of education. By the Renaissance, some schools were beginning to realize that unhealthy students were less able to learn, so they began to add physical activity to their curriculum.

Sport and Pleasurable Movement

As children, we learn that movement itself is pleasurable. As we get older and our skills advance, we find the simple pleasure of sporting movement. We learn the pleasure of controlling our bodies to improve our performances, yet there is a simple joy in the movement itself, the doing. Too often our field has overlooked or downplayed pleasure as a motivation or reward for movement and sport.[3]

Gregg Twietmeyer argues that

> *Kinesiology is, in an important sense, an evangelical profession; a profession which must be willing to proudly profess the joys of moving well, for those joys are learned. The degree to which pleasure and intrinsic satisfaction are found in kinesiology depends on how well we steward our inheritance.*[4]

His comments are an outgrowth of the argument made by Klaus Meier more than 30 years ago that "Anything worth doing is worth doing badly."[5] Pleasure does not necessarily require skill.

Changing Terms for Human Movement

Our field has been known by many other labels in the past. Most of them are now considered too narrow and exclusive to express the full scope of the field.

Gymnastics

Gymnastics was the earliest of those titles. During the 1800s, *gymnastics* referred to exercises or activities that took place in a gymnasium, rather than to the activities that today are part of that particular sport. The term was very popular with European programs, but in the United States it was used for only one phase of the total physical education program. Today, because its meaning is limited, the term usually includes an explanatory subtitle, such as Olympic gymnastics or corrective gymnastics.

Hygiene and Health

Hygiene, another popular term of the 1800s, referred to the science of preserving people's health. Its definition is similar to today's health education programs, which developed around 1900 when state legislatures passed laws requiring the teaching of basic health practices. Many of the early leaders in American physical education were physicians concerned with improving the overall health of students.

Exercise and Fitness

Physical culture, a popular term during the late 1800s, was often used with the term *physical training* to sell programs of personal health. Today, in the United States, physical training refers exclusively to conditioning exercises and programs—education only of the physical. The term is still commonly used to describe programs in the armed services, but it is a far too narrow concept of physical education to be used by today's educators.

Physical Education

Daryl Siedentop argues that "there is probably less agreement today on the basic meaning of physical education than there has been at any time in our professional history." However, he notes that the most widely accepted model is the "developmental" model, "education through the physical," which came from the progressive education movement in the first half of the twentieth century and emphasized fitness, skill, knowledge, and social development.[6] The model can be rephrased in this way: Physical education is education of, about, and through the physical.

One of the most lasting definitions for physical education was written by Jesse Feiring Williams: "Physical education is the sum of man's physical activities selected as to kind, and conducted as to outcomes."[7] He explains his definition by debating whether educating only the physical aspect of the body is sufficient to define the field:

> *When mind and body were thought of as two separate entities, physical education was obviously an education of the physical . . . with new understanding of the nature of the human organism in which wholeness of the individual is the outstanding fact, physical education becomes education through the physical. With this view operative, physical education has concern for and with emotional responses, personal relationships, group behaviors, mental learnings, and other intellectual, social, emotional, and esthetic outcomes.*[8]

Williams stresses the point that even though physical education teaches using physical means through physical activities, its goal goes beyond the physical. It seeks to influence all areas of educational development, including the mental and social growth of the student. While the body is being improved physically, the mind should be learning and expanding, and there also should be social development, such as learning to work with others.

The basic points that define the field are named consistently by different scholars:

1. Physical education is conducted through physical means; that is, some sort of physical activity or some type of movement is involved.
2. Physical activity is usually (though not always) moderately vigorous, it is concerned with gross motor movements, and the skills involved do not have to be very finely developed or of high quality for benefits to be gained.
3. Although the student gains these benefits by a physical process, the educational benefits for the student include improvements in non-physical areas, such as intellectual, social, and aesthetic growth, that is, the cognitive and affective domains.

In summary, the meaning is clear: Physical education uses physical means to develop each person's whole being. This is a characteristic that physical education shares with no other area of education. Because the educational results of the physical experience are not limited to the physical or body-improving benefits, the definition does not refer solely to the traditional meaning of physical activity. We must view the term *physical* on a broader, more abstract plane, as a condition of mind as well as body. Indeed, this physical education should bring about improvements "in mind and body" that affect all aspects of the person's daily living, and the whole person should benefit by the experience. This mind–body holistic approach includes an emphasis on all three educational domains: the psychomotor, the cognitive, and the affective. Indeed, Robert Gensemer refers to "the body as a place for the mind."[9]

Sport

In defining physical education, we must also consider its relationship to play and sport. Many scholars have studied play and its implications for our well-being. Many of their studies consider sport and physical education to be one and the same, but play, sport, and physical education are three different, yet overlapping, entities.

Play is essentially activity used as amusement. We think of play as non-competitive physical amusement, although play does not have to be physical. Play is not necessarily sport or physical education, even though elements of play may be found in both.

Sport is an organized, competitive form of play. Some people view sport simply as an organized form of play, which might put it closer to physical education as we have defined it. However, careful examination shows that sport traditionally involves competitive activities.

When we refer to sport as "organized" competitive activity, we mean that the activity has been refined and formalized to some degree—that is, some definite form or process is involved. Rules, whether they are written or not, are used in the activity, and those rules or procedures cannot be changed during the competition, although new rules may evolve from one episode to the next.

Sport is, above all, a competitive activity. We cannot think of sport without thinking of competition, for without the competition, sport becomes simply play or recreation. Play can at times be sport, but strictly speaking, sport is never simply play; the competitive aspect is essential to its nature.

Physical education has elements of both play and sport, but it is not exclusively either, nor is it a balanced combination of the two. As its title indicates, physical education is physical activity with an educational goal. It is physical and it seeks to educate, but neither play nor sport, even though both can be used in the educational process, always includes the educational aspect of the physical experience as a vital aim.

Play, sport, and physical education involve forms of movement, and all three can fit within the context of education if they are used for some educational purpose. Play can be relaxing and entertaining without any educational aim, just as sport can exist for its own sake without any educational aim. For example, professional sports (some people prefer the term *athletics*) have no educational goals, yet we still consider them to be sport. An activity does not need to be amateur to be considered sport. Sport and play can exist purely for pleasure, purely for education, or for any combination of the two. Pleasure and education are not mutually exclusive; they can and should coexist.

Allied Areas: Health Education, Recreation, and Dance

Our definition of physical education is concerned with the development or education of each person, both of their physical body and through physical means. To complete the description of this very broad concept, three areas allied to the field of physical education and sport must be introduced: health education, recreation, and dance.

Health Education

The old concept of health education has become more comprehensive over the last several decades. When we speak of health education, we use it most often in the sense of the total health-related fitness of the person: physical, mental, emotional, and social. The old model had three subareas: health instruction, health services, and health environment.

Today the Centers for Disease Control and Prevention's National Center for Chronic Disease Prevention and Health Promotion promotes a model that it calls a coordinated school health program (CSHP).[10] The CSHP model has eight components:

1. *Health education.* A K–12 school curriculum to address "the physical, mental, emotional, and social dimensions of health."
2. *Physical education.* A K–12 school curriculum "that provides cognitive content and learning experiences in a variety of activity areas. . . . Quality physical education should promote . . . each student's optimum physical, mental, emotional, and social development."
3. *Health services.* Services that "appraise, protect, and promote health."
4. *Nutritional services.* "Access to a variety of nutritious and appealing meals that accommodate the health and nutritional needs of all students."
5. *Counseling and psychological services.* Services "to improve students' mental, emotional, and social health."
6. *Healthy school environment.* "The physical and aesthetic surroundings and the psychosocial climate and culture of the school."
7. *Health promotion for staff.* Improvement of staff health should improve the staff's commitment to student health and their ability to serve as role models.
8. *Family and community involvement.* Involves the school, parents, and community together; uses community resources and services to meet health-related needs.

Recreation

We generally think of recreation as leisure-time activity. However, recreation can fulfill Jay B. Nash's earlier educational goal of "the worthy use of leisure."[11] In that view, activities are selected by the individual to serve a constructive nature, and they are not so much time consuming as time using. These activities are physically, mentally, and socially healthful.

Nash describes recreation as a complement to work and, therefore, a need of all individuals. The emphasis of recreation in this sense is the "re-creation" of the person, the revitalization of body and mind that results from getting away from the stressful things in life. Like physical education, recreation is a broad and rapidly growing field. The growth of park programs across the country led to an expansion of outdoor education and related activities. The educational base of recreation also has been broadened by the need to educate people in how to use their leisure time.

Dance

Dance does not have a large number of professionals, but it is quite large in terms of the popularity of its activities for people of all ages. Dance has been something of a stepchild of physical education because it hangs on the periphery of the field.

Although dance activities can definitely be a part of physical education, dance itself is strongly identified with the arts. Possibly, dance came into the realm of physical education as a natural result of its body movement orientation. Perhaps this bit of the arts can do much to temper the sometimes excessively athletic orientation of physical education with the aesthetics of art. However, most dance programs have now joined fine arts and performance arts programs.

Changing Focuses of Human Movement Studies

The focus of our field has varied over time. A brief look at the changes in focus, roughly in chronological order, shows that although the focus changes, there is still a constant underlying recognition of the value of human movement and exercise.

Health Focus

The first focus of our field was health, in particular, children's health. As discussed elsewhere in this text, physical activities were used even in ancient times to improve health and fitness. During the Renaissance, wealthier parents realized that their children's health was affected by a lack of exercise. The early programs of physical education were focused on improving health and developing social physical skills.

Education Focus

Eventually, educators realized that poor health and fitness was a major factor in students' poor academic performance. By the late 1700s, early private schools in Europe were adding physical activity as a way to improve student health, resulting in improved classroom performance.

Fitness Focus

By the late 1800s, the focus of physical education was increasingly on physical fitness. Though the underlying reason for that focus was the effect that it had on student learning, teachers were increasingly aware of the importance of fitness on long-term health.

Sport Focus

By the 1920s, sport had become a major factor in physical education programs. The reason for the change from educational gymnastics and calisthenics to sports

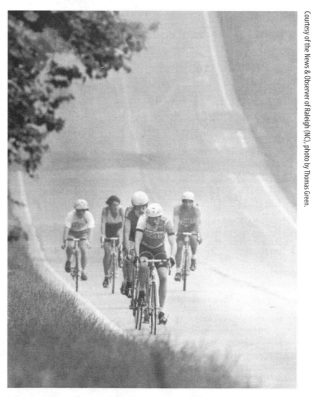

Courtesy of the News & Observer of Raleigh (NC), photo by Thomas Green.

The move of services from the public to the private sector limits many recreational opportunities to people with higher incomes.

was very simple: Students were more likely to benefit from the programs because they were more fun.

Lifetime Fitness and Wellness Focus

By the 1970s, the focus on popular competitive sports began to give way first to a lifetime fitness focus, and then to a lifetime wellness focus. Lifetime fitness still had a sport emphasis, but it shifted from the most popular competitive sports to sports that people could enjoy throughout their lifetime, such as tennis and swimming, rather than football.

The lifetime wellness focus was a shift from developing high-level fitness and sports skills to a focus on wellness for a healthy life. This meant a focus on levels of basic fitness through moderate exercise that would benefit even people of lower skill or fitness levels, resulting in a longer life span and fewer health problems during their lifetime.

Holism: The Unity of Mind and Body

One of the difficult questions over the ages has been the philosophical clash between the intellectual and the physical. A common belief is that the mind and the body are separate, with an emphasis on either one or the other. In most cases, this belief, called dualism, leads to a preference for the mind and a belief that physical activities are inferior to mental activities. We see this idea in the medieval Church, with its growing belief in the evil nature of the body. Because the body was considered evil, acts that the body enjoyed were discouraged. Even today we see this belief in the idea of the superiority (and separation) of mind over body.

The contrary philosophy is monism, a belief in the unity of mind and body. We trace the heritage of this idea to the ancient Athenians, with the concept of "a sound mind in a sound body." That motto is often considered an ideal statement of the goal of traditional physical education: the use of physical activities to develop all aspects of the person—mind, body, and spirit. It is consistent with Earle Zeigler's argument that the real focus of our field is developmental physical activities, rather than physical activity alone. There is a goal of developing the person in many ways.[12]

However, the real question is not whether we believe in a holistic concept; the question is whether that concept is now dominant in our society, or even in our field. In society, dualism still rules, even though our field stresses monism. Physical education programs are downsized or removed because physical classes are considered inferior to intellectual classes. The belief in the value of using physical means to develop the whole person has not captured the public imagination. Indeed, there is some question regarding whether the holistic concept is dominant even in the practices of our field. Too often people reject healthful activities by citing the lack of value or balance in their school's physical education classes. This difference between what we teach and what we do is a thorn in the side of the field of physical education.

Developing a Field: From Education to Science to Medicine

For the first roughly 80 years from the founding of American Alliance for Health, Physical Education, Recreation and Dance (AAHPERD) the field was physical education, and we were concerned primarily with teaching and coaching physical activity.[13] The original impetus for the teaching was the improvement of student health for the purpose of improved learning capabilities in the academic sphere. Many of the early leaders of AAHPERD were medical doctors, though medical education was more limited than it is for today's physicians.

By the 1960s, our field was suffering from decades of a feeling of academic inferiority. Professors at the growing research institutions feared that they were not sufficiently respected because they suffered the indignity that brought horror to research institutions—they were practitioners. Rather than focus on theoretical knowledge, they actually taught people to do things. The more practical or applied a field is, the more suspect it is to research university professors.

What was "physical education" has expanded massively in the last half century. Little side areas of interest became specialties, and then subdisciplines. Too often we stated our "area of focus" arguments too narrowly. Most fields do not change their names. The sad reality was that the primary problem with the name "physical education" was a long history of too many lazy teachers negatively affecting too many generations of students.

The discipline movement arose from the influence of concerned faculty at research institutions. Their expressed concern was that physical education "got no respect" because it was not sufficiently scholarly. It was not known for serious, rigorous research that expanded the bounds of knowledge. While we can successfully argue that a significant portion of the faculty's concern grew from a fear of seeming unimportant in their home institutions, still there was a solid core of truth to the charge. As an adjunct to Schools of Education, whose academic standards were traditionally among the lowest in most universities, the limited research that was done was usually applied studies aimed at solving particular (often small) practical problems.

This concern of research university faculty led to three things happening, each leading to the next:

1. Franklin Henry wrote a seminal article (taken from an earlier presentation) calling for the development of an academic discipline of physical education.[14]
2. In 1989, the American Academy of Physical Education recommended that the new discipline be called "kinesiology." The group renamed itself the American Academy of Kinesiology and Physical Education.
3. In 1990, a series of papers was produced and published in *Quest* arguing that kinesiology was the best name for our field, just because, and creating a field for it almost from the whole cloth.[15] This was received with enthusiasm primarily at research universities.

In that call for kinesiology as the name for our field, Karl Newell defined kinesiology as "the study of movement or, more generally, the study of physical activity."[16] We need to remember that this argument is based on kinesiology as the name at the college level rather than at every level of application. In fact, it is largely a creature of the largest research-focused universities. We can understand some of the reason behind this drive toward acceptance of the new name by a comment made while arguing the new name's value: "The word kinesiology in its present broad sense is an appropriate image that serves to market our field of study."[17] As Larry Locke put it,

> *I now will embarrass us all by noticing what we are really talking about. This program* [on The Evolving Undergraduate Major] *is about power and turf. It is about who will control the undergraduate major, not about what is in it or its present state of evolution. This program is about who will teach it and which students will be required to take it. . . . The disciplinarians still covet those captive, credit-bearing clients [teacher education majors] who still constitute the largest single population of undergraduate students passing through most of our schools.*[18]

A decade later, after listening to discussions of the future of the field in higher education, Locke remarked that

> *almost all of [this] discussion reflects the particular contexts of Research I and Research II universities. Whether lessons about prospering in those environments can safely be generalized to institutions in the other eight Carnegie categories is still unclear. The majority of kinesiology and physical education programs in North America are not in colleges or universities with research as a primary mission. Thus, in contemplating our professional and academic colleagues' good counsel, we should remember just how narrow and really peculiar the experiences behind these analyses and consequent advice have been.*[19]

The supporters of kinesiology argue that it is a superset of the discipline—a field of study, rather than a discipline. Or, as Waneen Spirduso writes, "a cross-disciplinary field of study rather than an academic discipline, strictly defined." As she emphasizes the value of the focus on studying physical activity, she argues that it "really is the common denominator of sport, exercise, ergonomics, biomechanics and all the other activities that kinesiologists study."[20]

Charles Corbin argues that "becoming a field is more than saying we are one."[21] He uses Myron Lieberman's characteristics of a profession to "provide a basis for developing criteria for establishing a field." Corbin states that a field must have the following:

1. A discipline (unique subject matter) that uses intellectual techniques
2. Disciplinarians with long training in the unique subject matter and its intellectual techniques, who should be dedicated to research that contributes to preparing professionals in the field and providing the field's social service

3. A subject matter related to the delivery of a social service (professional education)
4. Professionals with long training in the disciplinary and professional subject matter
5. A clarified code of ethics and an organization or organizations that govern the field and enforce the code
6. Agencies dedicated to preparing disciplinarians and professionals who have studied all types of knowledge and are dedicated to the field and the social service it provides
7. A clientele that needs and demands the field's services

Corbin argues that we are a discipline, but not yet a field. He says that we need more than simply an organization; we need to commit to the field's common goals.

This approach is similar to an earlier recommendation by Earle Zeigler when he described physical education as going through stages of being a multidiscipline, a cross discipline, and finally an interdiscipline as the subdisciplines begin to interact once again. He called for

> *a recognizable state of reunification within what we presently call the field of sport and physical education. We do need a new name, but it should be a name that reflects both the disciplinary and the professional aspects of our work. . . . We simply must figure out ways and means of unifying the various aspects of our own quasi-profession/quasi-discipline to at least a reasonable degree.*[22]

At the same time, some scholars questioned the value of the discipline movement. As Lawrence Locke points out and Elizabeth Bressan emphasizes, we did not develop disciplines—we simply declared that they are present. Locke says that disciplines do not appear by being declared or "proven." "They are created by the labor of inquiry, the accumulation of knowledge and theory, the fortunes of social recognition, and the accidents of history."[23]

Elizabeth Bressan writes that young scholars in the disciplines are, in fact, trained in the language and bases of fields other than physical education, so that

> *there is no real community of scholars who study physical education, or human movement or sport or whatever particular delineation of content upon which we might settle. A sound disciplinary structure is supposed to promote such communal identity and effort.*[24]

Jan Broekhoef suggests that a discipline is not as necessary as we originally believed:

> *The assumption . . . is that persons who have mastered the formal content of the academic discipline will be better prepared to teach than those who possess only professional and applied knowledge.* Unfortunately, there is no evidence to support such an assumption *[my emphasis]. . . . Theory and practice should stand in a reciprocal relationship.*[25]

Broekhoef argues that because the field is concerned with educating people, there is a need to place the disciplines into an educational context so they will contribute to the role of physical educators. He notes the weakness of a theory-based program that is not rooted in practice, saying: "I should like to throw in a Latin phrase of my own: *Primum vivere, deinde philosophari.* Freely translated this means that people have to live first before they can philosophize."[26] In other words, theory must be grounded in practice. His point is reinforced by Joan Vickers, who points out the problems caused by our trying to teach methods without having first taught an underlying basis of skills (or applied experience).[27]

Christopher Hopper joins in the call for increased emphasis on the professional side, arguing that "the emphasis in academic and research-related areas of knowledge and the neglect of personal competency in activities is leaving the prospective teacher inadequately prepared to offer a variety of physical education experiences to children and adults." He suggests a return to "pedagogical commitment," adding that "such a mission would facilitate the integration of knowledge from research to practice."[28] This integration of the theoretical with the practical is a critical mix because "the reflective physical educator, with an adequate knowledge base, is a better teacher than a non-reflective highly skilled one."[29]

This call for a return to the original mission of physical education—the concern for helping others in areas related to health and for teaching physical activities—has been increasingly echoed in the field, as it was in 1940 in C. H. McCloy's article of challenge and complaint, "How About Some Muscle?"[30] Indeed, we need to remember Charles Poskanzer's remark that

> *Having agonized for years over the proper title for my own academic department . . . I have come to an inescapable conclusion. Academic respectability is acquired and maintained through intellectual honesty and professional integrity. The name matters not, and the label is unimportant. The ingredients are the important things. It's the substance, not the style, that counts.*[31]

Physical Education: Developing a Profession

For many years physical educators have spoken of themselves as members of a profession: teaching. In 1915 Abraham Flexner suggested a set of criteria for professional status. His criteria are still the most commonly accepted in the field. Flexner described six characteristics that determine whether a field really is a profession:[32]

1. Intellectual activity (a "body of knowledge")
2. Practical use
3. Research resulting in new knowledge and ideas
4. Self-organization
5. Capacity for communication (internal and external)
6. Dedication to helping others (altruism and service)

First, a profession's activities are intellectual. Physical skills may be involved in performing the work, but the work must have an intellectual base, or "body of knowledge." The intellectual nature of the field must be one of the most important aspects of the work, rather than the physical or other skills used to apply the knowledge. This is the area where physical education has been most criticized by outsiders.

Second, a profession's work must be practical. It must have a genuine use. Even though it is based on knowledge, that knowledge has no value unless it is applied. Most physical educators agree that physical education has an intellectual base, and every physical educator will agree that the work is practical. The knowledge is applied to develop and improve people's fitness, skills, and health.

Third, a profession is concerned with research that results in new knowledge and ideas, which are then tested and applied in the professional work. This characteristic certainly is true of physical education, although some educators are dissatisfied with the limited amount of research and the tendency to experiment only in the most narrowly practical areas. Some critics argue that physical educators and coaches are the most resistant of all groups to change, even when research has shown that the changes are needed.

Fourth, a profession has a formal organization. Examples in physical education are the numerous professional groups, such as AAHPERD and the American College of Sports Medicine (ACSM). Organization is closely related to the fifth characteristic, the capacity for communication.

Fifth, a profession has formal means of communication among its members, not only to enable them to work together to solve common problems but also to distribute information. AAHPERD is the largest group that assists physical educators in meeting those communication requirements. It holds regular meetings at the state, district, and national levels and also sponsors many publications. The ACSM has a large annual convention and also sponsors publications.

Sixth, a profession practices altruism and service. That is, the members of the profession are dedicated to helping others. A profession shows concern for people's welfare, and it exists (at least in part) to help improve or protect others' lives. Few people would disagree that this characteristic applies to teaching.

Most physical educators consider their field a profession. It does meet all of Flexner's criteria to some degree, though some may disagree about the importance given to some of the criteria. However, 2 decades after Charles A. Bucher argued that physical education was not a fully matured profession but instead was an emerging one, Robert Gensemer echoed Bucher with his description of the field as "an emergent profession."[33]

Do people see physical educators as rendering a "unique and essential social service," one that could not be rendered by a non-professional? Some people believe physical educators are doing a job that most well-coordinated people could do. Are physical educators selective about the people admitted to the field? Research consistently indicates that the students majoring in the teacher preparation programs in our colleges rank low in intelligence and academic training among our nation's college students and that certification and licensure requirements sometimes vary so widely as to be almost meaningless. Are "rigorous training programs" provided for future members? There also are many doubts in this area. Finally, is physical education "self-regulatory"? Are unethical or ill-prepared members dealt with within the field? This has rarely been the case.

Bucher and Gensemer suggest, rightly, that physical education has not yet earned the full status of a profession but is still emerging. Though some educators argue that it has spent a long time emerging, its basic shortcomings as a profession are clear. Although physical education's goals equal the characteristics of a profession, its public status has not yet risen to that level. That is still a critical task for today's physical educators.

In the past, physical education was considered an applied field, one in which practical skills were gained through personal experience and then applied in teaching and coaching in the school setting. When the discipline movement grew in the 1960s and 1970s and advanced a more scholarly, research-based emphasis, that emphasis was largely defined as sport, though it was sometimes broadened to the less sport-centered term *movement*.

In the 1990s and with a shift toward a redefined kinesiology as the scholarly focus of a broader, more unified field of study, the idea of a research-focused subdiscipline of sport pedagogy has grown. During the early years of developing a discipline, many subdisciplines were proposed, debated, and justified, such as sport biomechanics or sport history. However, not every proposed subdiscipline found widespread acceptance.

A section on "The Academic Foundations of Exercise Science and Kinesiology," includes an overview of the subdiscipline of sport pedagogy. At this point, I simply want to emphasize the importance of physical education and sport pedagogy as a legitimate subject for scholarly study. The distinction between the two terms is that *physical education* traditionally refers only to school-related activities (though this book prefers a much broader definition), and sport pedagogy "is a broad field concerned with the content, processes, and outcomes of sport, fitness, and physical education programs in schools, community programs, and clubs."[34] Perhaps *movement pedagogy* would be a more accurate name for the subdiscipline. In short, movement pedagogy studies the organized teaching or learning related to human movement, regardless of where the activity takes place.

One factor in the development of a more scholarly focus in physical education was the Holmes Group report, which recommended a greater academic focus for all teacher education programs.[35] In a sense, it shone a light on weaknesses in the scholarly underpinnings of teacher education programs. Many state legislatures began to strengthen academic requirements for teacher education, and professional groups reacted by developing plans to raise their professional status with more academically oriented requirements. However, the legislatures have resisted the Holmes Group proposal to make teacher education a 5-year program, a proposal that was also recommended in the 1950s and 1960s.

Don Hellison points out that as the emphasis on scholarly research in physical education has increased since the mid-1960s, a consistent thread of whole-person emphasis is visible. The result is that "the personal and social development claims of the past have begun to be clarified and validated."[36] He adds that the more successful research approaches have been encouraged by this new emphasis on research. Hellison argues that the field is benefiting from the growth in scholarly research, in part because research is both establishing the value of educating through movement and showing us how to achieve the teaching outcomes that are our goal. As this chapter argues, those educational benefits are holistic, rather than just physical.

Scholarly research enables us to learn more about the effectiveness of modes of instruction to discover whether we can get the outcomes that we desire from the educational process. At the same time, new research is proving the value of the work done by physical educators. The original impetus for the formation of physical education programs was to improve the health of students, leading to improved scholarship on their part. Those holistic goals still exist, including the physiological benefits of physical activity, the socialization potential, the behavioral effects, and the original goal of better health.

Now scholars are closely examining the importance and role of physical education in achieving basic health objectives and in terms of the national educational strategy, Goals 2000: Educate America Act. Such research evaluates the impact on adults as well as schoolchildren. It is critical because we fear that American youth are losing the core of fitness and health that they once had. Even so, the standard was not a high one. The critical value of physical education in the schools and for the development of people as children, and even in old age, has never been more important than it is today.[37]

The Call for a Discipline of Physical Education

Scholars spent decades debating the status of physical education: Is it a profession or a discipline? Where does it fit in the academic scheme? However, our field has many dimensions. One of them is a body of knowledge, which is required by a discipline, and another centers on the field as a profession. To determine the status of the field, we must understand exactly what a profession and a discipline are, and then see whether our field has the characteristics of either one. However, a field does not have to be only a discipline or a profession.

When Franklin M. Henry called for a discipline of physical education in the 1960s, he envisioned it as a field with a broad concern, drawing from the expertise and methods of a range of outside disciplines—not just as a science, but as a field in the broader category of "arts and sciences," the study of all aspects of skilled human movement.[38]

What he got was something quite different. As different areas of interest became organized as subdisciplines, adding rigor to their research and focusing inward on their singular concerns, the pendulum began to swing toward a scientific field, rather than a broad one. Though these processes were happening in both the United

States and Canada, their driving forces were not the same. In Canada the move toward professionalizing sport to produce *high performance* success (such as at the Olympic Games) required administrators and sport scientists to operate the program. The knowledge of volunteers was not sufficient to gain success on the world stage. Many of the Canadian specialists did graduate work in the United States, where they encountered the other driving force: status in the research universities.

I defined a discipline as an area of knowledge and theory that can exist purely for itself with no need to show that it has a practical application. The interest in that side of the field began to develop in the mid-1960s, promoted by Franklin M. Henry's definition. The result was a flurry of discussion about whether physical education was a discipline, whether it had the required focus of attention and particular mode of inquiry. The question of whether physical education could demonstrate a body of knowledge caused particular concern.

Daryl Siedentop discussed the idea of a discipline by describing it as "value-free" because it tries to study "what is" rather than "what should be." He suggested that the difference between a discipline and a profession could be summarized by the idea that "a discipline describes while a profession prescribes."[39] A discipline avoids bias in research. On the other hand, a profession tries to solve a specific problem and must therefore study a specific group, which results in a biased study and results.

The interest in a discipline centered around Franklin Henry's 1964 article and its implications. While scholars tried to define a discipline and its area of study, AAHPER (as it was known then) worked to demonstrate the field's "body of knowledge." At the same time, scholars in the Big Ten Conference schools organized a series of annual conferences to discuss the different newly emerging disciplines or subdisciplines in sport studies. Meanwhile, the American Academy of Physical Education debated whether a new name was needed for physical education, one that would better demonstrate the true focus of its study.

In the years since Henry's article first appeared and spurred interest in developing a discipline, many changes in direction have affected our broad field. The first notable change was the split between groups focused on the profession and those focused on developing the discipline. Many conflicts seem to match physical education against exercise and sport science, "teachers" against "researchers." The more practical appearance of the profession side of studies has created problems for those interested in the discipline or research side because each group sometimes questions the other's validity or importance.

In truth, both groups contribute to our field in important ways. Their conflicts often seem to be little more than arguments over differing points of view, though often the real argument has been political rather than theoretical, a struggle for power or funding. However, the scholarly side of physical education is far more prominent today than it was then.

A second notable change has been the appearance of new professional societies representing the subdisciplines and their scholarly focuses of interest.

Those new groups have promoted scholarship in their areas by initiating national conferences and by publishing journals that offer more scholarly and specific outlets of research than those provided by the older organizations of physical education. By the late 1970s, AAHPERD recognized the growth of the scholarly interests and started discipline-focused academies within its own professional structure.

A third change in the direction of the field that has become evident over the last several decades is the great burst of scholarly research and writing. That growth of scholarship has been invaluable in revitalizing our field and presenting it to the outside world as an academically respectable field.

Our Field as a Discipline

The difference between a discipline and a profession can be confusing because a field can be a discipline, while its practitioners can be members of a profession. In essence, a discipline is an area of knowledge and theory that can exist purely for itself, but a profession must have a practical application. We have shown that our field has practical uses (such as developing people's fitness and health) and thus can be considered a profession. What, then, is necessary for the field to be considered a discipline? Franklin Henry defines an academic discipline as an organized body of knowledge collectively embraced in a formal course of learning. The acquisition of such knowledge is assumed to be an adequate and worthy objective as such, without any demonstration or requirement of practical application. The content is theoretical and scholarly as distinguished from technical and professional.[40]

Henry's definition (a synthesis of several other definitions of a discipline) makes it clear that to be considered a discipline, our field must have a "body of knowledge," that is, it must focus on some specific scholarly knowledge. Is this the case with our field? Henry and many others believe that it is.

We can think of a discipline as an area of basic science concerned with the discovery of new knowledge but not really obligated to find any use for that knowledge or to apply it in any way. The primary object of a discipline is to gain knowledge, while in a profession it is to apply that knowledge in a way that serves others.

Gerald S. Kenyon suggests that three criteria are necessary for a field to be a discipline:

1. A focus of attention
2. A unique body of knowledge
3. A particular mode of inquiry (research method)

Many authors suggest that the focus of attention of physical education as a discipline is the human movement phenomena, or as Kenyon puts it, the study of "man in motion." Although there is some argument over whether our field also possesses a unique body of knowledge, many people do feel that such a body of knowledge exists and that it has expanded vastly over the years. Kenyon suggests that our field's difficulty in becoming a discipline is in its use of a variety of research methods, rather than a single unique method. Kenyon writes that the field of study is still too broad and that the question of research methodology still must be settled.[41]

Perhaps the argument for a single particular mode of inquiry has been overstated as a requirement for a discipline. As a contrary example, historians use a wide range of methodologies in conducting their research. Historians have used methods from sociology, from econometrics, from archaeology, from psychology, even from art, to great effect and without criticism that they are failing to have a single method of inquiry or research method.

Research should be active in both a profession and a discipline. The difference in their research is that research in a profession focuses on solving specific questions or problems, so it is applied research. Research in a discipline focuses on the broader questions of advancing knowledge in the field.

In the early years of the discipline movement, Walter Kroll explained the need for research this way:

> Whether physical education [or exercise science] is only a profession or is both a profession and an academic discipline, its research efforts must be as much in evidence as its avowed dedication to good works. Only through research can a profession examine the basis of its practices and improve the quality of its services to society . . . it must be prepared to discover knowledge essential to its progress as a learned profession. . . . Regardless of how one chooses to think of [the field], research is essential to its progress and existence.[42]

Many people in our field see a discipline emerging not necessarily from the profession, but rather parallel to the profession. That is, the field is dividing into two groups: educators (the profession) and scholars (the discipline). Indeed, this has been the process for decades. Both the discipline and the profession have made great progress. However, we need to remember that one does not necessarily exclude the other, as the discussion of the proposed field of kinesiology shows.

Defining the Theoretical Base of the Discipline

The 1973 discussions of the theoretical base of physical education centered on four different areas: (1) human movement, (2) fitness, (3) sport, and (4) a multi-theoretical base.[43] In the case of human movement, movement is an open concept, more of a process than an absolute. In a discipline centered on human movement phenomena, there can be no physical education without movement. The definition of fitness included mental and physical fitness. Sport, the most widely accepted focus in the 1970s, was viewed broadly so that it covered sport for all, rather than elite sport only. The multitheoretical argument was that the field was too broad to focus on a single area of theory. In arguing for the multitheoretical approach, Celeste Ulrich noted that, even though each of the suggested areas was

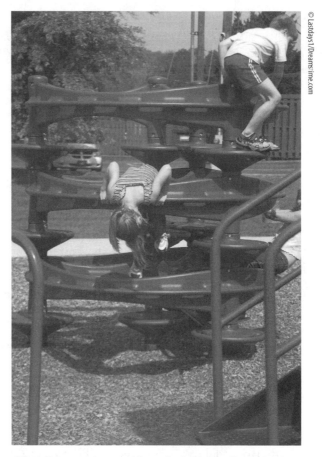

All children enjoy and benefit from quality exercise programs, increasing the job satisfaction of teachers.

called the base that lies at the heart of our field, each is actually part of a greater whole. In an argument that precedes the kinesiology movement of the 1990s, she pointed out that

> *the concepts cannot be isolated. One moves to be active. Sport is based upon specific patterns of activity. Fitness results from activity carefully "selected as to kind and conducted as to outcome." . . . But there may be a way of putting it all together. If [we] will stop seeking a uni-theoretical approach and agree that the uniqueness of [our field] is in its multi-theoretical approach.*[44]

From this point of view, our field draws from many areas of theory. In other words, people need not limit themselves to any single area of theory to say that they are working with the theoretical base of our field. That view is slowly emerging as the dominant one in the field.

Interestingly enough, all of those arguments are still strongly held. Though sport was the most widely accepted focus for much of that time, there has been a gradual shift toward human movement or physical activity as the preferred focus under an umbrella term, such as exercise science or kinesiology. We must recognize that in a way this is a return to the original umbrella fostered by AAHPERD, which was largely abandoned as an organization by the same groups of discipline specialists who now recommend that we have an umbrella field called kinesiology.[45] At any rate, as Linda Bunker notes,

> the profession . . . must refocus on the centrality of the study of human movement. [We] have too long diluted the basic field rather than emphasize the common mission of understanding human movement and the contribution it makes to human physical and mental health.[46]

Or, as Seymour Kleinman puts it, "The inherent and legitimate territory of our field, its uniqueness, is in the creation of, and engagement in, a variety of movement forms."[47]

Sport: The First Focus of the Emerging Discipline

Sport holds a prominent place in modern life. Millions of people participate in sporting activities, watch and read about them, and spend billions of dollars annually on sport-related activities and equipment. Though this massive interest in sport was noticed decades ago, the study of sport was largely ignored, except by sports journalists and the occasional scholar whose professional coworkers often considered the pursuit of such interests as scholarly "slumming."

But the impact of sport on modern society makes it clear that sport is a very legitimate field of academic study that has slowly crept into the academic mainstream. As Max Scheler noted in 1927,

> Scarcely an international phenomenon of the day deserves social and psychological study to the degree that sport does. Sport has grown immeasurably in scope and in social importance, but the meaning of sport has received little in the way of serious attention.[48]

We now see sport used at the international level for many blatantly political purposes: prestige, a show of friendship or of international acceptance, propaganda, and the influencing of public opinion. In the early 1970s, China invited a U.S. table tennis team to play as a sign of improving relations. Cuba used the 1976 Olympic victories of Alberto Juantorena as an argument that the Cuban political system had improved life there. Just as Hitler used the 1936 Olympics to show the "superiority" of his Nazi system, the Soviet Union used the 1980 Olympics to serve the same flagrant propaganda purposes for its communist system, and the United States used the 1984 Games to show the strength of its free enterprise system.

Sometimes we fail to realize the extent of our interest in modern sport. As Allen Guttmann notes:

One reason that sports are not understood is that familiarity has made their significance seem obvious when it is not. Another reason is that the philosophers, historians, sociologists, and psychologists who have concerned themselves with sports have only rarely written for the ordinary reader. They have communicated mainly with each other.[49]

"Sport science" was the discipline arm of physical education during the 1970s and 1980s. Though scholars were arguing that human movement is the focus of the discipline, sport was a more popular choice as the focus. Human movement was considered too broad because it could include such things as learning to hold a pencil or to walk, while sport is more specific to the type of activities that are actually used in the field. However, that idea was changing in the 1990s.

During the 1970s and 1980s, sport grew quickly as an area of study. Although it scarcely existed as a scholarly subject in 1970, it quickly became a large part of academic programs. Our basic areas of concern in sport studies are the meanings and relationships of play, games, sport, and athletics because their definitions are the focal points at which the study of sport begins. Hal A. Lawson calls them "ludic activities" because they are forms of playing.[50]

Sociologists have tried to define precisely the terms of sport studies. Play is described in many ways because the true meaning of play is not clear. Perhaps the most common definition of play is really a contrast, with play defined as the opposite of work, as in **Figure 1.1**. Because work is utilitarian (effort applied to a useful purpose), play is considered non-utilitarian. That is, play serves no useful purpose, at least according to the usual definition of "useful purpose." Not only is play non-utilitarian, but also it is pursued simply for its own sake. It is autotelic, too; that is, the pleasure of play is in performing the activity, rather than in the accomplishment (success or failure) of the activity. Performance (active participation) is the purpose of play. Because of this quality, play offers a type of freedom that is not available in daily work.

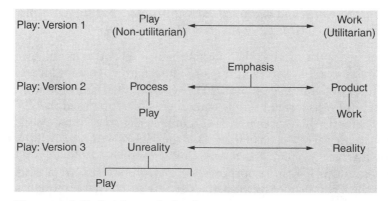

Figure 1.1 Definitions of play by contrast

Play can also be defined without contrasting it to work. Stephen Miller defines play in terms of the relative importance of means and ends.[51] In play, the means are more important than the end result. This can be rephrased by using the terms *process* and *product*. In play, the process is more important than the product. Klaus Meier suggests that play has two aspects: It is voluntary, and it is autotelic (pleasurable).[52] The voluntary aspect makes play different from work. The autotelic aspect (pleasure in the doing) does not necessarily contrast to work because work also can be pleasurable. Meier explains the major trait of play, however, when he states that "the prize of play is play itself."

Sigmund Freud defined play a third way, arguing that the opposite of play is reality.[53] Play is unreality; it is different from the real world. Thus, play is an escape from reality. This aspect of play can be both a strength and a weakness. Some escape from reality is useful in maintaining a balanced, harmonious life because it can act as a pressure release. On the other hand, a person can be too anxious to escape from reality and to seek that release too often, choosing instead to live in a dream world where the pressures of reality can be ignored.

In his work *Man, Play, and Games*, Roger Caillois defines play in terms of *paidia*, which might be called "child's play," and *ludus*, which might be called "complex play" or "adult play." He states that

> [games can] be placed on a continuum between two opposite poles.
> At one extreme an almost invisible principle, common to diversion,
> turbulence, free improvisation, and carefree gaiety, is dominant.
> It manifests a kind of uncontrolled fantasy that can be designated by
> the term paidia. At the opposite extreme, this frolicsome and impulsive
> exuberance is almost entirely absorbed or disciplined by . . . a growing
> tendency to bind it with arbitrary, imperative, and purposely tedious
> conventions . . . in order to make it more uncertain of attaining
> its desired effect. This latter principle . . . requires an ever greater
> amount of effort, patience, skill, or ingenuity. [This second component
> is called] ludus.[54]

Daryl Siedentop uses a paidia–ludus continuum to show ways of playing and their part in physical education. He explains that "as play moves from paidia to ludus, an ever increasing amount of skill, effort, patience, and ingenuity is required in order to be a successful player."[55] The free-spirited, no-limits play that is paidia has rules and structure forced on it, making it less free, yet much more complicated and challenging. The relatively formless play of children is not appropriate for organized education, but the more structured ludic form of play can be very useful in an educational setting.

Allen Guttmann explained the relationship of play, games, and sport with contrasting terms that show the elements forming each term, beginning with play. He defines play as "any non-utilitarian activity performed for its own sake," then subdivides play into two categories: spontaneous and organized.[56] Although we usually think of play as being spontaneous, Guttmann suggests that "most play is regulated and rule-bound." This is particularly true when play loses its individual characteristics and involves more than one person. Some organization becomes necessary when this occurs. In short, the more people who are involved in play, the higher the level of organization that is needed.

Organized play is called games, and to Guttmann "games symbolize the willing surrender of absolute spontaneity for the sake of playful order." He further divides games into competitive and non-competitive games, with competitive games called contests. He then divides contests into two categories, intellectual and physical, with the physical contests called sports. According to Guttmann, this distinction gives a final definition of sports as "playful contests which include an important measure of physical skill."

None of the subdivisions suggested in Guttmann's model is absolute; play is neither totally spontaneous nor totally organized. Contests are neither totally intellectual nor totally physical. Each category exists along a continuum, with different activities appearing at different points between the opposite ends. As an example, even a chess match, which is basically intellectual, has its physical side. The pieces must be moved, which requires physical effort. Furthermore, long periods of mental effort at a high level require physical stamina; even chess masters use much physical training to increase their stamina for a major match or set of matches in a championship.

A variation of Guttmann's model illustrates a different distinction between sports and contests and at the same time clarifies the distinction that philosophers make between sport and athletics. Although Guttmann presents sports as always being competitive, and therefore being contests, he cites Johann Huizinga's description of the intersection of games and contests that, when blended, can also be described as sport. Guttmann rejects this choice, but he notes that it does have its supporters. The contest can be viewed as a higher order of sport that is farther along the line toward organization and farther away from the "pure play" concept than sport because contests emphasize the victory (the ends) rather than the joy of competition (the means).

This brings us to the distinction that philosophers make between sport and athletics. The distinction is, at its core, one of emphasis. In athletics the emphasis is on the victory; the product or end (victory) is more important than the process or the means (play or sport) that leads to the end. Indeed, as David Young points out, the word *athletics* comes from a Greek word that means "to contend for a prize."[57] Obviously, the victory is the real goal, rather than the joy or spontaneity of the competition.

We often fail to distinguish between professional sports, which are purely goal centered and thus are athletics (if not entertainment), and intercollegiate athletics, which are supposedly genuinely sport and less goal centered. The term used for college activities probably is more accurate in philosophical terms than the term for the professional activities. Both are usually athletics rather than sport.

John McClelland offers a variation of this explanatory model.[58] His model adds warfare to the field of contrasts, arguing that sport and work can be described as productive activities, while play and warfare are wasteful (play in terms of time, and warfare in terms of time, money, and lives). At the same time, play and sport are ludic activities, contrasted to work and warfare, which are serious activities. His model expands the view of play and sport to fit into a broader outside world.

Of course, these definitions are open to considerable argument from both philosophical and semantic approaches. Play can be described as the opposite of work or by emphasizing process (the joy of participation). Games can be described as an organized form of play, and sport can be described as games with a primarily physical focus. The complexity of these concepts results in considerable overlapping of terms. Only when each concept is more clearly defined can we determine how each fits in real life and how each can be best used in the physical education program. At this time, the definition of each varies from person to person, from region to region, and from nation to nation. As Allen Guttmann puts it, "I shall be less intent on whether the sport appears than with how it appears."[59]

Modern society is more involved in athletics than in sport. As a result, philosophers such as John Keating and Paul Weiss have given more attention to the differences between sport and athletics. Keating describes the distinction as follows:

> *In essence, sport is a kind of diversion which has for its direct and immediate end, fun, pleasure, and delight and which is dominated by a spirit of moderation and generosity. Athletics, on the other hand, is essentially a competition activity, which has for its end, victory in the contest and which is characterized by a spirit of dedication, sacrifice, and intensity.*[60]

In his book *Sport: A Philosophic Inquiry*, Paul Weiss's theme for athletics is the pursuit of excellence.[61] Indeed, the first chapter of his book is called "Concern for Excellence." Harold VanderZwaag suggests that Weiss's book should have been entitled *Athletics* rather than *Sport*.[62] The theme of excellence and the idea of the pursuit of excellence as a major goal of athletics reappear throughout Weiss's work.

VanderZwaag maintains that sport and athletics cannot be contrasted as if they are exact opposites. He suggests another continuum, running from play to athletics, with sport between them and athletics viewed as an extension of sport. He further suggests that games can be placed along the continuum from play through sport and into the realm of athletics, although they do not reach the extreme end of the continuum. Instead, their nature changes as the activity moves toward pure play or pure athletics.

VanderZwaag also points out another contrast between sport and athletics. In sport, the spectator is unimportant, while in athletics the spectator is always important and may even become more important than the participant. An athletics event is frequently changed in some manner simply for the convenience of or appeal to the paying spectator. Thus, athletics differs from sport in both the importance of the outcome of a contest and the importance it places on the spectator, the source of the money that encourages the shift from sport to athletics.

Human Movement: The Current Focus of the Discipline

Under the brand of kinesiology, we argue that we are studying human movement. Because human movement is a very broad term, including the crawling of an infant, it may be more accurate to say that our discipline studies *skilled motor performance*. Traditionally, our field has not focused heavily on normal child development or basic movement patterns of elderly adults. Instead we have dealt with the improvement of performance, but through improved skill patterns and improved physiological capabilities, especially in a sport setting. Indeed, in 1964 Franklin Henry referred to "the development of personal skill in motor performance."[63]

Arguments were made for human movement as the focus of our discipline during the name debates published in the 1973 *Academy Papers*. In 1961, Eleanor Metheny and Lois Ellfeldt referred to physical education "as we prefer to call it 'movement education.'"[64] Although kinesiology broadens its definition to include medical aspects of movement beyond those traditionally part of our field, we are indeed concerned with human movement.

Formalizing the Subdisciplines

During the first decade of the discipline movement, scholars had two particular concerns. One was developing a definition of the field, along with a clearer name to represent the field. The other was developing the subdisciplines of the field. Each subdiscipline is a major subfocus of the field, such as biomechanics, exercise physiology, sport history, or movement pedagogy.

A university professor with a doctorate is trained with a primary focus on a single subdiscipline. Formally developing a subdiscipline followed much the same process as developing the larger discipline, except that it could be done more quickly. People interested in each subdiscipline worked to define more clearly what they studied and the methodology that they used in their research. At the same time, they began to form organizations devoted to their subdiscipline.

By the late 1960s, new subdiscipline organizations were holding their first academic meetings, and by the mid-1970s most subdisciplines had national organizations with annual conferences and scholarly publications.

Concerns About Our Field as a Science

In the United States, the drive was for status in the research universities, which required production of acceptable research and winning money for research grants. This was easier to accomplish in the sciences; sports groups and businesses spend little money on external research, but huge amounts are spent for medical research. Physical educators in the sciences followed the money.

In the early years of the discipline movement this was considered a good thing; we looked more academic, and we gained outside money through research grants. In the longer term, however, other related changes became noticeable.

The curriculum became more and more focused on science courses, and the sociocultural and educational focuses began to dwindle and even disappear.

Even 20 years ago concerns were expressed that our field had become "scientized" and too technocratic. As David J. Whitson and Donald Macintosh argued, in the new version of the discipline people were taught that their function was a technocratic one, the improvement of performance. Those goals were rarely challenged. As they argue,

> *Thinking differently about sport . . . requires exposure to alternative discourses, which allows the possibility of envisioning different roles for ourselves. That is why it is important that university physical education reconstruct a place for the humanities and for scholarship that is cognizant of questions that simply are not raised when improvements in performance are celebrated uncritically. If the purpose of the university is not only to train experts in a technical sense but to prepare them to play leadership roles in society, it is crucial that students are encouraged to think about the limits of their own knowledge structures.*[65]

They cite Linda Bain as expressing an alternative vision

> *in which physical activity (including sport but also dance and outdoor activities) is a medium for individual and collective exploration, and physical education is a discipline whose presupposed system goal is facilitating exploration and discovery. Here the discourse of physical education is articulated with those of empowerment and of emancipatory education. Physical education has a rich tradition of concern with such problems, but it is a tradition that is today in danger of being marginalized.*[66]

While some scholars have challenged the increasingly science-only focus of kinesiology in academic conferences, there had been a backlash against it in the field also. Many people have become concerned that kinesiology is so limited in its focus that its growth is a danger to our greater field. Scott Kretchmar wrote of this stage of the growth of the discipline, arguing that

> *in some ways the promise of science, and the unreasonable optimism that accompanied its early phases, has run its course. Science will not solve all the world's problems . . . not because science or scientists are inept, but rather because the typical reductionistic model on which science has operated cannot, in principle, produce a complete understanding of human behavior or fully predict it. . . . Worse yet, science done in the absence of moral research and reflection is dangerous. What can be done is not always what should be done, and a growing realization is emerging that "should" questions need the attention of specialists in philosophy and nonspecialists alike. . . .*
>
> *A growing disenchantment with the skeptical spirit that typifies much scientific inquiry also seems to be on the horizon. Oversimplified,*

the hard-nosed empirical attitude that is the target of some ire can be portrayed as follows: If it cannot be logically demonstrated, measured, or otherwise physically observed, it is not worth talking about. In physical education, some think that this attitude led to a curriculum top-heavy in courses like physiology, biomechanics, experimental psychology, motor learning, and other scientific bases of movement, but far too light in philosophy, ethics, history, and literature.[67]

In short, a completely science-focused field is too narrow in its view and methods to do justice to the broad range of valuable interests and concerns of our field.

Defining Our Field's Focus: Still an Issue

Rather than moving in a consistent direction, the focus of the field has bounced around like the ball in a pinball machine. We still have many issues debated within the field, things of greater importance than the significance of the field's best name. A critical one is how best to prepare students in the field. In the early years of the discipline movement, the common idea was to have students study an academic program unconnected to any professional goal. After 4 years of college, they could spend a year focusing on the professional side to qualify them for their workplace goals.

Ultimately this approach failed. It has been tried several times as an approach to preparing physical education teachers, with the fifth year being a master's degree program. Students (and their parents) have been resistant to the idea of a 4-year degree that does not qualify you for any kind of job. In related fields, such as physical therapy, bachelor's and master's degree programs have largely disappeared and have been replaced by 3-year doctoral programs, following an interdisciplinary undergraduate program, such as exercise science or kinesiology.

Walter Kroll addressed the dangers of overly theory-focused programs in the early years of the discipline movement, writing that

any graduate program [in an academic discipline] must provide for an optimum balance among teaching, service, and research emphases according to some goal. If, as in the case of medical and nursing education, a program over-emphasizes the scholar-research component then some deficit may arise in the service obligation. Such a deficiency in a profession could be disastrous. A similar deficiency can [also] result . . . in a program designed to produce an individual prepared to work in an academic discipline. In the case of those Ph.D.'s prepared in an academic discipline who find employment in institutions of higher learning, an extreme emphasis upon the scholar-research component may jeopardize the extent and quality of their teaching and service obligations. A point frequently overlooked is that an academic

discipline located in a university setting has both a teaching and a
service commitment as well as a commitment to scholarly research.[68]

In the years since that was written, medical education has been significantly changed because that field found that too many doctors were incapable of interacting and communicating with their patients. They were great in the lab, but poorly skilled in the hospital.

Many smaller colleges and universities (the producers of the majority of graduates in our field) have difficulty finding qualified doctoral faculty members. The problem has been an excessive focus in doctoral training on a single subdiscipline, such as exercise physiology, and a lack of wider exposure to the field as a whole. The result is one-subject teachers, when the colleges need people who can teach in more than one area and at the same time work effectively and knowledgeably with people who are trained in the other subdisciplines.

Jeffrey Ives and Duane Knudson address this concern in calling for greater disciplinary balance in exercise science. As they write,

> *[while] other allied health disciplines are adding areas in their scopes*
> *of practice, exercise science education and professional certifications*
> *remain narrow and limited. We can find no evidence that such a narrow*
> *scope of practice is beneficial, but rather that the omission of historically*
> *recognized and clinically relevant subdisciplines such as biomechanics*
> *and motor behaviour is a danger to the acceptance of exercise science*
> *as a profession. Just as importantly, an inability to integrate these*
> *disciplines as part of a holistic systems approach to human wellness*
> *and performance severely limits clinical decision making abilities.*
> *Strong interdisciplinary programs with an applied research base and*
> *field experiences to teach clinical skills are needed.*[69]

Diane Gill speaks of the need for integration within the field of kinesiology, meaning integration of multidisciplinary scholarship, focused on physical activity, integration of academic scholarship and professional practice, and work in public service "to serve the larger central mission." As she notes,

> *isolated multiple subdisciplines do not make for an integrated academic*
> *area, and a collection of cross-disciplinary areas that simply live together*
> *does not constitute an integrated kinesiology discipline. Inter-disciplinary*
> *implies actual connections among subareas, and an interdisciplinary*
> *kinesiology that integrates subdisciplinary knowledge is essential.*[70]

For years people in our field were dissatisfied with the term *physical education* because they felt that it did not clearly define the field. A related problem is that many people believe that the term recalls the close ties between physical education and school sports, which too often had little relationship to education. Some people wanted to drop the connection to sports, believing that only in this way could physical education show its true worth in the schools. For reasons such as these, people have long debated a new name for our field, one that will clearly tell people what the field is all about while giving a new image that is free of ties to the past.

Exercise science was first used at the University of Massachusetts Amherst in the 1960s and became widely used in the 1990s. It has the advantage of defining a wider area of emphasis than simply sport. Another of its strengths is that it is easier for people outside the field to recognize its focus. This trait is valuable when a major driving force for a new name is to improve the reputation (and name recognition) of the field among both the public and scholars in other fields. The term is sometimes combined into *exercise and sport science*.

Kinesiology is a title that some departments began using as early as the 1960s. Primarily research oriented, the term refers to the study of human movement or, more recently, physical activity.[71] However, in the sense that it refers to a particular study, it gives no indication of the breadth of what is taught. A student in physical education does not necessarily study movement. Teaching the strategy involved in playing a team game, for example, is definitely a part of physical education, but it is not kinesiology or the study of movement skill. Because practitioners are not always involved in studying the movement itself, kinesiology is too narrow in scope to define the whole field.

Although the American Academy of Physical Education selected *kinesiology* as its preferred title for the field in 1989, it recommended the title for academic units (in universities), not for teacher preparation programs.[72] However, the academy's members are scholars teaching at research universities, so they have their own bias toward that definition. They rarely include practitioners in their group. A major handicap of the name is that it is not one that the public understands.

Sport sciences or simply *sport* are too narrow to represent the whole field of physical education. We have discussed sport and what it represents earlier. The first description of a major sport science program was by Clark Whited in 1971.[73]

Some people prefer to keep the title physical education. Although many physical educators are not satisfied with this title, they realize that the public at least has some idea of what it means. They believe that developing a new image for the old term may be easier than trying to teach the public to recognize a new, unfamiliar title. However, it will not be easy to do, as the current reputation was developed over almost a century.

No matter what the final designation, we should keep in mind that each of the proposals depends heavily on individual interpretations of the focus within the field. Perhaps that diversity of opinion is a virtue in itself because it echoes the earlier definition of our field as a very broad area of work and study that includes many people who seem to have little relationship to each other in their interests and tasks.

In the future we may see the term *kinesiology* as the preference at research-oriented universities, *exercise and sport science* at the midlevel universities, and variations of names that include *physical education* with another term or terms to reflect the focus and mission of smaller college departments.

Our Field: No Consensus on a Defining Name

Today's Program Names: Divided by Focus

The different names used by academic programs today are based on their focuses, generally education, the disciplines, or medicine. Education primarily means teaching and coaching, which are the common focuses of physical education departments. The disciplines and applied programs usually use a variation of exercise and sport science or human performance as their names. Kinesiology as taught in the research universities is an adjunct of medicine or the health sciences.

Kinesiology: Unifying the Field or a Change of Focus?

For many decades the field has sought a better title for itself. The first reason for a new title was to better represent what the field is today; the title *physical education* essentially limits itself to teaching and coaching. Today the field is far broader in its reach than that old title indicates.

Franklin Henry's article "Physical Education: An Academic Discipline" called for the development of "*this cross-disciplinary field of knowledge*" [my emphasis], rather than the various separated subdisciplines we see today.[74] He specifically noted that it was *not* an amalgam of knowledge from other disciplines. The first program to try the discipline approach for its major was the "sport science" program at Brockport State. Clark Whited wrote that "Kinesiology, or the study of human movement, has long been an integral part of professional physical education curriculums, but it has never attempted to commandeer the field."[75]

A second motivation for a new title was the increasing emphasis on the scientific underpinnings of the field. Since the 1960s scholars have been conducting research leading to a higher-level understanding of the performing human body. Researchers wanted a name that reflected that more scholarly level of work.

A third motivation came primarily from faculty at the research-focused universities. They were concerned that the traditional title of physical education hurt their scholarly reputation among their fellow faculty in other fields. Some might consider this concern an example of social snobbery, but it was not an unjustified concern. Since the 1990s American research universities have in many cases dropped departments that train teachers, including physical education, as not sufficiently scholarly (in their opinion) for a research university. Beyond lip service, teaching is not respected in the research universities.

The search for a better name for the field is almost as old as the discipline movement. By the early 1970s, scholars were arguing for the adoption of a single academic focus and name for the field. Even after 40 years there is limited agreement, as seen by the large variation in current names used for departments across the nation.

By 1978, Franklin Henry was looking at the 14 years since his call for a discipline and finding that the picture was not as pretty as he had hoped. There was considerable discord, and an attempt to settle on a single descriptor for the focus of our field, published in *The Academy Papers* in 1973,[76] was unsuccessful. People could not agree. Indeed, a 1989 study by Stan Brassie and Jack Razor found something like 115 different titles for departments across the United States.[77] Even after 35 years, no term was dominant.

Also interesting is that just before the call by the research university for kinesiology as a name for the field, only one of 318 surveyed physical education programs reported that their department or unit was named "kinesiology," while 287 included "physical education" in their title.[78] Only 6 of the 52 units that were considering changing their title were considering kinesiology as their title.

Over the past decades, the subdisciplines were organized, devoted to the expansion of knowledge within their single subdisciplines. One of the problems created by the new groups was that many of the specialists turned their attentions away from the greater field and focused solely on their new subdiscipline groups. This caused the fracturing of the field. In 1985, Shirl Hoffman wrote of the danger that the specialization that was fragmenting the field could destroy our graduate programs.[79]

In the past, most people in the field were members of what today is AAHPERD. Many university faculty, especially those at research universities, were also members of the National College Physical Education Association for Men (NCPEAM) or the National Association for Physical Education of College Women (NAPECW), when men and women were loath to share roles across the sexual divide. At some point, reality (and perhaps Title IX) led them to unite in what became the National Association for Physical Education in Higher Education (NAPEHE), which later added kinesiology to its title, and then in 2012 dropped physical education. Some scholars were selected as members of the American Academy of Physical Education (whose name was also extended to include kinesiology).

In the early 1990s, several professors at research universities began to promote strongly the use of kinesiology as the name for the broad field, as well as the focus of its study. Numerous professional groups have added the term to their titles over the last 2 decades.

The picture is not as simple as that, however. Most university departments that took kinesiology as their title are in research universities. Few universities that put a greater focus on teaching than on research have converted to the new title. Several reasons can explain why, despite its popularity in the research universities, the new title has not largely replaced the old ones.

First, rather than truly representing the whole field, kinesiology was originally the name for a single area of study within the field. Thus, renaming the whole field kinesiology is much like defining the complete range of interests of the field as limited to motion analysis.

Second, although a major stated objective of the name change was so the public would more clearly understand what the field is, in reality the general public has no idea what *kinesiology* means. Almost every new title proposed for the field over the last 40 years is more recognizable to the public than *kinesiology* is.

Third, an unexpected thing happened in the kinesiology movement of the last 20 years: Although it supposedly started as a more scholarly name for the broad field that spreads around physical education, at some point it changed into a completely different field: health science. Kinesiology departments and major programs today act almost exclusively as preprofessional programs for graduate programs in the health sciences, such as physical therapy. They have turned into another version of biology premedical and preprofessional programs.

Since the foundation of the discipline groups, many members, mostly those in the science-focused subdisciplines, have moved to ally with the ACSM. Others stay largely within the confines of their subdiscipline group. The result is a field whose potentially contributing researchers are often involved in little or no collaboration for or contribution to the greater field of which they are ostensibly a part.

Rather than contribute to the scholarly development of the whole field, instead the new areas focused on self-aggrandizement of their subdiscipline and, in doing so, largely abandoned any interest in a unified greater field. We are human, and one of the human weaknesses is a tendency to view our personal interests as more important, more significant, simply because they are *our* interests. Instead of contributing to a greater field, each group tended to split away, mingling only with its own members.

In essence, the research university kinesiology programs left the field and became something only distantly related to their original field and its various subdisciplines. At colleges and universities that do not define themselves as research universities, kinesiology is most often found as one of several major programs within a larger, broader department with a title such as physical education or exercise and sport science. Meanwhile, the research university kinesiology programs are drifting toward absorption in larger units defined as health sciences.

The American Kinesiology Association was formed to promote kinesiology as a field. It worked with professors who are members of the National Academy of Kinesiology to gain recognition of kinesiology as a research field in the taxonomy of the National Research Council. After years of effort, in 2006 kinesiology was added as a "life science." In their presentation to the council, the group defined the field as

Kinesiology . . . examine[s] exercise and human movement at the cell level, in cultural practices, and everywhere in between. We use the tools of

biochemistry, physiology, engineering, anthropology, sociology, and other mainline disciplines to better understand human physical activity.[80]

This recognition makes it easier for university programs to get research grants.

The original Franklin Henry premise was cross-disciplinary research that would expand our knowledge of our field (with resulting improvement of academic programs and prestige of its professors). Instead, as medical research increasingly adapts that model, our field moves away from it.

One of the pitfalls of the effort by research university faculty to name our field kinesiology, and turn it into a health science, is that we often lose sight of what we are really studying and of what our students will do with it once they leave us. One of those problems is losing sight of the holism of the human. Don Hellison called for an integration of study, a return to an understanding that the body is not simply a sum of its parts.[81] Scott Kretchmar has spoken of our subdisciplines as silos, warning of the dangers of what he called "silo-limited, in depth graduate training."[82]

Jeff Ives and Duane Knudson have written of the need for greater disciplinary balance in exercise science, pointing out weaknesses of student preparation because of an overfocus on exercise physiology.[83] As they put it, *"The drift away from a balance and integration of academic preparation in exercise science represents a threat to the acceptance of exercise science graduates as exercise professionals."*

Along that line, Benoît Bardy in writing of the European perspective on kinesiology notes that the term is used almost exclusively in North America, that is, the United States and Canada.[84] The most common international terms are still "physical education" and "sport sciences" or "exercise science."

Names Reflect Program Focuses

Today there is no consensus on a name for our field, despite contrary statements by some professional groups. The following data are from fall 2009, collected from the websites of the universities themselves.[85] **Table 1.1** shows the complexity of naming patterns in the field. Almost two-thirds of departments in colleges and universities in the United States use more than one title in their naming, clearly demonstrating that there is no single name accepted by professionals as representing the whole field. This reflects Gilmour Reeve's statement, *"When will we acknowledge that an individual department does not (or can not) represent the entire discipline of kinesiology, rather than thinking whatever we do in our department is all that kinesiology is."*[86]

Table 1.1 Title Patterns of University Departments

Single Title	267	34.2%
Multiple Titles	490	62.7%
Not given	24	3.1%

Note: n = 781

Table 1.2 University Department Names

Name	Departments	
Physical Education	265	33.9%
Exercise and/or Sport Science	222	28.4%
Kinesiology	181	23.2%
Human Performance	95	12.2%

Table 1.2 shows the most common department names used in colleges and universities in the United States, in order of use. Because teaching and coaching are still popular goals, *Physical Education* is still the most widely used departmental title. Next most common are variations of *Exercise and/or Sport Science or Studies*. Third, at just under one-fourth of the titles, is *Kinesiology*, followed by *Human Performance*. Some departments use numerous other terms, but most of those titles are used by fewer than a dozen schools.

Table 1.3 shows the primary focuses of major programs offered in colleges and universities in the United States by the single word in major titles. One-third of the focuses are on education, with just under one-fourth each on exercise and science. Sport and kinesiology each have 7% of the major titles.

Table 1.4 shows the most common major programs offered in colleges and universities in the United States. One-half of the major programs are degrees in physical education, with another one-third in exercise and sport science. Kinesiology represents 10.7% of the major programs across the nation, followed by human performance with 4.3%.

Table 1.3 Terms in Major Program Titles Within University Departments

Education	582	34.1%
Exercise	406	23.8%
Science	378	22.1%
Sport	119	7.0%
Kinesiology	119	7.0%
Fitness	82	4.8%
Movement	21	1.2%

Table 1.4 Major Programs Within University Departments

Physical Education	582	52.4%
Exercise and/or Sport Science	362	32.6%
Kinesiology	119	10.7%
Human Performance	48	4.3%

Physical education, exercise science, sport, human performance, and kinesiology form a house of many rooms, and although communications between those working and studying within each of the rooms may sometimes be difficult, it is still one house, and its inhabitants have but one goal—that of our field, as I have broadly defined it.

Summary

Our field is a term used to represent a broad range of interests. We use physical activity, primarily in the play and sport settings, to produce holistic improvements in a person's physical, mental, and emotional qualities. We deal with the relationship between human movement and other areas of education—the relationship of the body's physical development to its mind and soul as they are being developed. No other single field is concerned with the total development of the human. Many names are used to describe our field. Our field today has its sometimes unclear focus as a result of changes that began half a century ago in the core field of physical education.

The motivations for human movement include (1) survival skills, (2) conformity conduct, (3) fitness and health, and (4) sport and pleasurable movement. The past terms for our field have included gymnastics, hygiene and health, exercise and fitness, physical education, and sport. The traditional allied areas are health education, recreation, and dance. Over time the focus of our field has moved from health to education to fitness to sport to lifetime wellness. The overall concern is with holism, the unity of mind and body, rather than dualism, the belief that the mind is superior to the body. Our field uses physical means to develop each person's whole being, mind, body, and spirit into "a sound mind in a sound body."

Over the past century or so, the field has gradually shifted its academic focus from education to science to medicine. Programs centered in education focused on developing a profession. In 1964, Franklin Henry called for the development of an academic discipline of physical education. A discipline is an area of knowledge and theory that can exist purely for itself with no need to show that it has a practical application. The discipline movement sought to improve scholarship by shifting the curriculum from education to science. In 1989, the American Academy of Physical Education recommended that the new discipline be called kinesiology.

When Franklin Henry called for a discipline of physical education, he envisioned it as a field with a broad concern, drawing from the expertise and methods of a range of outside disciplines, a field in the broader category of "arts and sciences," the study of all aspects of skilled human movement. Instead, as different subject areas became organized as subdisciplines, they divided into separate independent narrow interests, rather than joining a single broad one.

Defining the theoretical base of the discipline is still an issue. Early suggestions were (1) human movement, (2) fitness, (3) sport, and (4) a multitheoretical base. Sport was the first focus of the emerging discipline, but today the focus is more on physical activity or skilled human movement. Because *human movement* is a very broad term, it may be more accurate to say that our discipline studies skilled motor performance.

While some scholars have challenged the increasingly science-only focus of kinesiology, there has been a backlash against it in the field also. Many people believe a completely science-focused field is too narrow in its view and methods to do justice to the broad range of valuable interests and concerns of our field. A critical question is how best to prepare students for the field. Many smaller schools (the producers of the majority of our graduates) have difficulty finding qualified doctoral faculty because the graduate schools are training one-subject teachers, when the colleges need people who can teach in more than one area, plus work effectively and knowledgeably with people who are trained in the other subdisciplines. We need greater disciplinary balance.

The focus problem is reflected in the wide variety of department names in the field. We have no consensus on a defining name. Program names reflect their focuses, generally education, the disciplines, or medicine. Education primarily means teaching and coaching, which are the common focuses of physical education departments. The disciplines and applied programs usually use a variation of exercise and sport science or human performance as their names. Kinesiology as taught in the research universities is an adjunct of medicine or the health sciences.

A real question is whether today's kinesiology title unifies the field or represents a change of focus to the health sciences. Almost two-thirds of American university departments use more than one title in their names, clearly demonstrating that there is no single name accepted as representing our whole field. The most commonly used department names, in order of use, are (1) physical education, (2) variations of exercise and/or sport science or studies, (3) kinesiology, and (4) human performance. The research university kinesiology programs are drifting toward absorption into larger health sciences units.

Physical education, exercise science, sport, human performance, and kinesiology form a house of many rooms, and although communications between those working and studying within each of the rooms may sometimes be difficult, it is still one house, and its inhabitants have but one goal—that of our field, as we have broadly defined it.

Further Readings

Anderson, Douglas R. 2002. The humanity of movement or "It's not just gym class." *Quest* 54: 87–96.

Caillois, Roger. 1961. *Man, play, and games.* Trans. Meyer Barash. New York: Free Press.

Charles, John M. 1996. Scholarship reconceptualized: The connectedness of kinesiology. *Quest* 48: 152–164.

Clark, Jane E., ed. 2008. Kinesiology in the 21st century. *Quest* 60 (1).

Connor, Bill. 2009. What is a physical educator? *JOPERD (Journal of Physical Education, Recreation and Dance)* 80 (2): 6–7.

Corbin, Charles B., and J. Bradley Cardinal. 2008. Conceptual physical education: The anatomy of an innovation. *Quest* 60 (4): 139–153.

Dunn, John M. 2010. Kinesiology within the academy–thriving or surviving: An introduction. *Quest* 62: 1–3.

Ellis, Michael J. 1988. *The business of physical education: Future of the profession.* Champaign, IL: Human Kinetics.

Ennis, Catherine D. 2010. New directions in undergraduate and graduate education in kinesiology and physical education. *Quest* 62: 76–91.

Erb, Rachel. 2009. Exercise science: Integrating body and mind. *Choice* (October): 235–245.

Ernst, Michael P., Robert P. Pangrazi, and Charles B. Corbin. 1998. Physical education: Making a transition toward activity. *JOPERD (Journal of Physical Education, Recreation and Dance)* (November–December): 29–32.

Estes, Steven G., and Robert A. Mechikoff. 1999. *Knowing human movement.* Boston: Allyn and Bacon.

Gill, Diane. 2007. Integration: The key to sustaining kinesiology in higher education. *Quest* 59: 270–286.

Harris, Janet C. 1993. Using kinesiology: A comparison of applied veins in the subdisciplines. *Quest* 45: 389–412.

Hawkins, Andrew. 2011. Kinesiology for humans. *Quest* 63: 249–264.

Hays, Kate F., ed. 1998. *Integrating exercise, sports, movement and mind: Therapeutic unity.* New York: Haworth Press.

Huizinga, Johan. 1950. *Homo ludens: A study of the play-element in culture.* Boston: Beacon Press.

Ives, Jeffrey C., and Duane Knudson. 2007. Professional practice in exercise science: The need for greater disciplinary balance. *Sports Medicine* 37: 103–115.

Kretchmar, R. Scott. 2005. Why do we care so much about mere games? (And is this ethically defensible?). *Quest* 57 (2): 181–191.

Larsson, Håkan, and Mikael Quennerstedt. 2012. Understanding movement: A sociocultural approach to exploring moving humans. *Quest* 64: 283–298.

Lawson, Hal A. 2007. Renewing the core curriculum. *Quest* 59 (2): 219–243.

Morrow, James R., Jr., & Jerry R. Thomas. 2010. American Kinesiology Association: A national effort to promote kinesiology. *Quest* 62: 106–110.

Newell, Karl M. 2011. Physical education *of* and *through* fitness and skill. *Quest* 63: 46–54.

Ottosson, Anders. 2010. The first historical movements of kinesiology: Scientification in the borderline between physical culture and medicine around 1850. *International Journal of the History of Sport* 27: 1892–1919.

Park, Roberta J. 1998. A house divided. *Quest* 50: 213–224.

Reeve, T. Gilmour, ed. 2007. Kinesiology: Defining the academic core of our discipline. *Quest* 59 (1).

Sage, George H. 2013. Resurrecting thirty years of historical insight about kinesiology: A supplement to "What is kinesiology? Historical and philosophical insights." *Quest* 65 (2): 133–138.

Sawyer, Thomas H. 1992. The physically illiterate physical educator: What can be done? *JOPERD (Journal of Physical Education, Recreation and Dance)* (January): 7–8.

Seagrave, Jeffrey O. 1996. Scholarship in physical education in the liberal arts college. *Quest* 48: 190–199.

Twietmeyer, Gregg. 2010. Kinesis and the nature of the human person. *Quest* 62: 135–154.

———. 2012. The four marks of holistic kinesiology. *Quest* 64: 229–248.

———. 2012. What is kinesiology? Historical and philosophical insights. *Quest* 64: 4–23.

Wrynn, Alison. 2003. Contesting the canon: Understanding the history of the evolving discipline of kinesiology. *Quest* 55: 244–256.

Zeigler, Earle F. 1999. The profession must work "harder and smarter" to inform those officials who make decisions that affect the field. *Physical Educator* 56: 114–119.

———. 2011. A new "Principal Principle" (#14) of physical activity education is emerging. *Physical Educator* 68: 115–117.

Discussion Questions

1. **a.** Jesse Feiring Williams defined physical education as "the sum of man's physical activities selected as to kind, and conducted as to outcomes." Explain his definition, and give examples of how it would be interpreted in practice.

   b. How would you define physical education?

2. How has the philosophy of dualism affected the development of physical education through history?

3. How does a holistic field of physical education, exercise and sport science, and kinesiology contrast with the dualistic philosophy? What implications do those differences have for physical education programs?

4. Briefly define physical education, play, and sport. How does each compare to the others, and what is their interrelationship?

5. Briefly define *profession* and *discipline*, and explain how they are alike and how they are different. How can they come together within a field?

6. Discuss the criteria needed for a discipline. Show how physical education either does or does not meet the criteria, and why it would or would not be considered a discipline, as you interpret the criteria.

7. The question of the value of a discipline in physical education still arouses controversy. What are the good points of having a discipline? What do critics consider the not-so-good aspects of the discipline?

8. Compare and contrast the characteristics of a discipline (Flexner) with those of a field (Lieberman).

9. Discuss some of the models used to define play and sport, such as that of Guttmann. How does the paidia–ludus continuum fit into the models?

10. Compare and contrast the terms *sport* and *athletics*.

11. Using the various models suggested for defining play and sport, where would the following activities that are sometimes considered sports actually fit in?
   a. Billiards
   b. Sports car racing
   c. Horse racing
   d. New Games

12. The Holmes Group report called for a stronger academic core in the education of teachers. Why did it make that recommendation? If the recommendations are implemented seriously, what effects might they have on the field in the future?

13. What do you consider the most appropriate name for our field, and why?

References

1. Brassie, P. Stanley, and Jack E. Razor. 1989. HPER unit names in higher education: A view toward the future. *JOPERD (Journal of Physical Education, Recreation and Dance)* 60 (7): 33–40; and Brassie, P. Stanley, and Jack E. Razor. 1989. *A national survey of the changing structure and names of HPERD in higher education.* Reston, VA: ARAPCS.

2. Van Dalen, Deobold B., and Bruce L. Bennett. 1971. *A world history of physical education.* 2nd ed. Englewood Cliffs, NJ: Prentice Hall, 1.

3. Twietmeyer, Gregg. 2012. The merits and demerits of pleasure in kinesiology. *Quest* 64: 177–186; Booth, Douglas. 2009. Politics and pleasure: The philosophy of physical education revisited. *Quest* 61: 133–153; Pringle, Richard. 2010. Finding pleasure in physical education: A critical examination of the educative value of positive movement affects. *Quest* 62: 119–134.

4. Twietmeyer, Merits and demerits, 184.

5. Meier, Klaus. 1980. In defense of mediocrity: A re-visioning of play. Paper presented at the Ninety-Fifth Annual Convention of the American Alliance for Health, Physical Education, Recreation and Dance, Detroit, MI.

6. Siedentop, Daryl. 1994. *Introduction to physical education, fitness, and sport.* 2nd ed. Mountain View, CA: Mayfield, 216–218.

7. Williams, Jesse F. 1964. *The principles of physical education.* 8th ed. Philadelphia: Saunders, 13.

8. Ibid., 8.

9. Gensemer, Robert E. 1995. *Physical education: Perspectives, inquiry, application.* 3rd ed. Madison, WI: Brown and Benchmark, 6.

10. Centers for Disease Control and Prevention. Coordinated school health. http://www.cdc .gov/HealthyYouth/CSHP/.

11. Nash, Jay B. 1960. Education for leisure: A must. *JOHPER (Journal of Health, Physical Education and Recreation)* (January): 17–18, 62.

12. Zeigler, Earle F. 1997. From one image to a sharper one! *Physical Educator* 54: 72–77.

13. Portions of the following text are adapted from William H. Freeman. 2009. A new vision for the study and practice of skilled motor performance. Presented at the Annual Convention of the American Alliance for Health, Physical Education, Recreation and Dance, Tampa, FL.

14. Henry, Franklin M. 1964. The discipline of physical education. *JOHPER (Journal of Health, Physical Education and Recreation)* 35 (8): 32–33, 69.

15. Newell, Karl. 1990. Kinesiology: The label for the study of physical activity in higher education. *Quest* 42: 272–273.

16. Ibid., 269.

17. Slowikowski, Synthia S., and Karl M. Newell. 1990. The philology of kinesiology. *Quest* 42: 290.

18. Locke, Lawrence F. 1989. The name game: Power and turf at the 61st meeting. *Academy Papers* 23: 35–37.

19. Locke, Lawrence F. 1998. Advice, stories, and myths: The reactions of a cliff jumper. *Quest* 50: 238–239.

20. Spirduso, Waneen W. 1990. Commentary: The Newell epic—a case for academic sanity. *Quest* 42: 298–299.

21. Corbin, Charles B. 1991. Further reactions to Newell: Becoming a field is more than saying we are one. *Quest* 43: 224–229.

22. Zeigler, Earle F. 1989. Don't forget the profession when choosing a name! *Academy Papers* 23: 69, 76.

23. Locke, Lawrence F. 1979. Disciplines by declaration: Verities and balderdash. In *Proceedings, National Association for Physical Education in Higher Education Annual Conference*, 100.

24. Bressan, Elizabeth S. 1982. An academic discipline for physical education: What a fine mess! In *Proceedings, National Association for Physical Education in Higher Education Annual Conference*, 26–27.

25. Broekhoef, Jan. 1982. A discipline—who needs it? In *Proceedings, National Association for Physical Education in Higher Education Annual Conference*, 31, 33.

26. Ibid., 32.

27. Vickers, Joan N. 1987. The role of subject matter in the preparation of teachers in physical education. *Quest* 39 (August): 179–184.

28. Hopper, Christopher. 1984. Knowledge—toward an integration. *JOPERD (Journal of Physical Education, Recreation and Dance)* (March): 66–68.

29. Donna Woolard, personal note, August 21, 1995.

30. McCloy, Charles H. 1936. How about some muscle? *Journal of Health and Physical Education* 7: 302–303, 355.

31. Poskanzer, Charles. 1983. Editorial letter. *JOPERD (Journal of Physical Education, Recreation and Dance)* (February): 7.

32. Wade, Michael G., and John A. W. Baker, eds. 1995. *Introduction to kinesiology: The science and practice of physical activity*. Madison, WI: Brown and Benchmark, 123–125.

33. Bucher, Charles A. 1972. *Foundations of physical education*. 6th ed. St. Louis, MO: Mosby, 9–18; and Gensemer, *Physical education*, 3.

34. Siedentop, *Introduction to physical education*, 320.

35. Holmes Group. 1986. *Tomorrow's teachers: A report of the Holmes Group*. East Lansing, MI: Holmes Group.

36. Hellison, Donald. 1991. The whole person in physical education scholarship: Toward integration. *Quest* 43: 311.

37. McGinnis, J. M., Lisa Kanner, and Christopher DeGraw. 1991. Physical education's role in achieving national health objectives. *Research Quarterly for Exercise and Sport* 62: 138–142; Sadler, Wendell C. 1993. America 2000: Implications for physical education. *Physical Educator* 50: 77–86; Corbin, Charles B. 1987. Youth fitness, exercise and health: There is much to be done. *Research Quarterly for Exercise and Sport* 58: 308–314; and Haskell, William L., I-Min Lee, Russell R. Pate, Kenneth E. Powell, Steven N. Blair, Barry A. Franklin, Caroline A. Macera, Gregory W. Heat, Paul D. Thompson, and Adrian Bauman. 2007. Physical activity and public health: Updated recommendation from the American College of Sports Medicine and the American Heart Association. *Medicine and Science in Sports and Exercise* 39 (8): 1423–1434.

38. Henry, Franklin M. 1964. The discipline of physical education. *JOHPER (Journal of Health, Physical Education and Recreation)* (September): 32.

39. Siedentop, *Introduction to physical education*, 126–127.

40. Henry, Discipline of physical education, 00.

41. Kenyon, Gerald S. 1975. On the conceptualization of subdisciplines within an academic discipline dealing with human movement. In *Contemporary readings in physical education*, 3rd ed., ed. Aileene S. Lockhart and Howard S. Slusher, Dubuque, IA: Brown 343–347.

42. Kroll, Walter P. 1971. *Perspectives in physical education*. New York: Academic Press, 354.

43. Ulrich, Celeste, and John M. Nixon. 1973. *Tones of theory*. Reston, VA: AAHPERD; and Scott, M. Gladys, ed. 1973. Leadership: Focus on actions and alternatives. *Academy Papers* 7.

44. Ulrich, Celeste. 1973. A multi-theoretical crusade. *Academy Papers* 7: 19.

45. Trekell, Marianna. 1992. Umbrellas: Which way is the wind blowing? *Quest* 44: 127–134.

46. Bunker, Linda K. 1994. Virtual reality: Movement's centrality. *Quest* 46: 456.

47. Kleinman, Seymour. 1992. Name that discipline. *JOPERD (Journal of Physical Education, Recreation and Dance)* (May–June): 12.

48. Guttmann, *From ritual to record*, vii.

49. Ibid.

50. Lawson, Hal A. 1984. *Invitation to physical education*. Champaign, IL: Human Kinetics, 57–58.

51. Miller, Stephen. 1973. Ends, means, and galumphing: Some leitmotifs of play. *American Anthropologist* 75: 87–98.

52. Meier, In defense of mediocrity, 1980.

53. Slovenko, Ralph, and James A. Knight, ed. 1967. *Motivations in play, games, and sports*. Springfield, IL: Thomas, xxvii.

54. Caillois, Roger. 1961. *Man, play, and games*. Trans. Meyer Barash. New York: Free Press, 13, 27–33.

55. Siedentop, Daryl. 1980. *Physical education: Introductory analysis*. 3rd ed. Dubuque, IA: Brown, 261.

56. Guttmann, Allen. 1978. *From ritual to record: The nature of modern sports*. New York: Columbia Univ. Press, 9.

57. Young, David C. 1984. *The Olympic myth of Greek amateur athletics*. Chicago: Ares, 7.

58. McClelland, John. 2000. Athletics vs. sport in early modern Europe. Paper presented at the 28th Annual Convention of the North American Society for Sport History, Banff, AB.

59. Guttmann, *From ritual to record*, 11.

60. Keating, John W. 1964. Sportsmanship as a moral category. *Ethics* 75 (October): 25–35.

61. Weiss, Paul. 1969. *Sport: A philosophic inquiry*. Carbondale: Southern Illinois Univ. Press.

62. VanderZwaag, Harold J. 1972. *Toward a philosophy of sport*. Reading, MA: Addison-Wesley.

63. Henry, Discipline of physical education, 00.

64. *Academy Papers*. 1973. 7; cited in Gregg Twietmeyer. 2012. What is kinesiology? Historical and philosophical insights. *Quest* 64: 14.

65. Whitson, David J., and Donald Macintosh. 1990. The scientization of physical education: Discourses of performance. *Quest* 42: 48.

66. Ibid., 49.

67. Kretchmar, R. Scott. 1997. Philosophy of sport. In *The history of exercise and sport science*, ed. John D. Massengale and Rochard A. Swanson, 197. Champaign, IL: Human Kinetics.

68. Kroll, *Perspectives in physical education*, 20–21.

69. Ives, Jeffrey C., and Duane Knudson. 2007. Professional practice in exercise science: The need for greater disciplinary balance. *Sports Medicine* 37: 112.

70. Gill, Diane. 2007. Integration: The key to sustaining kinesiology in higher education. *Quest* 59: 270, 275.

71. Newell, Karl M. 1990. Physical education in higher education: Chaos out of order? *Quest* 42: 227–242.

72. Corbin, Charles B. 1989. AAPE resolution passed. *JOPERD (Journal of Physical Education, Recreation and Dance)* (September): 4.

73. Whited, Clark V. 1971. Sport science. *JOHPER (Journal of Health, Physical Education and Recreation)* 42 (5): 21–25.

74. Portions of the following text are adapted from Freeman, A new vision.

75. Whited, Sport science, 00.

76. *Academy Papers*, entire issue.

77. Brassie, P. Stanley, and Jack E. Razor. 1989. *A national survey of the changing structure and names of H.P.E.R.D. in higher education*. Reston, VA: AAHPERD.

78. Ibid., 84.

79. Hoffmann, Shirl. 1985. Specialization + fragmentation = extermination: Formula for the demise of graduate education. *JOPERD (Journal of Physical Education, Recreation and Dance)* 46 (6): 19–22.

80. Thomas, Jerry R., Jane E. Clark, Deborah L. Feltz, R. Scott Kretchmar, James R. Morrow, Jr., T. Gilmour Reeve, and Michael G. Wade. 2007. The Academy promotes, unifies and evaluates doctoral education in kinesiology. *Quest* 59: 190.

81. Hellison, Don. 1991. The whole person in physical education scholarship: Toward integration. *Quest* 43: 307–318.

82. Kretchmar, R. Scott. 2007. What to do with meaning? A research conundrum for the 21st century. *Quest* 59: 373–383.

83. Ives and Knudson, Professional practice, 103–115.

84. Bardy, Benoît G. 2008. A European perspective on kinesiology in the 21st century. *Quest* 60: 139–153.

85. Freeman, William H., and Donna L. Woolard. 2011. The quest for identity: Current department and major names in our field. Presented at the Convention of the Southern District of AAHPERD, Greensboro, NC; Freeman, William H., and Donna L. Woolard. 2012. Defining ourselves: Current major program names in the United States. Presented at the Annual Conference of the National Association for Kinesiology and Physical Education in Higher Education, San Diego.

86. Reeve, T. Gilmour. 2007. Kinesiology: Defining the academic core of our discipline. *Quest* 59: 2.

The Academic Foundations of Exercise Science and Kinesiology

This chapter briefly examines the academic focuses of our field and then provides an overview of the major subdisciplines. The term *sport* is commonly used as a modifier for many of the disciplines, such as *sport history*. That title arose during the 1970s as the disciplines were being formed, primarily because the commonly accepted focus of study for the disciplines at that time was sport.

Today we are left with titles that are inaccurate because they are too restrictive. For example, *sport pedagogy* is not accurate because many teachers of children use movement education and very little sport. Thus, I use the term *movement pedagogy*. Many psychologists now use the term *exercise and sport psychology* rather than simply *sport psychology*.

I have used many of the more traditional names—not because I consider them most descriptive of each discipline but because they are familiar and traditional. This is a variation of the same problem we have regarding agreeing on a single name for our field.

The Primary Subdisciplines of Our Field

In recent decades physical education, exercise science, and kinesiology have developed a three-tiered academic face. All three tiers are not present at every college, although most schools offer at least two of them. Karl Newell describes the tiers as academic program thrusts, identifying them as professional, disciplinary, and performance.[1] In essence, one major prepares teachers, another prepares scholars, and the third prepares performers (such as athletes). However, sport performance is not a widely accepted educational goal. It is seen only in a few nations that use international sport as a public relations and marketing tool, as American universities use their athletic departments.

A more realistic picture of American university programs today is shown in **Figure 2.1**, which illustrates the three types of major programs in our field:

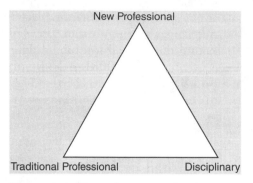

Figure 2.1 The primary academic thrusts of physical education

1. *Traditional professions*. Prepare physical education teachers and coaches, primarily for work in the school setting. Focus on the application of knowledge.
2. *Disciplines*. Prepare university students for research, medical, and health services jobs. Focus on research and the acquisition of knowledge. These jobs usually require further graduate or professional degrees.
3. *New professions*. Prepare students for jobs in exercise, fitness, and sport settings. This is the fastest growing area of the field.

The drawback of the discipline-based major has remained the same: There are few jobs for theorists, except in the research-focused university. Most students attend college to become trained for their life's work. Majors that do not offer that potential are losing students. The discipline may eventually gain more respect for the field, but it is the professions that will allow it to survive in its traditional range of interests.

The field of kinesiology takes a more limited view of our broader field, as reflected by its most accepted subdisciplines. As **Figure 2.2** shows, kinesiology generally includes only four primary subdisciplines, which were discussed in detail in an article titled "Kinesiology: Defining the Academic Core of Our Discipline," in a 2007 issue of *Quest*.[2] While kinesiologists will sometimes split the sociocultural foundations into sport psychology and sport sociology, sport psychology is the only subdiscipline commonly found in the kinesiology curriculum.

The fields of study or subdisciplines of our field are shown in **Figure 2.3**. Similar groupings have been suggested by other scholars. The figure shows the generally accepted subdisciplines within the academic field of exercise science and kinesiology and, at the same time, indicates their relationships to each other.

If we include movement pedagogy as a subdiscipline, we have eight recognized scholarly specialties within the field of physical education, exercise, sport, and kinesiology:

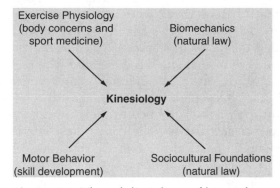

Figure 2.2 The subdisciplines of kinesiology

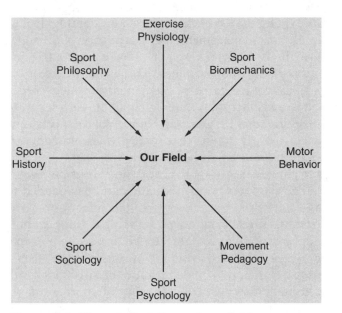

Figure 2.3 The subdisciplines of our field

1. Exercise physiology
2. Sport biomechanics
3. Sport psychology
4. Motor behavior
5. Sport sociology
6. Sport history
7. Sport philosophy
8. Movement pedagogy

These foundational areas of the field are its sociocultural, scientific, and pedagogical foundations. The focus of this chapter is not to summarize the content of each area, which is the function of specialized courses. Instead, it is to explain what each area studies, how that study is done, and why each area is important to an understanding of our field. The cultural foundations are our heritage in thought and deed, our philosophy, our history, our art, our literature. Physical education and sport are traditionally tied to the physical sciences, but the part played by the social sciences has become increasingly important. The scientific foundations are rooted in physical phenomena, and the social foundations are concerned with social phenomena. The most commonly accepted social sciences in our field are psychology, sociology, and history. The chapter also looks at motor behavior, which branches from psychology but includes aspects of the scientific foundations. Along with the science areas of biomechanics and exercise physiology, movement pedagogy is also considered.

Some writers expand the list of disciplines considerably, including such areas as sports medicine, sport management, and adapted physical education. I believe that the expanded lists simply reflect job options and subareas of disciplines, rather than new, separate subdisciplines. For example, adapted physical education can also be called a subarea of movement pedagogy because its focus is pedagogy applied to a distinct subgroup of people. If it is a separate subdiscipline, then so are elite sports, mature adult activities, youth sports, and kindergarten teaching. That view unfairly implies that some groups of people are more worthy of study or more important than other groups.

The cultural foundations are sport history and sport philosophy. These areas are sometimes called the sport humanities and can be expanded to include more specialized areas, such as sport art and sport literature. *Sport history* is the study of sport in the past. It shows us not only how sport developed, but also what was tried and either did not work or did not survive. It may help us to see better ways to do things, or at least help us to avoid the mistakes of the past.

Sport philosophy attempts to define and clarify sport and the sporting experience to determine the place and meaning of sport in our lives. The sport philosopher examines the sport setting so we can understand the circumstances under which sporting experiences take place. The critical elements of the experience itself are studied; that is, we study the elements that contribute to the experience. Finally, the broader meaning and implications of the experience are considered. In essence, the sport philosopher is concerned with what is significant about the sport experience.

The social foundations are sport sociology and exercise and sport psychology. Sport psychology and sport sociology examine human behavior in the sport setting. *Sport sociology* is concerned with the social behavior of people in the sport setting, both individually and in groups. This broad area is sometimes described as the sociocultural processes and institutions as they relate to and are affected by sport and sporting behavior. The sport sociologist focuses on the interaction of people with each other in a sport setting to determine how the process of sport affects their development and socialization or how they fit into society.

Sport psychology covers two areas of interest: motor skill learning and motor performance. At issue are the psychological factors affecting the learning and performance of physical skills and the impact of both internal and external factors on individuals.

Motor behavior deals with the learning and improvement of physical skills. It originally developed parallel to sport psychology, but eventually it grew to cover its own more specific area of interests.

The scientific foundations are sport biomechanics and exercise physiology. These are the areas traditionally considered the hard sciences of our field. *Sport biomechanics* is concerned with the effects of natural laws and forces on the human body during sporting activities. It has developed from the traditional subject area of kinesiology, which is also the study of movement. Traditional kinesiology has two basic components: anatomical kinesiology (the construction and working mechanisms of the body) and mechanical kinesiology (biomechanics or the mechanics of the human body). In sum, sport biomechanics is the study of the movement of the human body and how the effects of the laws of physics apply to it.

Exercise physiology is devoted to how the body functions during exercise. The effects of training are a critical facet of sport physiology research. This makes it perhaps the most important of the sport studies from a practical point of view because it is concerned with all aspects of how the body adapts to exercise. At the same time, this area may include sports medicine, an important and growing area of study. Sports medicine integrates the treatment and prevention of athletic injuries.

Movement pedagogy is concerned with teaching, particularly teaching play and the skills used in sporting situations. It includes the study of teaching methods and many other elements tied to the concerns of the profession of physical education. Daryl Siedentop is one who calls for the inclusion of pedagogy in the disciplines, calling it "the youngest of the sport sciences."[3] This implies a pedagogy that is a science, rather than an art, a technocratic system using computers, new technologies, and systematic instructional evaluation methods. Ann Jewett, speaking on research progress in curricular studies, noted that

> *influence on performance has been limited to some extent by the overwhelming need for theory-building. A substantial effort has gone into the business of conceptualizing curriculum as a field of scholarly inquiry. . . . Those who conceptualize the area [of curriculum and instruction] as pedagogy tend to include additional professional sub-areas so that pedagogy is viewed as including curriculum, instruction, supervision, and administration.*[4]

Charles Corbin commented that both Siedentop and Jewett have correctly noted that the root of criticism of pedagogy as a discipline has been caused by two factors, the "lack of sound research methodologies and basic theories."

However, he cautions that the results of pedagogical research must be usable by the practitioners if they are to be of true value.[5] Movement pedagogy has immense potential value to the field of sport studies and performance.

Exercise Physiology

Focus

Exercise physiology is concerned with how the body reacts and functions during exercise. The effects of training are a critical facet of exercise physiology research, which makes it perhaps the most important of the sport studies because it is concerned with all aspects of how the body adapts to exercise. Exercise physiology includes the function and contraction of the muscles, the workings of the nervous system during physical activity, the functions of the respiratory system, and the workings of the cardiovascular system.

Exercise physiology also encompasses sports medicine, an important and growing area of learning. Sports medicine is the treatment and prevention of athletic injuries. In turn, this broad interest in the health of the physically active body also can include adapted physical education or developmental activities for the physically or mentally handicapped or disabled. The sports medicine specialist deals with preventive training, treatment, and equipment that assist the performer in staying healthy; nutrition, drugs, and ergogenic aids; the treatment and rehabilitation of injuries; and ethical matters related to the training, exercise, and treatment of athletes.

Major Topics of Study

Exercise physiologists are interested in topics such as muscular function, the nervous system and its operation, respiratory function, cardiovascular function, muscular strength and endurance, cardiovascular endurance, the effects of exercise, defining and measuring physical fitness, the development of fitness, the physiology of performance, and the effects of ergogenic aids (drugs and hormones) on the body. The major areas of research emphasis include the following nine topics, which can overlap:[6]

1. Substrate utilization during exercise
2. Kinetics of oxygen uptake
3. Anaerobic threshold
4. Efficiency of physical exercise
5. Factors limiting performance
6. Environmental influences on performance
7. Mechanisms of muscular weakness and fatigue
8. Physiological adaptations to conditioning programs
9. The role of endurance conditioning in the prevention of and rehabilitation from disease

Method of Research

The exercise physiologist most often conducts research in a physiology laboratory, using equipment such as treadmills, exercise bicycles, oxygen-measuring equipment, and equipment that measures chemical characteristics of the body. Computerized monitoring and measuring equipment continues to develop rapidly and exercise physiologists are required to be familiar with the developing technologies.

The exercise physiologist works in areas related to chemistry. An increasing amount of research is being done in the field, testing athletes where and when they perform, just as some sport psychologists have begun to do. The research of the physiologist is important, for the work cuts to the heart of the training system: Unless an athlete is trained to a fine edge and to the highest level, good mechanics and well-planned psychological preparation will not be enough to result in high-level performances.

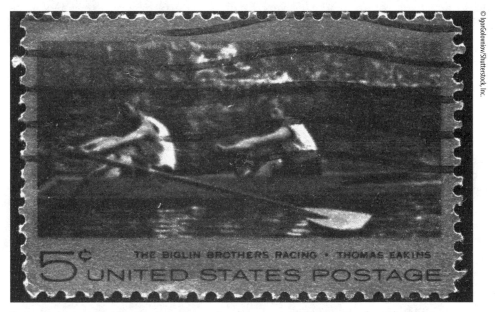

Sport has been vividly depicted by artists in a variety of ways and mediums.

Research Outlets and Sources of Information

Groups interested in the study of exercise physiology include the American College of Sports Medicine (ACSM), which encourages and publishes research in that area; the American Society of Exercise Physiologists; the National Strength and Conditioning Association; and the National Athletic Trainers' Association (NATA).

The American Medical Association Committee on the Medical Aspects of Sports actively works with physicians and keeps them informed of matters relating to sports problems, injury, and treatment. The work of this committee has become especially important because of the greatly increased participation in competitive sports and the related rise in sports injuries. Many of those injuries are treated by doctors who normally do not work with sport-related injuries and rehabilitation. New groups are developing for those interested in the fitness business field.

Publications in the field include the *Research Quarterly for Exercise and Sport* (published by AAHPERD), the *Journal of Applied Physiology*, the *Exercise and Sports Sciences Reviews*, *Physiological Reviews*, *Medicine and Science in Sports and Exercise* (published by the ACSM), the *Physician and Sportsmedicine*, the *Encyclopedia of Sport Sciences and Medicine* (also published by the ACSM), the *International Journal of Sports Medicine*, *Sports Medicine*, and the *Journal of Cardiopulmonary Rehabilitation*. Many national and international conferences on the subject are held each year by different groups interested in exercise physiology.

The future of exercise physiology will probably include more coordinated studies with coaches to determine and monitor optimal training levels in exercise programs. Those studies will utilize testing of the cardiorespiratory system and of the athlete's blood chemistry. Much work in this area has already been done in the Soviet Union and eastern Europe.

The question of training and certifying people who work in the rapidly expanding fitness industry has caused extended debate.[7] The ACSM has provided the major leadership in this area, beginning certification programs in cardiac rehabilitation in 1975. Many private groups have started their own programs, with widely varied quality of results. Subgroups of the American Alliance for Health, Physical Education, Recreation and Dance (AAHPERD) are working to create their own certification programs for people such as exercise specialists. The certification situation is chaotic, with many groups offering certifications of widely varying quality. However, such programs are still required by only a small number of employers, weakening the potential for barring unqualified workers from the fitness field. The ACSM standards are the most widely accepted in the field.

Currently, much research is being conducted by exercise physiologists on the prevention of athletic injuries, the development of better programs to prepare people for exercise programs, and helping people to recover swiftly from injuries. At the same time, specialists are working to prepare more athletic trainers and to educate more doctors in sports medicine so that prevention and treatment are raised to a higher level in the United States. Exercise physiologists are increasingly involved in medical research.

Biomechanics

Focus

Biomechanics studies the effects of natural law and forces on the body in sport. It developed from the traditional subject area of kinesiology, which is also a study of movement. Kinesiology has two basic divisions: anatomical (concerned with the construction and working mechanisms of the body) and mechanical (biomechanics, or the mechanics of the human body). Kinesiology in this context is a broad term because it studies both the body parts and the physical laws that govern their movement. For this reason, biomechanics is sometimes called "mechanical kinesiology."[8] In sum, sport biomechanics is the study of the human body and how the laws of physics apply to it.

Major Topics of Study

Topics that cover the core elements of the discipline include the following:[9]

1. The measurement of motion (how to make it more accurate)
2. Errors in data collection (because moving objects are hard to measure with much accuracy)
3. Kinematic analysis (studying an object's motion independent of the force causing the motion)
4. Kinetic analysis (of both internal and external forces affecting an object's motion)
5. Body segment parameters (developing more accurate estimates or measures)
6. Modeling and simulation (to predict actual behavior)
7. Analysis of sports equipment

Anne Atwater discusses the topics of biomechanical interest in terms of themes, by which she means the broad focus of the researchers.[10] Each of these themes has different concerns, thus different topics of interest: biological sciences, ergonomics and human factors, engineering and applied physics, health sciences, and exercise and sport sciences. Atwater predicts that the future growth in biomechanics research will be in the following three areas:

1. Biomechanical mechanisms that generate and control movement
2. Adaptive mechanisms of biological tissues to different stimuli
3. Biomechanics of injury prevention

Method of Research

Research in biomechanics falls into two large categories: either the fundamental study of the process of simple movements or the analysis of motor skills, which are more complex and thus more pertinent to sport skills. Seven means of conducting biomechanics research are the use of cinematography, stroboscopy, force platform studies, electrogoniometry, electromyography, telemetry, and computer-based studies.[11]

Cinematography uses motion picture photography to study movement. High-speed individual pictures are taken at timed intervals during a single continuing motion. *Stroboscopy* employs a similar photographic technique, except that an entire skill is captured in a single picture. A stroboscopic light flashes at preselected intervals of time during the performance. Only the positions of the action during the light flashes will show up in the picture, thus providing a representative view of the entire pattern of a motion.

A *force platform* measures the force pushing against it, such as the amount of push that a jumper uses in leaving the ground. It is used in studying the size and direction of forces, as well as their duration, and helps to give a clearer idea of the variables in performing skills such as the sprint start (measuring the time and amount of force exerted against the starting blocks and when each foot pushes and stops pushing).

Electrogoniometry records changes in joint angles using electrical instruments, giving a clearer idea of the sequence and ranges of motion that are used in performing a skill. *Electromyography* uses electrical instruments to record the work of muscles. It can tell what muscles are used in a skill, which muscles only assist with the skill, and what sequence of muscles is used in performing a complex skill.

Telemetry uses instruments to record electrical events in the body, which means any physical activity that can be converted into an electrical signal, such as a heartbeat. Small radio transmitters are then used to send the signal to recording instruments so that the performer can be studied while actually taking part in a normal performance, such as recording the heart activity of someone competing in a 1-mile race. The development of miniaturized electronics has allowed great advances in this type of research.

Computers can help to analyze complex skill performance. In fact, they can now be used to simulate skill activities. The mechanical characteristics of a performer, such as a discus thrower, can be fed into a computer and displayed on a screen, along with information on the thrower's performance. The computer can then simulate or predict how far the discus can be thrown if specific improvements are made in the thrower's technique. This gives the athlete a clearer idea of how a skill can be improved and the potential gain that might result from the improvement.

No description of studies in this area can be up-to-date because the research relies heavily on the instruments of current technology. Because that technology changes rapidly, it is impossible to describe the current capabilities in a textbook because a generation of a computer technology can begin and end between the start of writing and the actual publication of a book. As one example of the benefits of technology, we can manipulate the graphic images of a performance on-screen, seeing how much better the performer could have done under ideal circumstances.

The advances in the speed, power, and utility of microcomputers have gone far beyond our predictions; with the massive increases in memory and processing speed, we are increasingly able to simplify incredibly complex motion analyses. The speed with which technology advances makes predictions in this area meaningless. We can go far beyond the past in our capacity to record the actions of the human body, which allows us to monitor performance as it happens, analyze it, and give instant feedback.[12]

The motion analyses of biomechanics look at two aspects of motion study: kinetics and kinematics. *Kinetics* studies *what causes the movement of the body*, while *kinematics* studies *the resulting movement itself*. There are many other subareas within biomechanics, such as mechanics and dynamics, and even more specialized subdivisions, such as fluid mechanics, but these are better discussed in a biomechanics course. Kinetics and kinematics themselves are subdivisions of dynamics, which is simply the study of motion.

Early biomechanical research followed a qualitative model; that is, it tried to develop models of good technique, which people would then try to duplicate in their own performance. Of course, good is a value judgment, a subjective evaluation. Too often, the winning performer by objective standards (faster, farther, higher) was not best in terms of the good technique. Now research is along a quantitative model, using objective measures.[13] The performance is evaluated numerically, with specific points of measurement (not rating scales or other subjective measures). In terms of performance improvement, a person may have his or her movement patterns examined and tested by computer techniques, rather than compared to the model of another person's performance.

James Hay and Gavin Reid proposed a deterministic model of movement for analyzing performance.[14] The researcher first determines the performance goal or desired outcome. The researcher can then determine the factors that affect that outcome, then go on to determine the priority of those factors. Any factor may have component subfactors, which may themselves have subfactors. This model is increasingly used in research on elite performance because the factors can be interpreted in terms of training methods, as in periodization theory.

Research Outlets and Sources of Information

Many groups are concerned with sport biomechanics and hold meetings at the national and international levels to discuss research in the field. The International Society of Biomechanics (ISB) was founded in 1973, and the Olympic Scientific Congresses before each Olympic Games have offered a further outlet for research results. Members of the ACSM are involved in biomechanics research. The American Society of Biomechanics first met in 1977.

The ISB has a congress every 2 years and publishes the *International Series on Biomechanics*, with papers from each congress. The *Journal of Biomechanics* has been published since 1968. The *International Journal of Sport Biomechanics* (*IJSB*) began as a quarterly in 1985. The *International Series on Sports Sciences* (*ISSS*) includes volumes on biomechanical topics. The *Journal of Applied*

Biomechanics, *Journal of Human Movement Studies*, and the *Research Quarterly for Exercise and Sport* feature articles on biomechanics.

The future of biomechanics research will see more joint research projects with motor learning specialists, who are interested in determining how skills are learned and the most efficient teaching procedures, and with coaches, who are interested in improving the technical performances of athletes through scientific expertise and research capabilities. The sport training focus of biomechanics research was a conspicuous part of the successful eastern European athletics in the 1970s and 1980s, with the Soviet Union and the former East Germany leading the way in their application of research capabilities to athletic performance.

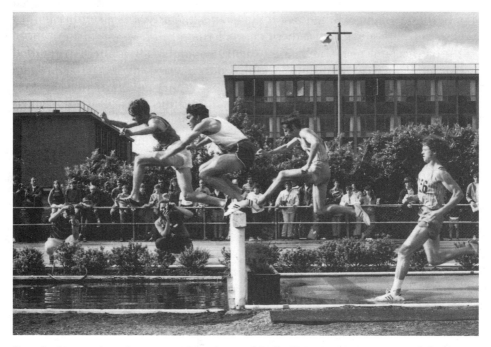

Steeplechasers show how sport has changed in facilities, organization, and the number of participants.

Sport Psychology

Focus

Sport psychology studies human behavior in the sport setting. In the realm of sport studies, psychology often has two aspects. Motor skill learning and performance (motor behavior) are common to both exercise science and sport. Sport psychology focuses on the psychological factors affecting the learning and performance of physical skills (how individuals are affected by both internal and external factors). It includes how people learn physical skills (motor learning) and also the effects of different stimuli on the performance of those skills (sport psychology). It studies the effect on performance of such aspects as motivation, arousal, anxiety, personality, and social factors.

Sport psychology is a field that has become very influential. Sport psychologists in the Western world now work directly with athletes and teams, just as specialists did in preparing high-level athletes in the eastern European socialist countries in the 1970s and 1980s. Coaches, teachers, and parents are now more concerned about preparing athletes for highly skilled performance and protecting their emotional and psychological health because the psychological stress level of elite sport is very high.[15]

Major Topics of Study

Sports psychology investigates issues such as the nature of motor skills, performance and learning, and the psychological characteristics of the performer. Specific topics can include personality, attention and arousal, anxiety and intervention, motivation, and social aspects of performance. The only difference between those factors in the teaching situation and the coaching situation is the level of skill and intensity of the performer. Other topics include problems of burnout, injury, and retirement (both voluntary and forced) from sport. The study may be from the point of view of the researcher or the applied use of psychology to improve performance.

When people think of sport psychology, they usually think of performance enhancement, especially performance enhancement for elite athletes. Some of the topics of interest in performance enhancement are arousal, stress and anxiety, burnout and staleness, career counseling (especially the end-of-career situation), coaching behaviors, concentration and attention control training, injuries, mental training techniques and effectiveness, self-regulation techniques, and substance abuse by athletes and coaches.[16]

A second area is health psychology, which has two goals: (1) to help athletes maintain their mental health and (2) to encourage the general population to enjoy the psychological benefits of exercise. This field includes exercise-related topics such as altered states of consciousness, exercise addiction, exercise initiation and adoption, exercise adherence, mood benefits of exercise, runner's high, stress reduction, the therapeutic benefits of exercise, and self-concept, self-esteem, and self-efficacy.

A third area is social psychology, which studies social interactions in sport and recreational settings and includes the interests of sport sociologists and topics such as aggression, drug use and social sanctions, gender issues, social dynamics within teams, and youth sport.

Method of Research

Some sport psychologists debate the direction to be taken in sport psychology research, particularly in methodology. Rainer Martens calls for more emphasis on "field" research; that is, research that studies performance where it takes place, on the track or playing field, rather than traditional laboratory research.[17] In the past, most research was done with individuals or groups in a laboratory setting that was carefully monitored, but today surveys and field observations are being used more often.

Standardized tests are used for many investigations of personality. Martens notes that sport psychologists spend little time actually studying sport or applied research. In response, he suggests the necessity of more theory-building work, which requires more time studying sport where and as it takes place. Martens does not call for the abandonment of laboratory research, but he is concerned about the ineffectiveness of sport psychology research on the world of sport:

> Have you not wondered why sport psychology, as we know it, has had little to no influence on the world of sport? It is not because the coaches and athletes are unreceptive to information from our field; indeed they are eager for such information. It is, unfortunately, because our insights have not been challenging, the issues studied have not been critical, and our data are not convincing to the vital issues in sport. Thus, experiential knowledge and common sense have been more appealing, and usually more beneficial, than knowledge from sport psychology research.[18]

Martens does add that field research can be just as erroneous as any other type of research, but he says that laboratory research often is not useful in the field situation. The essential problem is the complexity of human behavior. So many factors can affect a single situation that it may be impossible to determine how to change the factors if we want to increase or decrease some element of performance.

Daryl Siedentop agrees with Martens's suggestion that the field would be the best place for research in psychology and with the idea that new theories would be more likely to develop from field research that involves applied problems. However, Siedentop notes that "sport psychology will become more accepted in the 'field' if it adopts a more client-centered approach."[19] Sport psychologists reacted to this call for more applied research into the actual sporting practice instead of lab experiments that often bear little fruit in the field.

Sport psychologists still have much work to do in terms of field and laboratory research; actual work with coaches, athletes, and teams; the monitoring of programs, such as youth sports; and interpreting and teaching what they have learned to the teachers and coaches of the future.

Research Outlets and Sources of Information

The International Society of Sport Psychology (ISSP) was organized at the First International Congress of Psychology of Sport in Rome in 1965, and the North American Society for the Psychology of Sport and Physical Activity (NASPSPA) was founded in 1966. It first met at the 1967 AAHPERD convention, with

Arthur Slater-Hammel as its first president. The Association for Applied Sport Psychology (AASP) was founded in 1986.

Articles relating to sport psychology frequently appear in the *Research Quarterly for Exercise and Sport* and occasionally in *Quest*, but the primary scholarly publications are the *International Journal of Sport Psychology*, the *Journal of Sport and Exercise Psychology*, the *Sport Psychologist*, the *Journal of Applied Sport Psychology*, and the *Journal of Sport Behavior*. Studies also may appear in *Medicine and Science in Sports and Exercise*, the *Journal of Motor Behavior*, and *Perceptual and Motor Skills*. Research is presented at conferences and conventions of groups such as the NASPSPA, the AASP, the American Psychological Association (APA), and the ISSP. Occasionally, research may be presented at the conferences of related groups with a broader interest in sport, play, and exercise.

Motor Behavior

Focus

Michael Wade defines motor behavior as a subdiscipline that studies "how motor skill is produced."[20] It includes three subdomains: (1) motor control (how we control and coordinate our body), (2) motor learning (how we learn skills, including the variables that affect our learning), and (3) motor development (how our motor skills develop and change over time).

Motor development is concerned with physical ability and skill improvements that are primarily a result of maturation, and motor learning focuses on improvements that can be attributed primarily to practice and experience. Wade argues that the critical concept is skill because skill is what makes the difference between what we intend to do and what we succeed in doing.

Motor development is a branch of psychology, but it has developed several specialties. As Daryl Siedentop notes, "much of the early [research] was dominated by practical investigations. . . [since 1960], however, there has been much more theory-oriented research and gradual acceptance of an information-processing view of motor skill acquisition and performance."[21] Teachers were concerned with the most effective methods for teaching physical skills, so most of their earlier research tested specific methods or schemes of teaching. Gradually, researchers began to move toward formulating and testing theories of motor development and motor learning. The field of motor behavior is a very broad one, with a long historical background in psychology through its early interest in learning (not necessarily of physical skills). However, we are concerned primarily with physical skills, particularly those in the sporting situation.

Major Topics of Study

Numerous topics are important to the study of motor development and motor learning. Specialists in motor development study the following topics:[22]

1. *Heredity versus environmental influences in motor development.* This is the physical skill version of the traditional nature-or-nurture question. What is the influence of heredity on motor development, and what is the effect of the environment surrounding the learner?
2. *Relationships between age and sex and motor performance.* How does the expected motor performance level differ from one age or sex to another?
3. *Fundamental motor skill development.* What stages do people pass through when learning a given physical skill?
4. *Perceptual-motor development.* How does the coordination of a person develop, and what effect does coordination have on learning in other areas?
5. *Intelligence and motor performance.* Does the level of intelligence affect the speed of learning physical skills? Can the learning of physical skills raise a person's intelligence level?
6. *Cognitive processes and motor performance.* How does a person process information when learning physical skills? How much information can be processed?
7. *Physical fitness and children.* How does the fitness level of children differ from that of adults? Do exercise programs help children?
8. *Youth sports development.* What are the effects of youth sports programs on children? At what age are specific organized sports appropriate for children?

Research on motor learning includes the following topics:

1. *The stages of learning.* What are the steps and characteristics of the different stages of learning physical skills?
2. *Memory and motor performance.* What is the effect of memory on the learning of physical skills?
3. *Motor control.* How is the performance of physical skills controlled by the human body?
4. *Knowledge of results.* What is the most effective way to use knowledge of results in teaching physical skills?
5. *Practice conditions.* What are the most effective conditions for practicing physical skills?

Method of Research

Research in motor learning is becoming increasingly complex. Antoinette Gentile, in an overview of significant research during the 1970s, noted that the experimental tradition in motor learning in 1970 was still that of experimental psychology.[23] However, as more sharply focused theories and research topics appeared, experiments were based more on the methods of behavioral neurophysiology. For example, Michael Wade writes of the use of the "dynamical systems" approach that examines the person's motor control and coordination as a complex system "based on the concept that small changes in the organism can produce significant changes in motor behavior."[24]

Research Outlets and Sources of Information

Professional organizations concerned with motor behavior include NASPSPA and AASP. Some research is presented at meetings of the APA and of the ACSM. Publication outlets include the *Research Quarterly for Exercise and Sport*, *Human Movement Science*, the *Journal of Motor Behavior*, and *Perceptual and Motor Skills*. In addition, periodicals listed in sport psychology, and in some cases movement pedagogy, may feature some scholarly research in the field.

Sport Sociology

Focus

Sport sociology is concerned with the social behavior or organization of people in the sport setting, as individuals and as groups. This broad area is sometimes described as the sociocultural processes and institutions as they relate to and are affected by sport and sporting behavior. Sport is a significant part of our social order. It is often described as a "microcosm of society"; that is, a small-scale model of what the whole society is like. The sport sociologist studies "how the behavior of individuals and groups within sport is influenced by social relationships, past social experiences, and the social settings in which sport activities occur."[25]

Sociologists and sport sociologists make certain assumptions about the people whom they study; they assume that people are social beings, that their personal development is affected by social factors, and that they affect the social forms in which they live. In studying those assumptions in the sport setting, sport shows three patterns: It reflects culture and society, it reinforces social inequalities, and it is a vehicle for social conflict.[26]

Susan Greendorfer writes that

> *The subdiscipline. . . has undergone substantial transition during the past 30 years. . . research attention has shifted from the phenomena of play, games, and sport to more generic forms of physical activity as the study of body practices—from what was originally called sociology of sport to what some are now labeling "cultural kinesiology." What was once a discipline-based specialty (e.g., sociology) now appears to be shifting to an interdisciplinary approach where boundaries between the social sciences and the humanities (e.g., history, anthropology, literary analysis) are deliberately blurred. . . . Most sociologists of sport. . . agree that studies of sport and physical activity that are not also studies of societies where physical activity takes place are studies out of context.*[27]

Another direction in the focus of the subdiscipline is toward applied sport sociology, which was added as a research theme by the North American Society for the Sociology of Sport (NASSS) in 1985. The idea behind applied sport sociology is to make research more relevant and applicable to dealing with real-life problems and issues. Applied studies have the potential to help solve problems and develop methods for dealing with the conditions and practices of sport. This added research direction is not unusual in the sport subdisciplines. Areas of applied sport studies have grown in sport psychology, biomechanics, and exercise physiology.

Major Topics of Study

Early research in sport sociology studied three aspects of society: basic social units (both individual and group), social processes (such as the development of social status or prestige within a group or community), and organizational structure (such as schools or other sport-related organizations).[28] At the same time, the important part played by sport in the schools and in the community requires that we learn as much as we can about how sport affects the social aspects of the growing process. We need that knowledge so we can use sport in the most beneficial way to help children grow into healthy, socially useful adults.

Areas of research in sport sociology include sport and social institutions (such as schools and politics), social stratification (how people fit into social classes or are classified socially by others), and socialization (how people or groups interact and are affected by each other). Among the many subtopics that are studied are sexual differences and roles, racism, religion, values and ethics, economics, politics, leisure and work habits, ethnic groups, and social change.

Small group topics include interactions among people and subgroups, leadership, socialization, traits of delinquency and aggression, social mobility, the relationship of morale and self-concept to success, and the development of character. At the same time, sport sociologists are concerned with developing better theories to define and explain sport and its effects in and on society, along with improving research techniques used in the field.

Some of the areas of research interest in sport sociology include the following topics, which are among the functions of sport in society and which can become negative as well as positive:[29]

1. Emotional release (in a socially acceptable way)
2. Affirmation of identity (development of a sense of personal identity)
3. Social control (development of conformity and predictability)
4. Socialization (establishment of common values and acceptable behaviors)
5. Change agent (social interactions, assimilation, and upward mobility)
6. Collective conscience (enforcement of patterns of proper behavior)
7. Success (a way to attain success through participation or spectating)

Robert Gensemer contends that much past research in sport sociology described the negative aspects of sport. Because we now have a broad understanding of that side of sport, future research should focus more on the impact of sport on lifestyles, values orientations, and sport's place in today's high-tech world. Susan Greendorfer suggests that the subdiscipline's focus is "shifting from one whose attention was solely devoted to the study of sport to one more inclusive of a broad range of physical activity phenomena."[30]

Method of Research

Social aspects of life are difficult to research because they provide little truly objective data. Group and individual behavior are studied by using sources such as interviews, official statistics (which often are based on subjective judgments), library and archival research, questionnaires, surveys, documents, direct observation, and controlled experimentation.[31] Such sources are rarely objective because they require the opinion of an individual or group to determine a status or change. As a result, sociological research results often are controversial.

More recent research is falling into two categories: normative and non-normative. Traditional research is normative and is handicapped by being value laden. That is, the researcher assumes that certain conditions are correct or proper, then examines what the real conditions are. Examples are an attempt to prove that sport builds character or that sport is unfair. Non-normative sport is value neutral and seeks to describe what is, rather than compare it to an assumed ideal. Of course, this is not easy to do, and it does raise some questions beyond its accuracy:

> *A very serious problem of the value-neutral approach is that it does not take sides; it takes the way things are as a given entity (neither good nor evil). Thus, research in the name of value neutrality supports the status quo. If racism, sexism, and drug abuse exist in sport, and if the athlete is being abused, it seems to us [Eitzen and Sage] that the researcher cannot remain neutral. We cannot remain morally indifferent to injustice.*[32]

However, Stanley Eitzen and George Sage remark that "although [we] have taken the position that value neutrality is impossible in the social sciences, the issue is not a simple one and has encouraged considerable debate."[33]

Greendorfer suggests another research shift during the 1980s and 1990s, from the "natural science model" of research to more "interpretive and critical forms of theory." She explains that "research is always subject to the researcher's consciousness, prevailing ideological beliefs, and historical conditions."[34] Thus, research can never be truly objective and value free because the researcher has his or her own preformed biases and values that affect how data are interpreted.

Andrew Yiannakis describes research in the applied sociology of sport as having three phases of application.[35] The first is the Applied Research Phase, which has two levels: the Explanatory Phase (giving the foundation for more specific research), and the Operational Research Phase (giving specific solutions to problems). The second phase of application is the Knowledge Transfer Phase—identifying and defining a problem, reviewing and assessing possible solutions, then recommending specific solutions. The third phase of application is the Implementation Phase—putting the recommendations into effect. During the third phase the sport sociologist becomes a change agent. This different role can create problems for researchers because it can destroy the objectivity that a researcher must have to be effective.

Research Outlets and Sources of Information

The Committee for the Sociology of Sport was an early branch of the International Council of Sport Science and Physical Education (ICSSPE), and it was followed by the International Committee of Sport Sociology (ICSS) in 1964. The ICSS conducts regular international sport sociology seminars. Professional groups that have some sport sociology research presented at their conventions include the NASSS, the American Sociological Association, the American Anthropological Association, The Association for the Study of Play (TASP), NASSH, and the Popular Culture Association.

Publications focusing on sport sociology research include *Sociology of Sport Journal*, *International Journal of Sport Sociology*, *Journal of Sport and Social Issues*, *Arena Review*, *Journal of Sport Behavior*, *Quest*, *Research Quarterly for Exercise and Sport*, and *JOPERD*. Some sport history meetings and periodicals publish studies of sport sociology in a historical context, such as whether sports participation was widely used in blending early immigrant groups into the existing communities in the United States. Some sport sociology studies may also be found in meetings and publications relating to sport psychology, sport philosophy, and popular culture.

Sport History

Focus

Sport history examines sport (and exercise science) in the past. With its concern about the who, what, when, where, how, and why of our field, sport history helps us to put the present into context. It shows us where we have been and how we got to where we are today, and it may indicate where we are going and what we will see when we get there. It can illuminate sport problems that need to be solved.

History is also related to philosophy. Although historians try to follow scientific methods in studying history, their most vital concern is not the scientific process or the use of provable fact, but the subjective process by which they decide what is important—what facts they will use, what each fact means, how the facts fit together, and how to present and interpret the chosen collection of facts. Although the process of history is in many respects scientific and objective, the result is largely subjective because each person's interpretation of a fact may be different. Each historian has a philosophy that is reflected in the way the research is approached and in the conclusions that are drawn.

Method of Research

There are two types of historical research: descriptive and interpretive.[36] Descriptive historical research is the early phase of historical study because it simply determines the facts of the matter—the *what* of history—and reports them. The first historic works on a subject are usually descriptive. The more advanced (and more difficult) level of historical research is interpretive; it is an attempt to explain *why* something happened or what is important about an event or trend. Because evidence is both analyzed and interpreted, the issue of values and value systems is injected into the research process. Richard Swanson and Betty Spears divide the basic research questions into categories related to people (who and what), time (when and where), and curiosity (how and why).[37] As James Davidson and Mark Lytle point out, "History is rooted in the narrative tradition... it... remains dedicated to capturing the uniqueness of a situation." In short, they write, "good history begins with a good story."[38]

Sources for historical research can be primary or secondary. A primary source is the evidence of any person or thing that was present at the event being studied. It may be the diary of a person who was there, or it may be official records kept during the event. In short, it is firsthand information. A secondary source is someone who was not actually present when the event happened, such as a report by a person who interviewed one of the participants. Thus, it may be less reliable evidence.

Historical research involves three basic concepts: change, development, and progress.[39] *Change* is a simple concept, a difference from an earlier status or condition. Change can be documented easily because no values are involved. Either a rule did or did not change; the evidence is usually clear. *Development* is a series of changes in a direction; it, too, is simple to prove with evidence. The speed of change in a direction can range from slow (evolution) to fast (revolution). If it is consistent in a single direction, it can be documented to show a trend. Again, no values are involved. Simple facts can establish direction.

The third concept of historical research is *progress*, which requires value judgments and thus is less focused on facts. Change and development are descriptive ideas, but progress is always interpretive because it assumes that the change should be an improvement. One of the difficulties of historical research is that many ideas are based on the concept of progress, which Robert Nisbet says has been accepted for 3000 years of Western history. Yet, the validity of progress as a concept is beginning to be questioned because it is so value laden. As Robert Nisbet writes, "the idea of progress holds that mankind has advanced in the past—from some aboriginal condition of primitiveness, barbarism, or even nullity—is now advancing, and will continue to advance through the foreseeable future."[40]

This idea, clearly, is a value judgment, for one must first believe in the idea of progress. The concept is critical to sport because modern sport is concerned with records and breaking them. Only the belief in the idea of progress makes records worth keeping because they are goals to be surpassed.

Research Outlets and Sources of Information

The North American Society for Sport History (NASSH) was founded in 1973 and held its first convention at Ohio State University that same year. It meets annually and publishes online *Proceedings*, which contains abstracts of the papers presented at the convention, along with the *Journal of Sport History*, which is published three times a year.

The names of sport history publications have been cited at length by Ronald Smith, with a shorter list by Darrell Crase in *JOPERD*.[41] The most commonly seen journals are NASSH's *Journal of Sport History*, *Sport History Review* (formerly the *Canadian Journal of History of Physical Education and Sport*), the *International Journal of the History of Sport*, and *Sport in History*. Sport history articles occasionally appear in *JOPERD* and the *Research Quarterly for Exercise and Sport*. Many sport historians are listed, along with their research interests, in an online directory compiled for NASSH.[42]

Sport Philosophy

Focus

Students sometimes wonder, What does a sport philosopher do? Because the work of the philosopher is mental and is not easily observed, it is a difficult role to describe. The sport philosopher attempts to define and clarify sport and the sporting experience to determine the place and meaning of sport in our lives.

William Harper suggests three reasons for the philosophical study of sport, pointing out that these reasons do not exhaust the possibilities.[43] The first reason is to discover what there is to know. In essence, we want to learn what we really know about sport, including play, games, exercise, and athletics. Our culture has many beliefs about sport, but which beliefs are really proven? Many of the popular ideas about sport have rarely been studied closely, such as the relationship between sportsmanship or character development and sports participation.

The second reason for studying sport philosophy is to guide practical action. Serious thinking about sport can provide answers that will be useful in planning the future direction of sport. Knowledge should be applicable to some purpose, if possible. This is an important function of some of the answers we may gain from sport philosophy: They can provide guidance for the future of sport.

The third reason is to produce a deeper understanding. Many of our sport studies are better described as merely wading into the shallows of sport, rather than as dredging the depths of the subject. Our knowledge and understanding of sport are minimal in comparison to what we really need to know. A deeper understanding of sport helps us to learn more about humanity—the essential condition of the peoples of the earth, their wants, and their needs.

Major Topics of Study

Scott Kretchmar describes the major topics of philosophical study in terms of the types of questions that are asked. He suggests five questions, each dealing with a branch of philosophy:[44]

1. Questions having to do with the nature of things (metaphysics)
2. Questions having to do with what people know (epistemology)
3. Questions having to do with the value of things (axiology)
4. Questions having to do with good behavior (ethics)
5. Questions having to do with what is beautiful (aesthetics)

When we think of philosophy, we usually think of *metaphysics*, or the nature of reality and being. Metaphysics tries to answer questions about what is real and what really exists, questions that cannot be answered scientifically.

Epistemology is the study of the theory of knowledge. It is an examination of how knowledge is gained and what kinds of knowledge can be obtained, or what can be learned and how it can be determined. It involves the processes of perception (how we see and understand things) and knowledge, including the process of learning, which we sometimes call *the scientific method*.

Axiology is the study of values in general terms. It involves the nature and kinds of values. We are most concerned with two specific subareas of axiology: ethics and aesthetics.

Ethics is concerned with morals and conduct, or determining proper rules of conduct. It is a study of ideal conduct and the knowledge of good and evil. It examines what actions are right and wrong, or what people should and should not do.

Aesthetics deals with the nature of beauty, which is very subjective. Earle Zeigler defined aesthetics as the "theory or philosophy of taste" because beauty is very much a matter of personal taste.[45]

Method of Research

Scott Kretchmar writes that "philosophy is valuable not only for the theories and propositions it produces but also for the thinking skills it requires." He goes on to explain that

> *the philosophic process is the art and science of wondering about reality, posing questions related to that wonder, and pursuing answers to those questions reflectively. It is an art and a science because the philosophic skills of wondering, posing questions, and searching for answers are grounded partly on repeatable methods that can be objectified and explained (science) and partly on intuitions, tendencies, and flashes of insight that can neither be fully predicted nor accounted for (art).*[46]

The question of method in philosophical studies is often confusing to the beginner. Ultimately, any philosophical question is subjective; empirical research is not possible because the phenomena are not observable. Indeed, Harold VanderZwaag and Thomas Sheehan state that "there is no common methodology for sport philosophers" primarily because of the highly individual nature of the process, although they do suggest that analysis and synthesis are the "two pillars of integrity" in philosophical research.[47]

Kretchmar writes of three analytical or reasoning techniques of philosophers: induction, intuition, and deduction.[48] *Inductive reasoning* is based on going from the specific to the general; that is, taking a specific situation or fact and drawing more general conclusions about it. Intuitive reasoning is based on being able to recognize a situation or fact and describe it without gathering further information. With *intuitive reasoning*, you can create and analyze situations in your mind. *Deductive reasoning* is based on going from the general to the specific; that is, taking a broad principle and trying to develop more specific information or guidelines from it.

The three basic approaches to philosophical study are speculative (suggesting possible answers to a question), normative (suggesting guidelines or norms), and analytical (evaluating the ideas of others). The areas or methods of philosophical study are the historical background study, the varied interpretation method, the value judgment, the clarifying of the main issues, and the determination of relationships to similar concepts.

The philosophical and the scientific methods of organizing research studies are very similar. However, we need to look at several other research methods to provide a broader exposure to the many possible approaches to philosophy. Kathleen Pearson suggests two research approaches that can be used as part of a brief self-study program.[49] The first is called the "goodness-of-fit approach" because it is similar to the statistical study that compares how closely two statistical models agree. In this case, the researcher takes a suggested paradigm or model (such as those for the relationships of play, games, sport, and athletics) and determines whether another example actually conforms to the suggested one. The second method is the "implications approach," in which the researcher studies what something would be like if it did conform to a given model, or the researcher studies the implications of such a condition.

Robert Osterhoudt suggests that the basic method used in philosophical studies is a systematic "dialectic," or dialogue, of either of two types: speculative or critical. He believes that both types are valuable because "without the speculative, philosophy would be reduced to logic [and] without the critical, [philosophy would be reduced] to poetry. Philosophy is wholly neither."[50]

Seymour Kleinman has argued against the idea of developing a "correct" theory of sport.[51] He suggests that theories put structure and limits on sport that close it to anything beyond its imposed bounds, whereas sport demands openness. Kleinman discusses three methods of theorizing: formal description, logical description, and phenomenological description. Formal description relates the properties or characteristics of a phenomenon, logical description studies how a term is used in the language, and phenomenological description analyzes the experience itself. The latter method is Kleinman's preference because it concentrates on the phenomenon as it actually happens, without limits.

Research Outlets and Sources of Information

The International Association for the Philosophy of Sport (IAPS), formerly the Philosophic Society for the Study of Sport (PSSS), was founded in 1972 at a regional meeting of the American Philosophical Association. The society, with its annual meetings and the annual publication of its *Journal of the Philosophy of Sport*, has led the way in promoting the philosophic study of sport and sport-related activities.

The major research outlets in sport philosophy are the annual meetings of the IAPS, its journal, the journal *Sport, Ethics and Philosophy* from England, and *Quest*, which is published by the National Association of Kinesiology in Higher Education (NAKHE). Some papers are given at annual conventions of the AAHPERD and NAKHE, and some articles appear in *JOPERD* and occasionally in the *Research Quarterly for Exercise and Sport*.

The Sport Humanities

Focus

The sport humanities are the fine arts side of the discipline. Unlike sport history and sport philosophy (which are also in the humanities but are major subdisciplines), it is not yet considered a subdiscipline, but it is an important area of interest in the field. The primary focal areas of the sport humanities are sport literature and sport art. Robert Pestolesi and Cindi Baker also include sculpture, dance, and music in this area. As they remark, "the concept of the fully educated person goes beyond the ability of an individual to function in a specified career path. The connection between the liberal arts and technology has vast implications for the impact of sport on our culture."[52]

The study of sport literature became an organized area in 1984 with the formation of the Sport Literature Association at a meeting in San Diego, California. They named their first meeting the Coroebus Conference in honor of the first recorded Olympic champion in ancient Greece. As Susan Bandy writes,

> *This alliance of sport and the arts is a curious one, one that no culture or civilization prior to the Greeks or since has been able to achieve. The source of this alliance stems from the philosophy which matured and governed much of cultural life as the Greeks progressed toward the Golden Age. This philosophy placed humanity at its center as the principal source of all truth and the principal object of all truth. The importance placed upon the human being resulted in a philosophy and a cultural ideal which affected all aspects of Greek life. This philosophy. . . [required people] to strive to be good, noble, learned, and beautiful, and later matured with the inclusion of arete, the striving for excellence, and aidos, honor, respect, and modesty.[53]*

This interest of sports people in the arts is related to the growth of interdisciplinary studies in many other areas of education and scholarship. Bandy describes the interest in the sport humanities as being recent, writing in 1988 that

> *only within the last two decades have the creative and artistic dimensions of sport been recognized by scholars in physical education. Prior to this time, sport was viewed primarily from biological, psychological, or socio-logical perspectives. With the interest in sport philosophy which began in the early 1960s and the more recent interest in sport literature, however, the creative and aesthetic dimensions of sport are being recognized.*[54]

In that same period, people interested in sport art were building an interest in that area by sponsoring small exhibits of sport art at the annual AAHPERD conventions. Robert Sorani was a leader in encouraging this exhibit. An early leader in teaching sport art was Hal Ray of Western Michigan University.

Major Topics of Study

The primary topics of study in the sport humanities are the interpretations of meaning and significance of sport literature and sport art. Scholars study the use of the arts to depict sport and to demonstrate aspects of the sport experience: "This perspective reveals the distinguishing feature of humankind—the basic human need and inclination to play; that is, to engage in and value things in-and-for themselves apart from their extrinsic and instrumental worth. From this, one can argue that this distinguishing feature of humankind is the basic source of art."[55]

Both sport literature and sport art include a performance dimension. Thus, scholars may *study* each area, but others are instead *producing* sport literature, especially fiction and poetry, and physical works of sport art in various media, including sculpture, paintings, photographs, and films.

Method of Research

As Susan Bandy writes, "Sport literature. . . has offered to the scholarly investigation of sport a more subjective view than. . . the other subdisciplines. In doing so, it, along with sport philosophy, has revealed the perspective that only the arts can provide."[56] The research methodology in sport literature is that of the field of literature, although studies in sport literature tend to be less strictly structured than studies for literature-related groups such as the Modern Language Association.

In sport art we find two approaches. The first is the study of sport art, which is subjective and interpretive, reaching into the other methodologies, such as sport history (for art of the past and present) and sport philosophy (for an understanding of the meanings that underlie the art). The second is performance, rather than scholarly study; people produce sport art to interpret their views of sport to other people.

Research Outlets and Sources of Information

The primary publication in sport literature is *Aethlon: The Journal of Sport Literature*, produced twice a year by the Sport Literature Association, which meets annually on college campuses across the United States. At this time there is no scholarly publication in sport art.

Movement Pedagogy

Focus

With the 1990s shift away from physical education and toward a redefined kinesiology as the scholarly focus of a broader, more unified field of study, the acceptance of a research-focused subdiscipline in pedagogy has grown. The distinction between the terms *physical education* and *sport pedagogy* is that physical education traditionally refers to school-related activities only, while sport pedagogy "is a broad field concerned with the content, processes, and outcomes of sport, fitness, and physical-education programs in schools, community programs, and clubs."[57]

However, I prefer the term *movement pedagogy*, which seems a more accurate name for the subdiscipline. In short, *movement pedagogy includes the study of any organized teaching or learning related to human movement, regardless of where the activity takes place.*

Movement pedagogy was a late-developing subdiscipline and grew as a result of the discipline movement's focus on scholarly research combined with prolonged criticisms of the quality of teacher education in physical education. As other subdisciplines began to produce scholarly research, the teacher education specialists in some of the larger university programs began to do more research on teaching methods and procedures.

No national organization for movement or sport pedagogy has developed at this time. Movement and sport pedagogy are a focus area at many physical education and sport conferences and conventions around the world.

Major Topics of Study

Daryl Siedentop lists five areas of study as the most common in movement pedagogy: teacher behavior, student behavior, teacher effectiveness, teacher issues, and curriculum.[58] Movement pedagogy has two primary divisions: instruction (which deals with the process of teaching, including assessment) and curriculum (which deals with the content of the program, including its goals, implementation, and outcomes). Few specialists work entirely in just one area because their interests overlap.

Method of Research

The basic research methods of movement pedagogy developed from those of motor behavior, more specifically called *motor learning* or *motor skill learning* at that time. The proper method for research is not a matter of full agreement among specialists in movement pedagogy. For a fuller picture of the differing views on the methods of movement pedagogy, you should read a series of articles on the topic, "Research on Teaching in Physical Education," beginning with an overview by Stephen Silverman. The articles that follow all respond to Silverman's review, creating a forum for widespread discussion of research issues and methods.[59]

Research Outlets and Sources of Information

The movement pedagogy specialist has a wide range of research outlets, which also provide many sources of information. Many programs are held at the state, district, and national conventions of AAHPERD, including the several pedagogy-focused subgroups that meet at those conferences. Other conferences or conventions include research and presentations in movement pedagogy.

One such group is NAKHE. Another is the International Committee of Sports Pedagogy (ICSP), which is sponsored by four other groups that hold regular conventions: the International Association for Physical Education in Higher Education (AIESEP), the International Society for Comparative Physical Education and Sport (ISCPES), the International Federation of Physical Education (FIEP), and the International Association of Physical Education and Sport for Girls and Women (IAPESGW). Research is also presented at conferences on sport coaching education, coach certification, and the Olympic Scientific Congresses.

The first specialized research journal is the *Journal of Teaching in Physical Education* (*JTPE*), begun in 1981. Research on movement pedagogy also appears in the *Research Quarterly for Exercise and Sport*, as well as specialized journals such as those cited earlier in subdisciplines such as motor behavior.

Summary

This chapter examines the academic focuses of the field, then provides an overview of the major subdisciplines of kinesiology. The term *sport* is commonly used as a modifier for many of the disciplines because during the development of the disciplines in the 1970s, sport was the most accepted focus of study.

In recent decades physical education and kinesiology developed a three-tiered academic face. While they are often described as professional, disciplinary, and performance thrusts, a more practical picture of American universities shows three types of major programs: (1) the traditional professions (teaching and coaching careers), (2) the disciplines (research, medical, and health services careers), and (3) new professions (jobs in sport, exercise, and fitness settings).

Though scholars propose many subdisciplines, there are eight commonly recognized scholarly specialties within kinesiology: (1) exercise physiology, (2) sport biomechanics, (3) sport psychology, (4) motor behavior, (5) sport sociology, (6) sport history, (7) sport philosophy, and (8) movement pedagogy. Those areas are the scientific, sociocultural, and pedagogical foundations of the field. The chapter explains what each subdiscipline studies, how that study is done, and why each area is important to an understanding of the field; it also lists professional groups and publications for each area.

Further Readings

Andrew, David L. 2008. Kinesiology's inconvenient truth and the physical culture studies imperative. *Quest* 60: 45–62.

Bandy, Susan J. 2008. Blurring boundaries, crossing borders, and shifting paradigms: Embracing transdisciplinary in sport studies. *2008 NASSH Proceedings*: 48–50.

Charles, John M. 1996. Scholarship reconceptualized: The connectedness of kinesiology. *Quest* 48: 152–164.

Clark, Carol, and Allen Guttmann. 1995. Artists and athletes. *Journal of Sport History* 22: 85–110.

Clark, Jane E. 2003. The changing role of mentoring the future professorate with special attention to being a low-consensus discipline. *Quest* 55: 51–61.

———, ed. 2008. Kinesiology in the 21st century. *Quest* 60 (1).

Emra, Bruce. 1999. *Sports in literature.* 2nd ed. Lincolnwood, IL: NTC/Contemporary.

Erb, Rachel A. 2009. Exercise science: Integrating body and mind. *Choice* (October): 235–238, 240–245.

Fahlberg, Larry L., and Lauri A. Fahlberg. 1994. A human science for the study of movement: An integration of multiple ways of knowing. *Research Quarterly for Exercise and Sport* 65: 100–109.

Gumbrecht, Hans Ulrich. 2006. *In praise of athletic beauty.* Cambridge, MA: Belknap Press of Harvard University Press.

Guttmann, Allen. 2008. Does Clio need help? A plea for more extensive use of literary and visual texts. *Sport in History* 28: 104–122.

———. 2011. *Sports and American art: From Benjamin West to Andy Warhol.* Amherst: University of Massachusetts Press.

Hellison, Donald. 1991. The whole person in physical education scholarship: Toward integration. *Quest* 43: 307–318.

Ives, Jeffrey C., and Duane Knudson. 2007. Professional practice in exercise science: The need for greater disciplinary balance. *Sports Medicine* 37: 103–115.

Lacerda, Teresa, and Stephen Mumford. 2010. The genius in art and in sport: A contribution to the investigation of aesthetics of sport. *Journal of the Philosophy of Sport* 37: 182–193.

Larsson, Håkan, and Mikael Quennerstedt. 2012. Understanding movement: A sociocultural approach to exploring moving humans. *Quest* 64: 283–298.

Lowe, Benjamin. 1977. *The beauty of sport: A cross-disciplinary inquiry.* Englewood Cliffs, NJ: Prentice Hall.

MacLean, Malcolm. 2010. Where the "real" meets the "conceptual": The uncomfortable boundary between histories of sport and cultural studies. *Sport in History* 30: 489–500.

Maguire, Joe. 1991. Human sciences, sport sciences, and the need to study people "in the round." *Quest* 43: 190–206.

McKibbin, Ross. 2011. Sports history: Status, definition and meanings. *Sport in History* 31: 167–174.

Mangan, J. A. 2011. Prologue: New agendas and new questions for the history of sport. *International Journal of the History of Sport* 28: 1087–1088.

Massengale, John D., and Richard A. Swanson, eds. 1996. *The history of exercise and sport science.* Champaign, IL: Human Kinetics.

Patterson, Jan. Why teach physical education history? *JOPERD (Journal of Physical Education, Recreation and Dance)* 75 (7): 39–42.

Perry, Phyllis J. 1998. *Exploring the world of sports: Linking fiction to nonfiction.* Englewood, CO: Libraries Unlimited.

Polley, Martin. 2007. *Sport history: A practical guide.* New York: Palgrave Macmillan.

Reeve, T. Gilmour, ed. 2007. Kinesiology: Defining the academic core of our discipline. *Quest* 59 (1).

Reid, Heather L. 2009. Sport, philosophy, and the quest for knowledge. *Journal of the Philosophy of Sport* 36: 40–49.

Silverman, Stephen, ed. 2009. The Academy Papers: Advancing research in kinesiology. *Quest* 61 (1).

Tinning, Richard. 2008. Pedagogy, sport pedagogy, and the field of kinesiology. *Quest* 60: 405–424.

————. 2010. *Pedagogy and human movement.* New York: Routledge.

Discussion Questions

1. Give a brief description of the discipline of exercise physiology. Include a description of the area it studies, how it studies it, and the major topics it studies.

2. Give a brief description of the discipline of biomechanics. Include a description of the area it studies, how it studies it, and the major topics it studies.

3. Give a brief description of the discipline of sport psychology. Include a description of the area it studies, how it studies it, and the major topics it studies.

4. Give a brief description of the discipline of motor behavior and its three subareas. Include a description of the areas it studies, how they differ from each other, how the areas are studied, and the major topics of study.

5. Give a brief description of the discipline of sport sociology. Include a description of the area it studies, how it studies it, and the major topics it studies.

6. Give a brief description of the discipline of sport history. Include a description of the area it studies, how it studies it, and the major topics it studies.

7. What is the difference between descriptive and interpretive history? Why is interpretive history more advanced and difficult to do?

8. Three basic concepts involved in historical research are change, development, and progress. What are they, and why are they important concepts to the sport historian?

9. Give a brief description of the discipline of sport philosophy. Include a description of the area it studies, how it studies it, and the major topics it studies.

10. Give and discuss three of the characteristics of the sport experience, as suggested by VanderZwaag and Sheehan.

11. Give a brief description of the sport humanities. Include a description of the area it studies, how it studies it, and the major topics it studies.

12. Give a brief description of the discipline of movement pedagogy. Include a description of the area it studies, how it studies it, and the major topics it studies.

References

1. Newell, Karl M. 1990. Physical education in higher education: Chaos out of order? *Quest* 42: 227–242.

2. Reeve, T. Gilmour, ed. 2007. Kinesiology: Defining the academic core of our discipline. *Quest* 59 (1).

3. Siedentop, Daryl. 2009. *Introduction to physical education, fitness, and sport.* 7th ed. New York: McGraw-Hill, 367.

4. Jewett, Ann E. 1982. Most significant curriculum research in the past decade. *Academy Papers* 16: 71.

5. Corbin, Charles B. 1982. Applications. *Academy Papers* 16: 95–96.

6. Faulkner, John A., and Timothy White. 1981. Current and future topics in exercise physiology. In *Perspectives on the academic discipline of physical education*, 76–89. Champaign, IL: Human Kinetics.

7. Powers, Scott K., and Edward T. Howley. 1994. *Exercise physiology: Theory and application to fitness and performance.* 2nd ed. Madison, WI: Brown and Benchmark.

8. Alexander, Marion J. L. 1994. Biomechanics: The mechanics of human motion. In *Physical education and kinesiology in North America: Professional and scholarly foundations*, 237–239. Champaign, IL: Stipes; and Gensemer, Robert E. 1995. *Physical education: Perspectives, inquiry, application.* 3rd ed. Madison, WI: Brown and Benchmark, 138.

9. Cavanaugh, Peter R., and Richard N. Hinrichs. 1981. Biomechanics of sport: The state of the art. In *Perspectives on the academic discipline of physical education*, 137–157. Champaign, IL: Human Kinetics.

10. Atwater, Anne E. 1991. Biomechanics: An interdisciplinary science. *Academy Papers* 24: 5–14.

11. Carr, J. Ann. 1978. The biomechanical perspective. In *Foundations of physical education: A scientific approach*, 103–110, 125–129. Boston: Houghton Mifflin.

12. Gregor, Robert J., Jeffrey Broker, and Mimi Ryan. 1992. Performance feedback and new advances in biomechanics. *Academy Papers* 25: 19–32; and Hay, James G. 1992. Response to "Performance feedback: Advances in biomechanics." *Academy Papers* 25: 33–37.

13. Hamill, Joseph. 1995. Biomechanics. In *Introduction to kinesiology: The science and practice of physical activity*, ed. Michael G. Wade and John A. W. Baker, 47. Madison, WI: Brown and Benchmark.

14. Ibid., 47–48.

15. Rotella, Bob, and Bob Cullen. 1995. *Golf is not a game of perfect*. New York: Simon and Schuster.

16. Berger, Bonnie G. 1995. Exercise and sport psychology. In *Introduction to kinesiology: The science and practice of physical activity*, ed. Michael G. Wade and John A. W. Baker, 83–91. Madison, WI: Brown and Benchmark.

17. Martens, Rainer. 1979. About smocks and jocks. *Journal of Sport Psychology* 1: 94–99.

18. Ibid., 95.

19. Siedentop, Daryl. 1980. Two cheers for Rainer. *Journal of Sport Psychology* 2: 24.

20. Wade, Michael G. 1994. Motor behavior. In *Physical education and kinesiology in North America: Professional and scholarly foundations*, 151–154. Champaign, IL: Stipes.

21. Siedentop, Daryl. 1980. *Physical education: Introductory analysis*. 3rd ed. Dubuque, IA: Brown, 112.

22. Colfer, George R., Keith E. Hamilton, Richard A. Magill, and B. Jean Hamilton. 1986. *Contemporary physical education*. Dubuque, IA: Brown, 99, 102.

23. Gentile, Antoinette M. 1982. Most significant research of the past decade: Motor learning and control. *Academy Papers* 16: 29–39.

24. Wade, Motor behavior, 166–168.

25. Coakley, Jay J. 1990. *Sport in society: Issues and controversies*. 4th ed. St. Louis, MO: Times Mirror/Mosby, 2.

26. Eitzen, D. Stanley, and George H. Sage. 2003. *Sociology of North American sport*. 7th ed. Boston: McGraw-Hill, 4–5; and McPherson, Barry D., James E. Curtis, and John W. Loy. 1989. *The social significance of sport: An introduction to the sociology of sport*. Champaign, IL: Human Kinetics.

27. Greendorfer, Susan L. 1994. Sociocultural aspects of kinesiology. In *Physical education and kinesiology in North America: Professional and scholarly foundations*, 100, 116. Champaign, IL: Stipes.

28. Ibid., 102.

29. Wilkerson, Martha, and Richard A. Dodder. 1979. What does sports do for people? *JOPER (Journal of Physical Education and Recreation)* (February): 50–51.

30. Gensemer, *Physical education*, 138; and Greendorfer, Sociocultural aspects of kinesiology, 113.

31. VanderZwaag, Harold J., and Thomas J. Sheehan. 1978. *Introduction to sport studies: From the classroom to the ball park*. Dubuque, IA: Brown, 175–176.

32. Eitzen and Sage, *Sociology of North American sport*, 13.

33. Ibid., 20.

34. Greendorfer, Sociocultural aspects of kinesiology, 112.

35. Yiannakis, Andrew. 1992. Toward an applied sociology of sport: The next generation. In *Applied sociology of sport*, ed. Andrew Yiannakis and Susan L. Greendorfer, 3–20. Champaign, IL: Human Kinetics.

36. Jable, J. Thomas. 1980. The types of historical research for studying sport history. In *Getting started in the history of sport and physical education*, 13–14. Brockport, NY: History of Sport and Physical Education Academy.

37. Swanson, Richard, and Betty Spears. 1995. *History of sport and physical education in the United States*. 4th ed. Madison, WI: Brown and Benchmark, 3–7.

38. Davidson, James West, and Mark Hamilton Lytle. 1992. *After the fact: The art of historical detection*. 3rd ed. New York: McGraw-Hill, xiv.

39. Nisbet, Robert. 1980. *History of the idea of progress*. New York: Basic Books.

40. Ibid., 4–5.

41. Smith, Ronald A. 1980. Presenting and publishing sport history. In *Getting started in the history of sport and physical education*, 24–31. Brockport, NY: History of Sport and Physical Education Academy; and Crase, Darrell. 1985. Current periodicals in physical education and the sport sciences. *JOPERD (Journal of Physical Education, Recreation and Dance)* (October): 76–80.

42. Wright, Jerry, Ying Wu, and Ronald Smith, eds. 1992. *Directory of scholars identifying with the history of sport*. 5th ed. University Park: Pennsylvania State University/North American Society for Sport History.

43. Harper, William A. 1978. The philosophical perspective. In *Foundations of physical education: A scientific approach*, 45–46. Boston: Houghton Mifflin.

44. Kretchmar, R. Scott. 1994. *Practical philosophy of sport*. Champaign, IL: Human Kinetics, 16–17.

45. Zeigler, Earle F. 1964. *Philosophical foundations for physical, health, and recreation education*. Englewood Cliffs, NJ: Prentice Hall, 22.

46. Kretchmar, *Practical philosophy*, 1, 4–5.

47. VanderZwaag and Sheehan, *Introduction to sport studies*, 142.

48. Kretchmar, *Practical philosophy*, 19–25.

49. Pearson, Kathleen. 1978. A self-study guide: Two approaches to doing philosophy of sport and physical education. In *A self-study guide for the philosophy of sport and physical education*, 10–18. Brockport, NY: Sport Philosophy Academy.

50. Osterhoudt, Robert G. 1978. *An introduction to the philosophy of physical education and sport*. Champaign, IL: Stipes, 8–9.

51. Kleinman, Seymour. 1968. Toward a non-theory of sport. *Quest* 10: 29–34.

52. Pestolesi, Robert A., and Cindi Baker. 1990. The humanities in physical education. In *Introduction to physical education: A contemporary careers approach*, 106. 2nd ed. Glenview, IL: Scott/Foresman/Little, Brown.

53. Bandy, Susan J. 1988. *Coroebus triumphs: The alliance of sport and the arts*. San Diego: San Diego State Univ. Press, 3–4.

54. Ibid., 4.

55. Ibid., 5.

56. Ibid., 4–5.

57. Siedentop, *Introduction*, 366.

58. Ibid., 369.

59. Silverman, Stephen. 1991. Research on teaching in physical education. *Research Quarterly for Exercise and Sport* 62: 352–364.

PART 2

Our Cultural Heritage in History

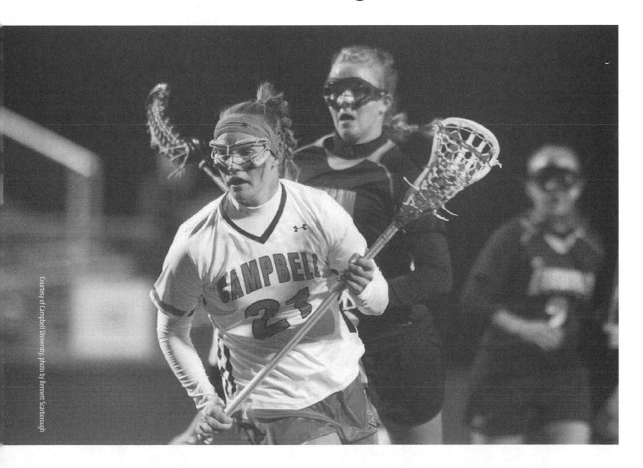

Physical Education and Sport in the Ancient World

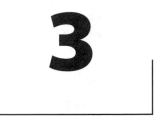

Scientists have difficulty determining where humans originated; that is, whether life began in a single area of the world. Scholars theorize that humans evolved from simpler forms of life, but they have been unable to find concrete examples of all stages of the evolutionary process. Traces of early humans have been found scattered across Africa, Asia, and Europe.

During prehistoric times, the world went through eras of great changes in climate, which varied from periods of tropical conditions to great ice ages and back to tropical conditions. In time those changes forced early people to disperse gradually across the face of the earth in search of a haven from nature's harshness. Primitive people eventually reached all of the continents and appeared on many of the earth's islands. Because of the differences in the level of the seas, many areas that are now below water level were at one time dry land. Those dry areas may have provided land bridges to areas that are now islands. A prominent site for this land bridge theory is the Bering Strait, which may have been a dry land connection used by Asian people to migrate to North America.

Primitive Times and Survival Sport

Primitive people lived in a harsh environment. To survive constant battles with nature, they gradually developed crude tools, such as axes, knives, and bows and arrows that elevated them above other forms of animal life. The primitive humans' cranial capacity (which was larger than that of other creatures in relation to their body size) permitted the full development of their ability to reason, improving their chances of survival.

More advanced speech patterns developed as people became able to understand shades of meaning. Greater precision and refinement in communication skills were necessary steps toward civilization because they allowed people to work together to improve their group lives. Only the toughest and fittest individuals could survive the harsh life, but the formation of larger groups eased the difficulties of survival for the individual members, who could then improve their defenses.

Early humans gathered first into family groups. Next, groups of different families banded together into tribes with strong leaders or chiefs. The tribe overcame the difficulties of providing food by learning to plant and harvest crops. Thus, they led a more settled life than earlier people, who constantly migrated while searching for food.

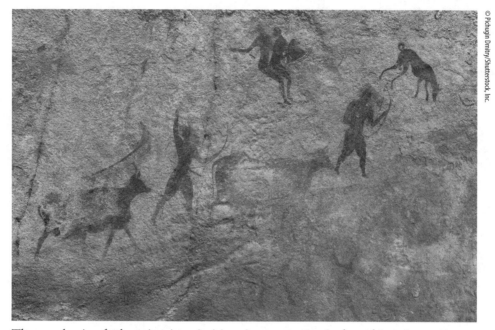

The emphasis of education in primitive times was survival; prehistoric cave paintings often depict hunting and warfare.

As farming developed and people were able to live and feed in one area for a much longer time, villages grew and society became more stable. Because their food sources had expanded, people were no longer forced to move when game animals became scarce. Settlement in villages sped up the process of civilization with improvements in the crude standards of living and a gradual change in the type of education provided for the young.

Dance activities and other ceremonial forms had meaning in primitive societies as prayers or ways to communicate with forces that could not be explained. Primitive people both feared and worshipped the forces of nature. Because they tried to influence what they could neither understand nor explain, they gradually developed religious beliefs and customs. Early humans used dance for religious communication and experience.

Among the physical activities of primitive people were the hunting skills of archery, spear and rock throwing, and stalking animals. Survival skills included such activities as running, jumping, and swimming; hand-to-hand combat (primarily wrestling) represented the fighting skills.

As societies grew more complex and life became easier, recreational activities developed. Those activities often grew from earlier survival skills (such as archery and running contests), but they were intended more for children or for adults as entertainment. As games and sports developed, ball games became popular activities in early societies. Despite differences caused by climate, local customs, and available natural materials, the games that developed around the world were basically similar because they often served as training methods in skills that children would need as adults.

The character of education changed with the appearance of more complex cultural patterns. As civilizations grew, the world moved closer to the state concept. Large groups of people who shared similar characteristics (such as racial group, language, customs, and mode of living) developed loose governmental forms and leaders. Rather than directing education, which had been primarily physical education in primitive cultures, toward the survival of the individual and small groups, the new states oriented the educational process toward state strength and survival and often toward their expansion.

The essential characteristic of primitive physical activities was survival skills, practicing the skills needed for defense against natural enemies. Similarly, sport was essentially survival sports, or natural sports, because many of the sporting activities came from the same basic skills as the physical activities.

The sporting activities of primitive people fell into the category of games and sports, but they also included dance activities, which were very important to early cultures. The three types of primitive games were the games of chance, games of dexterity and skill, and children's games.[1] The games of dexterity and skill included ball games and games such as archery, hoop and pole, and snow snake. Although the competitions were most often between two or more people in a village or tribe, some were held between different villages and tribes. Most often these were ball games roughly similar to modern lacrosse or soccer.

When we look at the early forms of sport used by primitive people in Western cultures (European prehistory), we often see a warlike basis for the activities. Success in sport required a mastery of the basic skills of war. We have traditionally considered this warlike basis of sport to be a common trait, but it is not true for all primitive societies. However, even though prehistoric sport was not always warlike or war oriented, it was taken seriously.

Before the Greeks

Ancient China

Chinese civilization was the major civilization of East Asia, though it had no effect on the development of Western civilization and its patterns of education. Chinese history extends more than 2000 years before the present era. Chinese civilization remained stable well into modern times, making it one of the longest-lasting civilizations.

Early China was a society of agrarian people governed by tradition. Everyone fulfilled assigned tasks exactly as those tasks had been carried out before their birth and would be performed long after their death. The very strong societal organization was based on a strong family unit, which was controlled by its eldest member. Every individual had strong family ties and followed the tradition of ancestor worship. Obedience and subservience to the family or group were stressed, rather than individuality.

The nation's feudal system was based on a group of major lords who had the allegiance of many vassals. The dominant interest of the government was to maintain the status quo, keeping things as they had been in the past.

The educational process, which was primarily for the upper classes, gradually became book oriented and formal. The emphasis on memorizing ancient writings required oral tests in which entire passages were recited from memory. The result was a system of rigorous examinations that left no time for physical activities. Many of the ancient writings or teachings were based on the works of Confucius and Buddha. Education attempted to develop a student's intellectual, moral, and aesthetic senses. During the earlier period of China's history, the educational process included physical training, but as that process became more ritualistic, there was less time for physical activities.

In many societies the nation's military needs are the reason for developing a program of physical training. That reason was not generally true for the ancient Chinese because they had developed a policy of isolationism. Their country had many natural barriers that made invasion by outside forces extremely difficult. The towering Himalaya Mountains, which were almost impossible to pass, block many of the southern approaches to the land. The Gobi Desert forms a great barrier to the west. The Great Wall (completed about 200 BCE) was built to protect much of the open northwest border of China.

Many social problems resulted from the static nature of Chinese society because it could accept no innovations unless they were justified by ancient authorities. Moreover, the system of respect for the past and honor of family elders was implemented and upheld by the teachings of Confucianism, which stressed the self-restraint and moderation necessary in such an unchanging society. As religions developed, the teachings emphasized a life of contemplation as the ideal.

The nature of those aspects of Chinese life made vigorous physical exercise a practice that drew little interest in the society. However, early versions of soccer, polo, chess, and competitions in archery and wrestling were practiced by the people. A program of mild physical exercises, similar to gymnastics-oriented calisthenics, was developed and called *cong fu*. The objective was to prevent disease, which the Chinese believed could result from a lack of physical activity. Dancing was also popular. Although it was primarily ceremonial, there were both religious and popular forms. The popular forms were informal recreational dances.

Ancient India

India was not a major influence on the development of Western civilization, but it represents an important civilization almost as ancient as China's. The primary religion was Hinduism, which was also a social system and thus a factor of importance in the development of Indian culture. The people were divided by the system into castes (social classes). The caste system became very rigid, severely limiting the social mobility of people in Indian society. Because they could not move to either a higher or lower caste, people's positions in life were unchanging.

The primary aim of a Hindu was to be virtuous. Asceticism, which was also stressed, could take almost any form, from a simple moderation of a person's wants to self-torture (only rarely), depending on the strength and direction of the person's religious views.

Education was based on a person's caste, and the castes limited the type of occupation that its members could follow. The choice of occupation had no relationship to a person's talents or abilities. No stress was placed on individuality; the emphasis was on the future life. Hindus believe in reincarnation; that is, the soul of a person returns to earth (after the body's death) to inhabit another body. The body can be human or animal, depending on how well the person's previous life was lived.

There was little interest in physical education, although there were some recreational sports and games and some dances that were used for ceremonies and religious observances. Some physical training was provided for members of the military, who entertained themselves with hunting activities when there was no war. Physical exercises were sometimes used to promote health, but the care and exercise of the body were not major concerns of Hinduism.

Ancient Egypt

Western civilization started in the ancient Middle East, an area that spreads inland around the eastern end of the Mediterranean Sea into the area of the ancient Fertile Crescent along the valleys of the Tigris and Euphrates Rivers. Egypt furnished a natural place for an ancient civilization to flourish. The annual floods of the Nile River provided a rich soil for farming, and water was always available for irrigation.

Although the civilization of ancient Egypt arose thousands of years in the past, it reached its peak around 1500 BCE, when it controlled large areas of the Middle East. The Egyptian people had a very complex civilization. They developed writing and paper, accomplished great feats of engineering, developed a 12-month calendar, and made many advances in the sciences, farming, and the arts. Egyptians were very religious, believing in many gods and a life after death. This civilization was also one of the earliest to give women a role and status roughly equal to those of men. Egyptian women had many more rights and powers than did women in other early societies.

Education in early Egypt was primarily professional training, particularly for the position of scribe, which required the important skills of reading and writing. Education was directed toward the practical aspects of learning a trade. Students often served apprenticeships.

There was little interest in physical education. Because the Egyptians were not usually militarily oriented, there was little urging for physical training from that direction. Although physical education was not a major part of Egyptian life, physical activities were very important to the Egyptians. They enjoyed many games and sports, and women frequently participated. Swimming was popular (Egyptian civilization was based on the Nile River), as were gymnastic activities, hunting, games involving the skills of fighting and war, and many types of ball games. Harold Evjen cites "a centuries-long involvement in sports and physical activities including wrestling, stick fighting, acrobatics, boxing, archery, equestrian events, boating, and ball games."[2] The Egyptians also had a great love of dance activities.

The Ancient Middle East

The Middle Eastern civilizations included the Sumerians, Babylonians, Assyrians, Persians, and Macedonians. Their area of the world spread eastward from the Mediterranean Sea across the Tigris and Euphrates valleys and ranged northward to present-day Turkey, southward to the Arabian peninsula, and eastward almost to modern India's border.

The Assyrian civilization began before 2000 BCE and reached its peak of power about 1200 BCE. Thereafter, one civilization followed another until about 100 BCE when the Macedonians faded from the scene.

Much of the emphasis within those successive civilizations was on military conquest. Because of this military focus, physical education in those cultures consisted primarily of war-related activities, such as handling weapons and developing skills in hand-to-hand combat. Much of the fighting of the Persians was done on horseback, so their culture stressed good horsemanship. They also placed a strong emphasis on swimming.

The physical education process for men began in early youth, lasted well into the adult years, and was very rigorous. Because little emphasis was placed on intellectual development, the process was more training than true education. Dance, which was largely a part of ceremonial exhibitions, was discouraged as a recreational activity.

Donald Kyle, in his summary of our current understanding of sport in the ancient Middle East, writes:

Although the evidence invites multiple interpretations, the Late Bronze Age Minoans, Hittites, and Mycenaeans all had physical sporting activities as well as [used] physical performances [in public spectacles]. Whether or not they had athletics per se remains a matter of definition and criteria . . . but sport and spectacle had a long Bronze Age history in lands around the Mediterranean. . . . The historical imagery of the male leader as champion, athlete, wrestler, hunter, or hero, someone possessed of strength, skills, and virtues evocative of superhuman elements or divine favor . . . is at least as old as Mediterranean civilization. That imagery of physical performance also pervades the mythology, legends, and epics of Dark Age and Archaic Greece.[3]

Ancient Greece: The Golden Age of "Pure" Physical Education and Sport

The first Greek-speaking people were the Achaeans. They were invaders who settled in the northern areas of the Greek peninsula about 1900 BCE and replaced the society and culture of the Minoan civilization of Crete. By about 1500 BCE, the Achaeans controlled most of the peninsula and had established Mycenae as their capital. Their economy was based on trade, and they established a number of commercial alliances with other prominent cities and states of the eastern Mediterranean area, such as Troy, Cyprus, Palestine, and Egypt.

After several hundred years, however, prolonged warfare and a declining economy allowed another invasion of the Greek peninsula. Those northern invaders, the Dorians, referred to themselves as Hellenes and to the area they had invaded (the peninsula of modern Greece) as Hellas.

The period of the Achaean or Mycenaean culture, from about 1500 to 800 BCE, is often called the Age of Homer. Descriptions of Greek life and customs at that time appear in the two epic writings attributed to Homer, the *Iliad* and the *Odyssey*. The *Iliad* includes the first written accounts of sport competitions, along with the first coaching advice, from Nestor to his son.[4]

Political rule was by an oligarchy; that is, by a small group of male aristocrats. Women were not accepted as equal to men in this society; they were considered property. The education of males was military in nature. There was no formal education as we think of it today. The emphasis was on developing military skills with such activities as running, boxing, and wrestling.

Funeral rituals were similar to those of the Egyptians. Indeed, recent discoveries show Egyptians using Greek competitions and even competing in the Olympic Games in the third century BCE.[5] Games had some religious functions because the people also developed funeral games to honor their dead. Such games were usually held close to the burial place of the honored person.[6] Prizes were given to the winners of contests in foot racing, boxing, wrestling, and chariot races. Most other contests and sports at this time were informal, rather than regularly occurring, organized events.

As the Mycenaean influence declined, the Greek peninsula gradually split up into a number of small city-states, which were independent political units. Within each city-state, a town controlled the territory in its immediate area but had no ties or obligations to any other city-state. As the city-states grew in strength, the classical Greek civilization with which most modern people are familiar gradually began to appear. During the Hellenic period, the major city-states were Sparta and Athens. Those two city-states, though similar in many respects, were in marked contrast in their forms of government and in their philosophies of education.

Spartan Education

Sparta, located in the southern Peloponnesus, was a totalitarian society; individuals existed for and were controlled by the state. The state was oriented entirely toward military life. Weak children were abandoned to die in the wilderness so that the strength of the state would not be threatened by weak citizens.

Education, which was controlled by the state, was a harsh process of training for males. The educational process was almost entirely physical. The emphasis on preparing male children for military life included diligent programs of running and throwing activities (javelin and discus), swimming, wrestling, boxing, and gymnastics. Dance was popular in Sparta because, although it imitated military movements, it was also part of ceremonial and recreational occasions. Music was also important, and much of the exercise was performed to music. Many songs were composed to honor dead heroes, and the laws of the state were set to music.

The male children went through three stages of military training. At the age of 7 years, they left their homes to live in barracks and trained in packs under an older youth until they were about 14 years of age. They then underwent more intensive military training until they were about 20 years old, at which time they became regular members of the military. As military men, they continued to live in the barracks until they were 30 years old. At that age they could marry and leave the barracks, though they still were required to eat their meals with the other soldiers.

The education of girls was not neglected. It also was controlled by the state from the time a girl was 7 years old until she was about 18 years of age. The training emphasized weight control and conditioning to prepare the girls for motherhood, and it included many of the same activities performed by the boys. The girls participated regularly in athletics, just as the boys did. Many memorial markers honoring girls' athletic feats were put up by their proud fathers and brothers. Unlike the men, however, when a woman married, her athletic activities ended, and she was expected to stay in the home. Even so, Spartan women did enjoy greater freedom and rights than other Greek women did.[7]

The Spartans were important participants in the games and sports at many festivals, but they discouraged boxing and pankration (a sort of freestyle, no-holds-barred fighting) because the fighter had to admit defeat to prevent death or severe injury. Spartans were taught never to admit defeat; they considered victory to be very important. Indeed, the records of their victories provide many of our earliest clues to the nature of sport in ancient Greece.

Because of their emphasis on military training, the Spartans developed the best war machine in Greece, but they did not develop the political ability to rule well. The boundaries of the areas that they ruled successfully were never very large, even though they did defeat the Athenians in the Peloponnesian Wars.

The Spartans placed little emphasis on intellectual forms of education. They were trained for war, but they were not equipped for a successful peace. Their inability to rule well in times of peace eventually led to the fall of the Greek people, who were conquered first by the Macedonians and then by the Romans. The Spartan failure emphasized the severe shortcomings of their unbalanced approach toward education.

Athenian Education

The Athens of classical times has long been our model for the theoretical balance necessary in education because of its emphasis on physical education. Athens contrasted strongly with Sparta in many ways. Although Athens began as an oligarchy, it developed a democratic society oriented toward the individual rather than toward the state. Its concept of democracy, however, was basically one for the men rather than for the women, who had few rights.

The Athenian education system was the first that we consider modern. It was concerned with the all-around development of the individual, both mentally and physically. The old motto that stresses the goal of education as "a sound mind in a sound body" (*mens sana in corpore sano*) expresses the essential balance that was the best quality of Athenian education. The process emphasized physical training, public worship (which included music), public speaking, and learning the traditions and customs of the state. Later, book learning was added to this list, as reading and writing became necessary skills. Athenian education valued *paideia*, which means the "beautiful and the good."[8] This represented the ideal characteristics of the Athenian citizen: aesthetic sensibilities, knowledge, physical skills, and a strong sense of ethics.

The educational system in Athens, like its government, was primarily for men; women were educated in the home and had few rights. Plato suggested that the educational process for boys should begin with physical education at about the age of 6 years, with grammar added at the age of 10 years, and music added at the age of 13 years. In reality, however, all three portions of the process began at about the same time and continued until a boy reached the age of 18 years and entered the military.

The program of physical education for older males was concentrated at the *gymnasium*. The name for this type of training school came from the Greek word meaning "naked" because the Greek males exercised and performed in the nude. The gymnasium was relatively elaborate, and because space was needed for running and throwing activities, it was built outside the city. A smaller version of the gymnasium, the *palestra* (or wrestling school), was located within the city and used primarily for training schoolboys.

A teacher of physical exercise at the palestra was called a *paidotribe* and was similar to today's physical education instructor. The men who coached or trained athletes for competition were called *gymnastes*.[9] These instructors were often retired champion athletes. Their duties were similar to those of today's coaches.

The basic aim of the educational process at the gymnasium and at the palestra was not physical development for its own sake. Instead, the goal was to develop the qualities of each individual through the use of physical means. The activities used by the Athenians at the palestra and the gymnasium were essentially the same as those used by the Spartans, with the addition of exercises designed to improve their movement skills, such as posture and the mechanics of graceful movement. Spartans stressed the development of the man of action, but the Athenians sought a harmonious development of the individual across physical and intellectual lines. Physical activities were more fully integrated into the Athenian educational process than in any other civilization before or since Athens.

The Greeks and the Leisure Ideal

The Greeks gave us our first coherent sense of the leisure ideal. That ideal implied some wealth (otherwise one had no time for leisure), and it was a complex goal. Leisure required free time, intellectual ferment, and the pursuit of an ideal. "To the ancient Greeks, education was the ultimate justification of human life and human communities. . . . The Greeks set out to produce, through education, a higher order of men."[10]

Paideia referred to culture, to education, and to self-improvement. The ideal of Greek culture was *arete*, which meant virtue or excellence. Knowledge came from virtue, and limits were implied. Delphi's two inscriptions, which represented Greek ideals, were "Know thyself" and "Nothing in excess."

The Greeks saw life in collective terms: The community was critical. Thus, they needed to have good citizens. They tried to develop the character of the individual because those individuals produced the character of the community. This was critical to their ideal of culture and leisure. Without good citizens, neither ideal could be found. Also critical was their belief in free will. Everyone had the power to make choices. The reason for gaining knowledge was to prepare you to make the right choices. These basic ideals are a critical foundation for our modern concepts of education, leisure, and citizenship.

Greek Athletic Games and Contests

The religious games and festivals held by the Athenians and other Greeks from 1000 to 300 BCE were generally celebrated by athletic contests, dances, and music. Some of the festivals were celebrated within a single city-state and by only one sex, as in the case of honoring local gods. Other festivals, however, were broader in appeal and sometimes were celebrated by all of the Greek people.

The major festivals appear to have evolved from earlier funeral games, though scholars do not agree on the issue.[11] This funerary origin was not rare in ancient times; the great Irish festival, *Aonach Tailteann*, may be older than the Olympic Games. Indeed, the Irish claim that it was the inspiration for the Greek games.

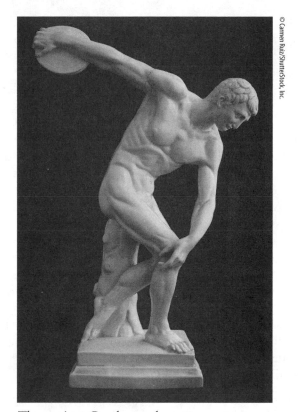

The ancient Greeks used sport as art to depict the ideal body.

The greatest of the Greek festivals was the Olympic Games, celebrated in honor of Zeus, their chief god. The festival lasted for 5 days in late August and was held in every fourth year (thus the term *Olympiad*, meaning a 4-year period).

The traditional date for the start of the Olympic Games is 776 BCE, although there were undoubtedly irregular contests as early as 1000 BCE. However, recent research suggests that the first of the regularly scheduled games started between 700 and 600 BCE.[12] The games took place near the village of Elis in western Greece. They may have been held originally to honor Herakles, an early traditional hero, with the worship of Zeus appearing in the sixth century.[13] Women were banned, perhaps because Herakles was a warriors' hero and because the presence of women was thought to diminish the warriors' power.

Manfred Lammer presents a view of Greek sport that is different from our traditional beliefs. In writing of the Greek concept of *agon*, often translated as *contest* in the phrase *agon olympikoi*, he notes that the word can as easily mean *war* and *battle*, and in fact the games translation comes to us from the Romans, who thought the Greek festivals *looked* like Roman *ludi*, or games. He stresses that the early competitions were exercises by the upper classes in the skills of war, and the gymnasium was "a military training centre for the heavily-armed sons of middle-class citizens who had acquired wealth and political influence during the period of colonization and expanding trade."[14] Lammer notes that the earlier champions were warrior–athletes; only later do we find victors with no ties to the military.

Contrary to our traditional beliefs, the most successful Greek athletes were extremely serious about their training. This is evident in part by the length of some of their careers and the vast number of contests cited for those athletes, which imply weekly competitions for up to 6 months of every year. Professional coaches appeared early, as did the coordination of the athletes' training program with medical advice.[15]

We have assumed that the early Greek athletes were aristocrats simply because those people had the money and leisure to undergo serious training. However, the common people were not barred from the competitions, nor are we entirely sure that all successful athletes were from the upper class. That too is a tradition handed down (usually with little evidence) from the late nineteenth century.[16]

Another false teaching of the nineteenth century was the idea that the ancient Greeks were interested more in well-fought competition than in the actual outcome. In rejecting that belief, David Young quotes Pindar's description of the losers in a sporting contest:

> For them was judged no pleasureful trip home. When they came back
> to their mothers, no joy burst forth, none of that laughter that gratifies.
> No. Rather, down back roads, hiding from their enemies, they skulk,
> bitten by their calamity . . . the most hateful homecoming of all,
> greetings of dishonor, a road to be travelled in secret.[17]

In short, to the Greeks the Olympic Games were not a frivolous affair. As David Young writes,

> Greek athletics were a serious business. . . . The more we recognize their
> essential nature and their distinctive character the better we will under-
> stand both the Games and the Greeks. . . . No other people in history
> until our own day ever organized such athletic contests into large-scale,
> international, adult competition. . . .
>
> Nobody, not even a Roman, hated public humiliation more than
> an ancient Greek. To an important degree Greece was a shame culture,
> and athletic defeat was . . . public humiliation. But a Greek would run
> that risk when others would not, and for one overpowering reason. The
> chance to win was worth risking all. . . .
>
> Yet behind the Greek willingness to run the risk lay something more
> complex, more specifically Greek than the almost universal thirst for
> money, glory, and fame. It was a love of competition, and a desire to be

first; a compulsion to surpass ordinary human limitations and achieve what other men cannot. It was the Greek's nature to put himself and others to the test. . . .

The physical athletic contests remained the exemplar, human competition par excellence. They represented elementally and in microcosm the general Greek struggle to rise above man's essentially ephemeral, abject condition and do what a man cannot ordinarily do. To compete in the nude underscored this symbolic test of the individual man. The man and all he could do were laid bare for all. Only performance and achievement counted . . . in the readiness of adult men to run the naked risk of public dishonor for the chance to achieve distinction, there we find what separated the Greeks out from other people.[18]

Every fourth year a month-long peace (the *pax Olympica*) was declared around the time of the games. Each city-state was required to cease fighting with any other city-state and allow all athletes passage through its territory. Lammer maintains that the Olympic peace was really more a treaty of immunity during the games than a true declaration of peace. The city-states agreed to the truce so that no local war would interfere with the competition. Until later years, women were not allowed to view or compete in the games, and by custom, the athletes competed in the nude.

The games may have been the greatest cultural exchange among the Greeks of that time. Many people who came to watch the games mingled during the week of competition, and all of the athletes were required to spend their last month of training prior to the games in a common training camp with all of the other Olympic competitors.

The games originally were held on a field beside a statue of Zeus, with the foot races starting at its base. Later, over a period of years, a stadium was constructed. The primary foot race of the games was the *stade*, which ran the length of the long, narrow stadium, or about 192 meters.[19] A second race was twice that long, and other races up to 5 kilometers in length were held at some festivals. However, the shortest race was the most important one. Starting places were carved into stone for the sprinters, and javelins (later replaced by stone pillars) were used to mark the turning points and finishing lines.

Other events in the Olympic Games included the discus throw, the javelin throw (thrown with the aid of a leather strap), the long jump (with hand weights to assist the takeoff), wrestling in several different styles, boxing, the very rough *pankration*, chariot and horse racing, and the pentathlon. The pentathlon consisted of five events: a sprint, the long jump, the discus and javelin throws, and wrestling. We do not know how the winner was chosen, although H. A. Harris suggests that victory was required in three of the five events.[20]

In addition to the Olympic Games, there were many other Greek festivals that included athletic competitions. The most prominent ones were the Pythian Games at Delphi (honoring Apollo and awarding a laurel wreath), the Isthmian festival at Corinth (honoring Poseidon and awarding a pine wreath), and the Nemean festival at Nemea (honoring Zeus and awarding a celery wreath). They were the other three members of the Big Four circuit. There were also many less important local festivals.

Evidence is clear that there also were athletic competitions for women. Records indicate that a festival of Hera was held every 4 years at the Olympic stadium at a time separate from the Olympic Games. In this competition the racing distance for the women was shortened by one-sixth. Apparently the women's competitions were expanding by the first century AD because their events were being recorded as part of the other competitions that have been mentioned.[21]

Women's competition may have appeared at least as early as men's competition in Greece, and the Heraea (games of Hera, the sister–wife of Zeus) at Olympia may have begun before the Olympic Games. Women's sport was present very early and occasionally had highly skilled participants. However, because there is so little evidence for it, it was probably still considered unimportant, reflecting women's place in Greek society.[22] Other games for women and for youth appeared in later years.

Although many of the competitions were during religious holidays, H. A. Harris suggests that this had little actual religious significance in terms of the origin of the games. He theorizes that the holidays simply provided a convenient leisure time for the competitions, just as the American football bowl games were not founded as religious celebrations of Christmas and New Year's Day.[23] Indeed, we will see that this was also true during the late Middle Ages.

The Question of Amateur and Professional Athletics in Greece

Because the Greeks held many local games in addition to the Olympic Games, interest in athletic competition became widespread. The presence of a coach's handbook on training, by Philostratus in the third century BCE, shows that the coaching profession was well established by the Golden Age of Greek sport.[24] The athletic games developed from ceremonies to worship the gods and from games that were held to honor the dead at their funerals. During earlier times, the prizes were small, usually tokens representing the importance of the god or the person who had died. As time passed, however, the size and nature of the awards changed.

The prize for an Olympic victory was traditionally a wreath or crown formed from an olive branch and its leaves. It was a symbolic prize, rather than a valuable one, although in earlier years valuable prizes may have been common. However, the city-states began to offer additional prizes to their citizens who won Olympic victories. At the vale of Olympia a man received only an olive wreath, but when he returned home he might be given enough wealth to last a lifetime. The victorious athletes usually were feted by their city-states when they returned home. Triumphal parades were held, and many privileges were given to the victors. Often statues of the Olympic champions were erected. Gifts of food, money, and civic honors were common and worth winning, so more competitors entered the games.[25]

The ancient Greeks are the source of many of our traditional Western ideals. Whenever our ideals are based on writings from another language, the accuracy and tone of the translation are critical. In many cases translators convey more accurately what they want to find, rather than what is actually there. So it is with the early Greeks and their sport. Their ideals and practices were explained to us by scholars who sought to show the value and honor of their late-nineteenth-century Victorian gentleman's code—the social code of aesthetes and social climbers, of nouveau riche and of snobs—a code based not on honor, but on wealth and privilege. They presented the athletes of ancient Greece in the guise of Victorian upper-class wannabes.

That ideal took hold, despite its unreality. The amateur Greek was a fiction, like the later creation of Abner Doubleday as the inventor of baseball—yet another fake created by men trying to stake a claim (in that case the false claim that baseball was a completely American invention).

Scholars who studied Greek sport took up that fiction, the idea that the Greeks preferred amateur sport. It was not true; in fact, the Greeks had no word for amateur until the late 1800s, and that word was adapted into Greek from French. Indeed, the ancient Greek word *athletes* (*athlete*) means "competitor for a prize," though the contrasting term (*idiotes*, or layman) translates roughly as "wholly unskilled" or "non-participant."[26] For the Greeks, the distinction was in the level of training and skill, not in the idea of reward or lack of reward. As David Young writes,

> *Ancient amateurism is a myth. No victor in the Olympic Games of classical Greece would ever be eligible in their modern counterpart. [This changed in the 1990s.] Ancient athletes regularly competed for valuable prizes in other games before they reached the Olympics, and they openly profited from athletics whenever they could. . . . The truth is that "amateur" is one thing for which the ancient Greeks never even had a word.*[27]

Indeed, the record suggests that it was not uncommon for the best Olympic athletes to change city-states when offered large enough rewards. David Young cites the sudden disappearance of the Italian colony of Croton from the list of cities with victors at the same time that its wealth vanished.[28]

Donald Kyle writes about the importance of wealth for competing athletes. In his description of sport in ancient Athens he writes that

> *given the natural physical inequalities of men and the fact that physical potential was a prerequisite, athletic success tended to favor the few who had the leisure, finances and inclination to train and travel. . . . At Athens athletics demonstrably were related to wealth and social prominence. . . . In actual competition men won by merit, but socio-economic factors affected one's chances of competing. Men of limited resources were*

*limited to local and lesser contests and to modest celebrations and dedi-
cations. . . . In the fourth as in earlier centuries, the mass of the Athenian
population watched and enjoyed the athletic endeavors of a minority.*[29]

Our modern concept of the amateur athlete is largely a creature of the
Victorian age, a leftover remnant of a class-conscious, racist nineteenth-century
society whose social ideas were reflected in their institutions, such as sport, just
as ours are today.

The Olympic Games were finally abolished in AD 394 by Theodosius I,
the emperor of the Byzantines (the Eastern Roman Empire), primarily because
Theodosius, a Christian, considered the games to be a pagan event because they
were held to honor the Greek gods. At the same time he abolished other similar
games for the same reason.

Greek Physical Education and Sport Revisited

Although we think of the time of the ancient Greeks as a time of pure sport,
genuinely amateur athletic competition was never the true state of affairs.
The Greeks had neither the word *amateur* nor the concept. H. A. Harris argues
that the decline of sport came when the emphasis was shifted from participation
to the winning of prizes and the amusement of spectators.[30] The Greek athletes
competed for prizes offered by the city-states, the city-states offered the prizes
to attract the athletes, and the games were staged to bring fame and business to
the city-states. Sport became more of a business than an amusement for both the
organizers and the competitors. This may have been a problem, but it is unclear
whether it contributed to a decline in sport or in the public interest in sport.

Greek civilization, particularly as represented by the Athenians, was a high
point in the history of education. This period marked the first time in Western
civilization that the educational process developed beyond simply meeting mostly
military or trade needs. For the first time, education had a balanced goal: the
development of a whole man, a person who was well and equally developed in
mind and body, a man who met the military needs of his day, but who, unlike the
Spartans, could also fulfill the civic or governmental needs of his time. Unfortunately, that concept was not yet extended to women.

Philosophy became a part of education during this period. People such as
Socrates, Plato, and Aristotle debated the ideal educational process that would
produce the well-rounded product. The balanced educational process of the Athenians was not to be seen again until the Renaissance, and when it did appear, it was
a deliberate attempt to copy the newly rediscovered Greeks. As Greek civilization
declined and Roman civilization grew to replace it, much of the glory of its culture
was lost to Western civilization. The power of the Greek people declined (largely
because of the prolonged wars between the city-states), and they were conquered
by the Macedonian empire of Alexander the Great. When Alexander died around
320 BCE, his empire broke into smaller nations. Greek civilization went through
a process of blending with the civilization of the Middle East over the next two

centuries. The resulting diluted Greek culture was encountered by the Romans, who became powerful in the eastern Mediterranean between 200 and 100 BCE.

The Greeks and Modern Society

Westerners feel close to the ancient Greeks for many reasons. They see the Greeks as the first people to express our modern concept of democracy, and they still think of their theoretical educational system as one of the best balanced systems of all time. Their philosophy of the harmonious relationship between the mind and the body lies at the heart of most contemporary Western philosophies of physical education.

The Greek society was similar to modern societies in many respects, but one common link was the strong interest in athletic competition. Sport was an important part of life for the Greeks. It was supported by most Athenians as a significant part of the educational process in the sense that it assisted in their search for bodily perfection to accompany their training of the intellect. Sport was supported by the government, as in Sparta, because it produced a population that would be prepared to serve in the army if the need arose.

The Athenians were also like modern societies in raising sport to an artificially high level of importance. Under the laws of Solon the values of monetary awards to winners at the Olympics and other games were set at levels that raised the champions to membership in upper-class society.[31] Those legal decrees were the precursor of today's state-run systems of sport.

The Age of Utility and Spectators: The Roman Empire

Roman civilization first appeared at a hilly point on the Tiber River in the central part of the Italian peninsula. Founded by shepherds and traders, Rome began as a republican society with the government of the state shared by its citizens. The small city-state gradually expanded its control of the surrounding territory until it had conquered the entire peninsula of Italy. It then looked to other parts of the Mediterranean, always with the excuse that Rome was only protecting itself against potential invaders.

The essential characteristic of Roman civilization was practicality: What would work in a given situation? While the Greeks had been thinkers and philosophers, the Romans were doers. The Greeks built philosophies, and the Romans built roads.

The Roman society of the early years was a strong one. It stressed strength, patriotism, religious faith, and character or morals. Women were more important and more equal in the Roman society than they had been in Greece.

Roman Education and Physical Education

The object of early Roman education was to produce children who would be true to the Roman ideals and religion. During a child's early years, education took place in the home. Physical training for the boys was directed almost entirely toward military goals. Unlike the Greeks, the Romans had no real interest in beauty, harmony, or the balanced development of the individual, although a strong sense of morals was considered important. The study of literature came from the memorization of the Twelve Tables, Rome's codification of the laws.

As the power and influence of the Romans grew and they gained control of more provinces in the eastern Mediterranean, they saw a greater need for education that would enable them to administer their territories. There was a trend away from the military orientation of physical training as the old part-time army of citizens became more of a full-time army of mercenaries, non-citizens who were paid to serve in the army.

Education in the home had made early Rome strong, but as the Empire grew, schools were developed outside the home. The majority of instruction was given by Greek slaves, who had a broader education than the Romans.[32] These Greeks provided the grammar studies of their traditional education, but as the Romans saw no practical use for gymnastics or music, those studies were not included in the program. The educational program was unbalanced because the Romans were interested primarily in education that had practical uses. Their contributions to civilization were notably in the practical areas of law and engineering.

The Romans also were very interested in baths. Ruins of old Roman baths, many of which were built and operated by the government, can be found in many areas of the Western world today. Some facilities were provided for exercise at the baths, but not on the scale seen in Greece. Exercise was only a minor part of the experience at the Roman baths. The emphasis was the sedentary pleasures of hot and cold baths and massage. The baths were more like health spas or social clubs today.

The great wealth that came into the Roman Empire from the conquered nations, along with the many slaves who did much of the work previously done by the poorer Romans, led to a breakdown of the societal morals of the Roman people. A Roman did not have to work to survive because the state provided free food. Political corruption grew with this luxury, and the old Roman ideals of patriotism and self-sacrifice died.

The later Romans saw little reason for physical training. Rome became a nation of spectators. The people would go to the circus or the amphitheater and watch chariot races or gladiatorial fights to the death. As people demanded more variety in the death struggles, there were fights between animals and men, between larger groups of men, and eventually, by flooding the arena, even small sea battles were waged. The Romans were known for their rabid support of the colors of their favorite professional chariot-racing teams, the most popular sport throughout the Empire.[33]

This preference for being spectators had a weakening effect on the strength of Roman society. The moral and educational values of the Romans gradually disappeared. The Romans were more interested in the violent sports (but only as spectators), and they had little interest in personal competition or in personal excellence.

Roman Sport

A number of advantages aided the survival of sport (particularly track and field) in Greece. The Greeks had centuries of experience in sport. Sport had religious ties because it had ceremonial uses, it had been a pastime of the wealthy, and it was still a part of the educational experience for Greek youth. Sport did not have the same advantages in the Roman world.

As mentioned, the Greeks were more philosophical than the Romans, who were more practical minded. The Greeks had a philosophical basis for sport as a cultural activity, but the Romans saw sport in only two ways, both of which were basically practical: as military training and as entertainment. The Romans were not interested in the educational value of sport, except as preparation for war.

Unlike the Greeks, the Romans were primarily spectators, rather than participants. For the most part they did not compete in sports; they watched others take part. Many questions have been raised concerning whether we should more accurately call the Roman spectacles *athletics*, or even *entertainment*, rather than *sport*. This change also would include our calling the participants *competitors* or *participants*, rather than *athletes*. The Roman pattern of going to sporting events to be entertained is a trend that is clear in today's athletics.

The most notable characteristic of Roman sport was its element of cruelty, with the gladiatorial bouts (occasionally including female gladiators),[34] the fights between man and beast, the mass executions—all apparently featuring the death of humans as public entertainment. These spectacles were held regularly, but the "performers" were usually condemned criminals and slaves. It was a case of "spectacle is the opiate of the masses" because it was a way of entertaining an idle population, distracting them from the less pleasant realities of their own lives. The Romans did not generally consider the spectacles cruel because they did not involve free people. The Romans saw those who died more as object lessons than as real people. To the Romans, allowing a condemned man to become a gladiator was giving him a second chance at survival.[35]

As William Baker notes, the difference between the Greek and Roman approaches to sport can be seen in their choice of words used to describe it. Although the Greeks used *agon*, roughly translated as *contest*, the Romans used the word *ludi*, which meant *game* but with the meaning of an entertainment or amusement. This difference shifts the emphasis from the competitors to the spectators, which the Romans did.[36] Also, the individualism of Greek sports did not appeal to the Romans. Greek athletics did not produce good soldiers.

The changing religious ideals under the Romans helped to destroy what strength remained in the Greek sports system. The new religion of Christianity opposed many sports as pagan because of their ceremonial use in honoring the gods. At the same time, the concept of the mind–body balance was lost, as was the idea of all-around bodily development. The age of specialization had come to the ancient world, and we can see its ill effects in sport even today.

The emphasis of sport originally had been the honor of victory and the joy of competition, but over a period of centuries it changed until there was only one real emphasis: victory—and few sought it. Most people preferred to watch and place bets on the outcome. This overemphasis on victory and reward carried into the early medieval period, when it (and much of sport) lost favor in a Christian reaction against the pagan elements of sport. As the Roman Empire dissolved, as the wealth vanished, the rich prizes were no longer available on a regular basis, and the traditional organized sports of the Greeks and Romans gradually disappeared.

The wealth and sedentary decadence of the Romans eventually brought down the empire. When the barbarians attacked, the Romans no longer had the internal strength to oppose a strong outside force. Although the Romans had gained control over most of western Europe, the Mediterranean, and the Middle East, the conquests began to reverse as the barbarians nibbled at the edges of the empire. By AD 400 the Romans were in full flight; they withdrew their outlying garrisons to return home to defend Rome, but to no avail. Wealth and moral laxity had made Roman culture too weak for a successful defense. Although the last true Roman emperor passed from the scene in AD 476, the empire continued, controlled by the newcomers and split into two parts: the western empire, centered around Rome, and the eastern empire, centered at Constantinople. From that time, the Roman Empire had little influence. Most of its former territories had fallen to various barbarian groups who had hoped to get a piece of the rich Roman life for themselves.

Summary

Ancient physical education was concerned with survival skills and conformity conduct. Early games were games of chance, games of dexterity and skill, and children's games. We often see a warlike basis for the early forms of sport, though ancient sport was not always war oriented. The first records of sport competitions are from the ancient Greeks and showed an emphasis on military skills. Funeral games honored their dead; prizes were awarded for prowess in foot racing, boxing, wrestling, and chariot races. The major city-states were Sparta and Athens. Sparta was a totalitarian society where the education was primarily physical and conducted in a military setting. This is an example of dualism, the separation of mind and body in education.

The Athenians are our model for a balanced education. Athens was a democratic society. Their education valued *paideia*, the "beautiful and the good." This represents the ideal characteristics of an Athenian citizen: aesthetic sensibilities, knowledge, physical skills, and a strong sense of ethics. Spartans stressed the development of the man of action, while the Athenians sought a harmonious development of the individual across physical and intellectual lines. The Greeks also had the first leisure ideal, as *paideia* to them also referred to self-improvement. The ideal of Greek culture was arete, which meant virtue or excellence. They believed everyone had the power to make choices. The reason for gaining knowledge was to prepare you to make the right choices.

The major Greek festivals apparently evolved from funeral games. The greatest was the Olympic Games, but there were also competitions for women, such as the festival of Hera. The symbolic prize for an Olympic victory was a wreath of olive leaves, but the city-states offered valuable prizes to their citizens. The ideal of the amateur ancient Greek is fiction created in Victorian England. For the Greeks, the distinction was in the level of training and skill, not in the idea of reward or lack of reward. The Olympic Games were abolished as pagan by the emperor Theodosius I in AD 394.

While the Greeks were thinkers, the Romans were doers. The Greeks built philosophies, the Romans built roads. Roman society stressed strength, patriotism, religious faith, and character or morals. Physical training for the boys was primarily for military goals. The Romans used public baths much as we use health spas or social clubs today. The later Romans became a nation of spectators preferring the violent spectator sports and having little interest in personal competition or excellence. The Greeks described sport as *agon* (contest), while the Romans used the word *ludi* (game), meaning entertainment or amusement. This shifted the emphasis from the competitors to the spectators.

The Greek ideal of a sound mind in a sound body reappeared during the Renaissance. It became the modern model for physical education, the concept of developing the whole person through physical means. The basic Greek ideals are a critical foundation to our modern concepts of education, leisure, and citizenship.

Further Readings

Athletics and philosophy in ancient Greece and Rome. 2010. *Sport, Ethics and Philosophy* 4: Entire issue.

Briers, Audrey. 1996. *Sporting success in ancient Greece and Rome.* Woodstock, NY: Schwartz.

Crowther, Nigel B. 1996. Athlete and state: Qualifying for the Olympic Games in ancient Greece. *Journal of Sport History* 23: 34–43.

_____. 2001. Visiting the Olympic Games in ancient Greece: Travel and conditions for athletes and spectators. *International Journal of the History of Sport* 18 (4): 37–52.

Dombrowski, Daniel A. 2009. *Contemporary athletics and ancient Greek ideals.* Chicago: University of Chicago Press.

Faulkner, Neil. 2012. *A visitor's guide to the ancient Olympics.* New Haven, CT: Yale University Press.

Finley, M. I., and H. W. Pleket. 1976. *The Olympic Games: The first thousand years.* New York: Viking.

Forbes, Clarence A. 1929. *Greek physical education.* New York: Century.

Futrell, Alison. 2006. *The Roman games: A sourcebook.* New York: Wiley-Blackwell.

Golden, Mark. 1998. *Sport and society in ancient Greece.* Cambridge: Cambridge Univ. Press.

Harris, H. A. 1972. *Greek and Roman sport.* Ithaca, NY: Cornell Univ. Press.

Hawhee, Debra. 2005. *Bodily arts: Rhetoric and athletics in ancient Greece.* Austin: Univ. of Texas Press.

Kyle, Donald G. 2007. *Sport and spectacle in the ancient world.* Malden, MA: Blackwell.

Lehmann, Clayton Miles. 2009. Early Greek athletic trainers. *Journal of Sport History* 36: 187–204.

Lindsey, Peter. 1991. The funeral games of Virgil's *Aeneid*. *Canadian Journal of History of Sport* 22 (2): 1–22.

Lunt, David J. 2009. The heroic athlete in ancient Greece. *Journal of Sport History* 36: 375–392.

McClelland, John. 2008. *Mind and body: Sport in Europe from the Roman Empire to the Renaissance*. London: Routledge.

Mechikoff, Robert A. 2009. *A history and philosophy of sport and physical education: From ancient civilizations to the modern world*. 5th ed. Boston: McGraw-Hill.

Miller, Stephen G. 2004. *Ancient Greek athletics*. New Haven, CT: Yale Univ. Press.

Newby, Zahra. 2006. *Athletics in the ancient world*. Herndon, VA: Duckworth.

Nicholson, Nigel J. 2006. *Aristocracy and athletics in archaic and classical Greece*. New York: Cambridge Univ. Press.

Papakonstantinou, Zinon. 2012. The athletic body in classical Athens: Literary and historical perspectives. *International Journal of the History of Sport* 28 (12): 1657–1668.

Papantoniou, G. 2008. Religiosity as a main element in the ancient Olympic Games. *Sport in Society* 11 (1): 32–43.

Potter, David. 2011. *The victor's crown: A history of ancient sport from Homer to Byzantium*. New York: Oxford Univ. Press.

Puhvel, Jaan. 2002. Hittite athletics as prefigurations of ancient Greek games. In *The Archaeology of the Olympics*, 6–31. Madison: Univ. of Wisconsin Press.

Reese, Anne, and Irina Vellera-Licoh. 2002. *Athletries: The untold history of ancient Greek women athletes*. Costa Mesa, CA: Nightowl.

Reid, Heather L. 2007. Sport and moral education in Plato's *Republic*. *Journal of the Philosophy of Sport* 34 (2): 160–175.

————. 2011. *Athletics and philosophy in the ancient world: Contests of virtue*. New York: Routledge.

————. 2012. Athletic beauty in classical Greece: Literary and historical perspectives. *Journal of the Philosophy of Sport* 39: 281–297.

Scanlon, Thomas. 2009. Contesting ancient Mediterranean sport. *International Journal of the History of Sport* 26 (2): 149–160.

Sinn, Ulrich. 2000. *Olympia: Cult, sport and ancient festival*. Trans. Thomas Thornton. Princeton, NJ: Markus Wiener.

Spivey, Nigel. 2004. *The ancient Olympic Games: A history*. New York: Oxford Univ. Press.

Swaddling, Judith. 1999. *The ancient Olympic Games*. 2nd ed. Austin: Univ. of Texas Press.

Young, David C. 1984. *The Olympic myth of Greek amateur athletics*. Chicago: Ares.

————. 2005. *Mens sana in corpore sano*? Body and mind in ancient Greece. *International Journal of the History of Sport* 22 (1): 22–41.

Discussion Questions

1. Discuss the roles of physical education and sport in ancient and early cultures. What part did they play? Did those roles change as the societies became more advanced?

2. Compare and contrast the Athenian and Spartan systems of education and physical education.

3. Explain how Greek culture and philosophy affected the development of the leisure ideal.

4. Briefly describe the origin, development, and end of the ancient Olympic Games.

5. How did the Greek concept of athletics compare to the concept of amateurism from 1880 to 1992? Are any of the problems in ancient Greek athletics similar to today's problems in athletics?

6. Compare and contrast the Athenian and modern ideas of education and physical education.

7. Compare and contrast Athenian and Roman physical education and sport. Can we find any lessons for today in the differences between their practices?

8. "The Greeks were also like modern societies in raising sport to an artificially high level of importance." Explain what the author means by that statement, giving examples to demonstrate your points.

References

1. Hackensmith, C. W. 1966. *History of physical education*. New York: Harper and Row, 7.

2. Evjen, Harold D. 1992. The origins and functions of formal athletic competition in the ancient world. In *Proceedings of an International Symposium on the Olympic Games*, ed. William Coulson and Helmut Kyrieleis, 96. Athens: Lucy Braggiotti Publications for the Deutsches Archaologisches Institut Athen.

3. Kyle, Donald G. 2007. *Sport and spectacle in the ancient world*. Malden, MA: Blackwell, 51–53.

4. Semotiuk, Darrell. 1982. Human energy in sport coaching: Historical perspectives from ancient Greece. *Canadian Journal of History of Sport* 13 (December): 20–21.

5. Kyle, Donald G. 2011. Ancient sport: Recent discoveries and developments. *2011 NASSH Proceedings*, 56–57.

6. Lunt, David. 2009. Games for the living and games for the dead: The convergence of life and death in ancient Greek athletics. *2009 NASSH Proceedings*, 40–42.

7. Kennard, June, and John Marshall Carter. 1994. In the beginning: The ancient and medieval worlds. In *Women and sport: Interdisciplinary perspectives*, ed. D. Margaret Costa and Sharon R. Guthrie, 15–26. Champaign, IL: Human Kinetics.

8. Weimer, Herman. 1962. *Concise history of education*. New York: Philosophical Library, 8.

9. Gardiner, E. Norman. 1910. *Greek athletic sports and festivals*. London: Macmillan, 468, 503.

10. Goodale, Thomas, and Geoffrey Godbey. 1988. The roots of the leisure ideal. In *The Evolution of Leisure: Historical and Philosophical Perspectives*, 18. State College, PA: Venture.

11. Evjen, Origins and functions, 104.

12. Christensen, Paul. 2009. Whence 776? The origin of the date for the first Olympiad. *International Journal of the History of Sport* 26 (2): 161–182; and Kyle, *Sport and spectacle*, 15–16.

13. Mouratidis, John. 1984. Heracles at Olympia and the exclusion of women from the ancient Olympic Games. *Journal of Sport History* 11 (Summer): 41–55.

14. Lammer, Manfred. 1984. The Greek agon—war or game? Paper presented at the Olympic Scientific Congress, Eugene, OR.

15. Young, David C. 1984. *The Olympic myth of Greek amateur athletics*. Chicago: Ares, 142–146.

16. Ibid., 147–157.

17. Ibid., 167.

18. Ibid., 172–176.

19. Ibid., 139.

20. Gardiner, *Greek athletic sports*, 359–371; and Harris, H. A. 1972. *Sport in Greece and Rome*. Ithaca, NY: Cornell Univ. Press, 34–35.

21. Sweet, Waldo E. 1987. *Sport and recreation in ancient Greece: A sourcebook with translations*. New York: Oxford Univ. Press, 238–239; and Harris, *Sport in Greece and Rome*, 40–41.

22. Miller, Stephen G. 2004. *Ancient Greek athletics*. New Haven, CT: Yale Univ. Press, 150–159.

23. Harris, *Sport in Greece and Rome*, 17.

24. Semotiuk, Human energy in sport coaching, 20–21.

25. Young, *Olympic myth*, 113; and Matz, David. 1991. *Greek and Roman sport: A dictionary of athletes and events from the eighth century B.C. to the third century A.D.* Jefferson, NC: McFarland, 6.

26. Young, *Olympic myth*, 7–8.

27. Ibid., 7.

28. Ibid., 139–142.

29. Kyle, Donald G. 1987. *Athletics in ancient Athens*. Leiden, Netherlands: Brill, 122–123.

30. Harris, *Sport in Greece and Rome*, 17.

31. Thompson, James G. 1988. Political and athletic interaction in Athens during the sixth and fifth centuries B.C. *Research Quarterly for Exercise and Sport* 59: 183–190.

32. Weimer, *Concise history*, 11–16.

33. Humphrey, John H. 1986. *Roman circuses: Arenas for chariot racing*. Berkeley: Univ. of California Press.

34. Manos, Alfonso. 2011. New evidence of female gladiators: The bronze statuette at the Museum für Kunst und Gewerbe of Hamburg." *International Journal of the History of Sport* 28: 2726–2752.

35. Auguet, Roland. 1972. *Cruelty and civilization: The Roman games*. London: Routledge; and Wiedemann, Thomas. 1992. *Emperor and gladiators*. London: Routledge, 105.

36. Baker, William J. 1988. *Sports in the Western world*. Rev. ed. Urbana: Univ. of Illinois Press, 31.

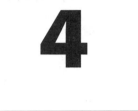

CHAPTER

4

Physical Education and Sport in Medieval and Early Modern Europe

The Roman Empire fell because most of the Romans made little effort to prevent its fall. The incoming barbarians wished to share in the advantages of the empire and had considerable respect for Roman traditions, but they did not really understand the Roman culture and were unable to preserve it. The rapidly growing Christian church was the only stable institution in Europe after the fall of the Roman Empire. The strength of the Church lay in its uncompromising dogmatism and its rigid organizational structure. Consequently, it was the strongest political force in Europe during the medieval period.

Medieval Society and Physical Education

The Middle Ages is a period that many people misunderstand. It is often called the Dark Ages in the belief that little is known about the period or that the people of the times were uncivilized or unenlightened. Those beliefs, however, are incorrect. Essentially, the Middle Ages was a transition period between a time when a large, unified nation or civilization (the Roman Empire) had disappeared and a later time when nations regained strength and stability (the Renaissance). However, the people of the Middle Ages did seem to be retreating from civilization.

The feudal system was the dominant form of social and political organization. Some scholars have suggested that the system had Germanic origins and developed from a form of tribal organization that tied the fighting men to a single chieftain. In the pyramidal structure of feudalism, the greater partners (lords) furnished financial or political support to the monarch and protection or some manner of making a living to their many lesser partners (vassals). The vassals provided military and political support for their lords and the monarch.

A vassal owed a stated period of military service for each landholding that he was given. The monarch owned all of the land and had the right to evict any person who broke his oath of fealty or loyalty. The landholdings were not hereditary, so the monarch could disown the heirs of a vassal (lords were considered vassals to the monarch). In this system, the land was divided into large manors or farms. The lords possessed the domain and all its products, plus a share of the products of the tributary lands that were worked by their vassals (in this case, similar to tenant farmers).

The towns were decaying because of the economic decline that took place from the fifth to the eighth centuries, the early Middle Ages. Trade in the Mediterranean Sea area was hampered by the rising Muslim tide. Its converts, at their peak of power, had gained control of the sea from Turkey around the south shore across Africa and upward into Spain. Travel was risky because of pirates at sea and barbarians and highwaymen on land. No strong, protective governments existed to assist free trade.

As Muslim strength declined, trade became more open on the Mediterranean. Towns gradually began to grow in areas where there was protection, such as beside castles and monasteries, and trade fairs sprang up across Europe. During the ninth to eleventh centuries, the signs of a stable civilization began to reappear, and the growing trade across the face of Europe led to the peak of medieval development around the twelfth to thirteenth centuries.

During this time, the need for money to wage wars led many monarchs to sell charters for towns, giving them the rights of a lord. Those towns, surrounded by walls for safety, became growing commercial and industrial areas. Traders and skilled artisans developed guilds, or trade unions, designed to ensure the quality of their products, to train apprentices in the skills of the trade, and to maintain price levels by limiting their competition in the field.

Between 1096 and 1270 a series of eight crusades, or military expeditions, were called for by the popes of the Catholic Church. Those campaigns were in response to several recurring problems: The Holy Land (around Jerusalem) was captured by the Muslims, who hated the Christians; the Western world was threatened by the Turks; and the papal strength and control were challenged by the Holy Roman Emperor, whose territories were concentrated in the area of today's Germany.

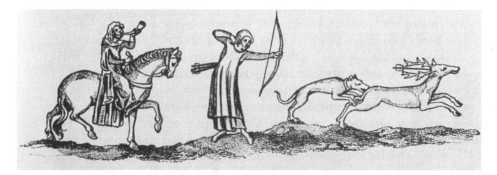

Hunting was a popular sport among the nobility during the Middle Ages.

Men responded to the call for the crusades for many different reasons, some of them religious. Men went on the crusades to protect the Church, or they went simply to gain salvation. Other men were greedy. They sought their fortune in the booty of victory or sought fame or adventure. However, as later crusades were called, their religious appeal diminished until they amounted to little more than self-seeking expeditions of greedy knights. A major effect of the crusades on late medieval Europe was the reestablishment of contact with areas beyond Europe.

Perhaps the best known tradition of the Middle Ages is chivalry, or the tradition of courtly love, which is based on heroic fancy and romantic notions. The fiction that chivalry ruled the world resulted primarily from a thirst for honor and glory and the nobility's desire for praise and lasting fame. It implied the qualities of compassion, piety, austerity, fidelity, heroism, and love.

The Catholic Church frowned on chivalry because of its erotic elements. The romantic ideal was actually adulterous, as the knight was expected to worship a married woman. The Church did approve of some of the other ideals of chivalry, such as the ascetic tendencies implied in suffering for one's faith.

Education during the Middle Ages usually was limited to members of the nobility. What little education there was for the common people was aimed toward learning a trade and surviving. The male nobility was educated for knighthood. Females received little formal education.

A young nobleman was trained in the house of another noble, rather than being trained by his own family. At about the age of 7 years he became a page. Until the age of 14 years he was trained by the women and household workers. Women were not usually rated very highly in the Middle Ages, although among the nobility they were expected to organize and administer large households and estates, particularly during the frequent absences of the men.

Following the page phase of training in which emphasis was on learning to serve people, a boy became a squire, usually by serving a knight or group of knights until he was 21 years old. During this period, he concentrated on learning the arts of war, developing his body, and performing acts of obligation to his lord.

Around the age of 21 years, perhaps earlier in cases of exceptional bravery, a young man became a knight. Knighthood was usually bestowed in a serious religious ceremony. A ceremonial bath, followed by an all-night religious vigil in the company of the young man's lord and a bishop, preceded the investitures, which often were held on major religious holidays and were accompanied by tournaments or other festivities. Physical education lay at the core of the training for knighthood at all stages, with the goals of acquiring military prowess and developing social graces and sports skills.

Much confusion surrounds the question of the Catholic Church's ideas on physical education in the late Middle Ages. No clear definition of its position has emerged from what is known about the Church and civilization at that time, but the traditional view is that the Church was usually opposed to physical education for three reasons. First, in the early years the Church was disturbed by what it considered the debased character of the Roman sports and games. Second, it closely associated the Roman games with pagan religions (the Church was extremely intolerant of other faiths). Third, the Church was developing a growing belief in the evil nature of the body. The body and soul were becoming viewed as two separate entities. The soul was to be preserved and strengthened, but the body should not be catered to in any way. It should not be given entertaining or beneficial physical exercises. The Church attempted to suppress many games and sports at this time because they were considered frivolous and perhaps tinged with sin. Dance was also strongly discouraged because of its sensual appeal.

However, this position was not universal. A number of churchmen, such as Saint Thomas Aquinas, were advocates of physical education prior to and during the Middle Ages. Usually those men had been exposed to a classical education and thus viewed the body as a unity of parts, rather than as separate and perhaps antagonistic parts. In the first several centuries of the Church's existence, and again after the Middle Ages, physical education was not opposed. As Aquinas explained it in the late 1200s:

In order to achieve happiness, perfection in both the soul and body are necessary. Since it is natural for the soul to be united with the body, how is it credible that perfection of the one (soul) should exclude the perfection of the other (body)? Let us declare, then, that happiness completed and entire requires the well-being of the body.[1]

During the Middle Ages, however, the dominant view of the Church, and of much of society, was very otherworldly. The primary concern of the immediate life was to prepare for the afterlife. A future life of justice and peace was promised. Thus, asceticism (the denial of the pleasures or needs of the body) was a popular concept among the more religious people.

This position came from the blending of the Roman and early Christian influences, "the stoic acceptance of good and bad fortune . . . accepting God's will." The Romans required discipline and careful regulation "because the good life must be imposed upon human nature that desired evil." The early Christians frowned on wealth, believing it was a sign of a person's "lack of Christian faith and service." This early position was influenced by Saint Augustine, who wrote that Rome fell as God's punishment for its corruption and sinning, and by Saint Benedict's rules for monasteries, which stressed work and taught that "idleness was . . . an enemy of the soul," both of which were positions that were echoed later by the Puritans.[2]

We have difficulty understanding the philosophies of these people because the difficulties they faced are beyond our experience. As Thomas Goodale and Geoffrey Godbey observe, "for several centuries the encompassing mood was one of pessimism, doom and gloom."[3] Life was filled with hard physical labor; millions died in a series of plagues so deadly that they were similar to having 75 million people die in the United States in a period of a few years. We cannot easily imagine such scenes, with whole towns wiped out by a disease with no known cause or cure. It is hardly surprising that people believed they were being punished for their sins.

At the same time, the monasteries began the move toward the modern concept of time, of governing our activities by the clock. Their rules of work and their concept of dividing and measuring the day's productive activities were a change from past customs, which often did not even consider work a virtue. Their vows of poverty, chastity, humility, obedience, and silence embodied the Christian ideal of that time. The monasteries also preserved classical writings and supported teaching and learning.

At this time, the Church was the savior of education because education as an intellectual process was generally conducted by the Church. Usually the educational process was purely intellectual and had no physical side. The common system consisted of the seven liberal arts, composed of the *trivium* (grammar, rhetoric, and logic) and the *quadrivium* (arithmetic, geometry, astronomy, and music). The monasteries preserved much of the learning that survived the Middle Ages and played a major role in education at that time.

In the fourteenth and fifteenth centuries, medieval civilization began to fade in the light of the new forces it had created. Europe was waking up and progressing rapidly. Its culture was flourishing, the towns were becoming strong, and education and the arts were developing in new directions. Kings and queens began to consolidate their power and form nations similar to those we know today. This period of rebirth for civilization led to the term by which we know the era: the Renaissance.

Medieval Sport: Source of the Sport Dichotomy?

The sport dichotomy is a characteristic of sport that has been noted as far back as the ancient Greeks: the growth or control of sport by the upper classes of a society.[4] The Homeric games involved primarily the upper classes because the lower classes either were not permitted to compete or had too little time to train for competitive success. Some scholars suggest that this trait of the Greek games disappeared rather early, and they do not consider it a common characteristic.

We next see this dichotomy, or class split, in sport during the Middle Ages. When we think of physical education or sport in the Middle Ages, we usually think of the activities of the upper classes. The age of chivalry, with its tournaments, was an upper-class phenomenon only; no chivalric tradition existed for the majority of the people. Accepted sports, that is, sports that were considered worthwhile, were always the sports of the upper classes. This tradition has continued to a marked degree to the present day. Even today the modern Olympic Games are completely controlled and dominated by a small group of wealthy men who are self-appointed custodians of the spirit of the Games. Their requirements, until recently, still reflected the same upper-class prejudice that was prevalent in the fourteenth century against allowing the general populace a part in sport.

Knight Sports: The Haves

We have already discussed the tradition of chivalry. Most of what we think of as sport of the medieval upper classes falls into this area. We commonly think of the tournaments at which the knights would fight to prove their strength and prowess.[5] The tournaments can be traced back to the tenth century, though elements of their activities go back to Roman times. They originated as military exercises, with some emphasis on the safety of the knights, but over a period of centuries they degenerated until they either were banned by the Catholic Church or became pointless after gunpowder was invented.

The tournaments, like the tradition of chivalry, were strictly for the upper class. Other segments of society could be spectators at a tournament, but only the upper classes could participate directly. As the Renaissance drew near, other activities developed that cut across such class boundaries. Also, the middle and lower classes began to develop their own sports activities separately from those of the upper classes.[6]

Middle-Class and Lower-Class Sport: The Have-Nots

The lower classes of the Middle Ages, the vassals and farmers, can be described as being almost outside society. Although they might be lowly spectators at the tournaments, that was their only involvement in that type of sport. As a result, they had their own games, most of which had ancient origins. Activities emphasized running, jumping, and throwing objects. The middle class, which began to develop with the rebirth of the cities after the tenth century, also was interested in sports activities. The people developed their own variations of the knights' tournaments as they trained themselves to defend their cities. They imitated upper-class sport in many respects, but they also were involved in adding democratic elements. Heiner Gillmeister maintains that many modern ball games were patterned by the lower classes on the characteristics of the tournament, with goals representing the city gates that were defended by the knights.[7]

One such influence was a French ball game, similar to rugby, called *soule*. Contests were held between many different competitive units, including cities, and the primary democratizing element was that people from every class (farmer, burgher, clergyman, and nobleman) might be on the same team. After the contest, both teams had a communal meal (which might not be a bad tradition to bring back to today's sport). People were beginning to discover that sports gave them opportunities in equality that were not available anywhere else.

In his struggle for recognition as an individual, man discovered in sport a meeting ground where he could prove himself under fair conditions. The respect for democratic practices and the self-esteem of the burgher, combined with the desire for fair play, may well be one of the most important contributions that the Middle Ages made to our heritage.

More recent research on medieval sport looks at literature and governmental records for evidence of sporting practices. We could use more research on the towns, which began to grow in size and importance during this period, as competitive sport usually begins to grow as towns grow. Our discussion of medieval sport is largely of sport in England. In describing the sporting activities shown on the Bayeux Tapestry (which illustrates the Norman Conquest of England in 1066), John Marshall Carter argues that the activities show that there was less distinction between the sporting activities of the nobles and peasants than we have believed in the past. Discussing the accounts of sport in London written by William Fitz Stephen, a twelfth-century religious clerk, Carter notes that "it is the idea that play is ritualized aggression and that play is training for war that provides a consistent thread through his ludic [playing activities] tapestry."[8] Fitz Stephen wrote of cock fighting, mock battles imitating the battles of the armored knights, archery, wrestling, stone and javelin throwing, bear and bull baiting, hunting, ice-skating, and football.

Indeed, Carter sees a precedent for the nineteenth-century Muscular Christianity movement during the medieval centuries, as the Church accepted more worldly recruits into the newer religious orders. Examining the sports of the nobility in the fourteenth and fifteenth centuries, Thomas Hendricks suggests that the distinctions between the classes were becoming more rigid, rather than less so, with more emphasis by the upper classes on maintaining class distinctions in sport.[9]

William Baker studies the development of medieval sport in the context of the Church, which he maintains did not discourage sport until the late Middle Ages. He suggests that the Church, in effect, followed the Romans' policy of adopting or accepting many of the customs of the people in the new countries, Christianizing many pagan holiday dates and even many activities of worship or ritual. Unintentionally, the Church popularized ball games by blending the Muslim spring ball games with Easter activities. They provided a natural time for these games and other recreational activities through their insistence on setting aside Sunday as a day of rest from work activities.[10]

The growing number of religious holidays during the Middle Ages provided a large number of days with recreational potential. Indeed, there are accounts of clergy complaining of people playing early versions of three-wall handball against the outside walls of the churches, using the corners formed by the buttresses to make their shots harder to return. One of the nineteenth-century public school handball games required a room designed exactly like the space between two particular buttresses of the school's chapel, including a similar drop off at the rear of the court.

In the later Middle Ages, both church and state began to make rules and laws against sporting activities, partly because of the civil disturbances and occasional deaths that resulted from sports. Both church and state feared social unrest by the common people. At the same time, the government was concerned about national defense. Men needed to practice their archery regularly, in case an army was needed, but they preferred other activities, such as playing football (soccer).

Times were changing, as seen by the decline in some of the traditional chivalric activities. The tournament sports of the knights began to disappear (as did many of the knights), and the activities in which they participated became outmoded, largely a result of the changes in weaponry. The widespread use of the English longbow, which could drive an arrow through a knight's heavy armor, combined with the appearance of gunpowder and early forms of guns, made the knight obsolete. The tournament as an upper-class activity became too dangerous when its functional value as a training ground was lost. After all, knights were sometimes killed in tournaments. By the early 1500s, the tradition of armored knights at the tournament was largely gone, after a spectacular last gasp in 1520 at the Field of Cloth of Gold with Henry VIII.[11]

The Church was developing a more negative view of the human body, which perhaps reached its peak with the Puritans in the seventeenth century. The Church wanted a more strict observance of religious occasions and fewer activities that catered to the pleasure of the human body, regardless of the type of pleasure. However, all of the rules, laws, and threats made little difference. Although the Church opposed play, many clerics themselves played as avidly as did the common people. A peasant had little freedom and few possessions in life, but sport was still free and there for the taking.

Physical Education in the Renaissance and Reformation

The Renaissance was a period of rebirth and transition in Europe. It began in Italy around the thirteenth century and spread gradually to the north and west across Europe for the next 2 centuries. It was a time of vast growth in learning and culture. Through contacts with the Arab world, the Western world was rediscovering many long-lost classical writings of the Greeks and Romans. Islamic scholars had preserved many of the ancient writings, and European scholars retranslated them from Arabic and shared them across Europe. The classical writers became very popular, and many of their teachings were imitated by the Europeans.

The universities, which were first established during the late Middle Ages, were growing into a potent intellectual force. Major centers of learning were located in Paris, Bologna, Salerno, Oxford, and Cambridge. Universities also were developing in other areas of Europe, especially in Germany, as the preference for Church-controlled education weakened and secular education grew. Along with the growth of the universities came the growth of humanism, which emphasized the development of man's being human, his essential humanity. The humanist scholars studied the classics closely because the ancient writings expressed humanistic ideas about education. This study of ancient writings (which the Church considered to be clearly pagan) created many problems for scholars in reconciling the humanities, or humanistic studies, to religion, which was still a dominant force in European life. "The Renaissance became perhaps our clearest example . . . of the necessity of a balance between freedom and order, individual interests and social and political stability, rights and obligations, power and responsibility."[12]

Europe also was making the transition to modern times. The political institutions were changing gradually from feudalism to more powerful monarchies, and the belief in the monarch's divine right to rule was growing. Europe was changing from a system of many small personal alliances between nobles to one in which the nation was the dominant unit. The governments were gradually being centralized, and the people were beginning to think of themselves as English, or French, or German, rather than as Londoners, or Parisians, or Hessians. The birth of nationalism changed the complexion of European affairs. Towns were becoming the new centers of life as the economy began to edge away from its old feudalistic, agrarian orientation.

The invention of gunpowder changed the face of feudalistic military tactics. It helped to thrust Europe into modern times, for with it a smaller force of men was vastly superior to a much larger force of bowmen.

The discovery and spread of knowledge were enhanced by Johannes Gutenberg's invention of movable type. The increased availability of books allowed knowledge and information to spread rapidly across Europe, providing a great impetus to education. The need to be literate increased immensely.

The oldest printed book on physical culture and sports was *De Arte Gymnastica*, written in 1569 by Hieronymous Mercurialis, an Italian physician. Terry Todd states that

> *Mercurialis's book was extremely influential when it was written, and almost all books on gymnastics—which in Mercurialis's day meant exercise—that followed are based on this standard work. He was the first Renaissance writer to address the connection between sport and health, and he was one of the first "medical professionals" to assert that exercise could be beneficial or harmful depending on its duration and intensity.*[13]

The Renaissance was a period of discovery of the outside world as well. People began to question the old teachings about the nature of the world and what lay beyond Europe and northern Africa. They undertook voyages west across the Atlantic Ocean and south and east around Africa to India and beyond. The circumnavigation of the world showed how limited human knowledge had been.

The education of the period began to develop along the lines of the Greek ideal: It stressed a classical education combined with physical education. A major early leader was Vittorino da Feltre (1378–1446). His school for the children of nobility imitated the Athenian model of classical studies taught according to the model set by Quintilian.[14] The subjects included Greek and Latin literature, swimming, fencing, riding, and dancing. Education was primarily for men, though women were treated as relative equals in Italy.

The Renaissance ideal was *l'uomo universale*, the universal or all-around man, who had many talents and interests in the arts and literature, politics, games and sports, and the social graces. He was supposed to be interested and moderately skilled in almost every aspect of contemporary life. The goal of Renaissance educators was to develop an all-around person with a balanced education.

Education was beginning to be accepted as valuable for its own sake, regardless of whether it was immediately practical. The barriers between separate areas of learning were beginning to break down because the Renaissance ideal stressed training across narrow divisions between areas of learning. The ideal was similar to the modern concept of interdisciplinary studies, in which the student tries to avoid the hazards of overspecialization that might result in an educational imbalance. Following the Renaissance, that trend reversed and students moved back toward specialization.

The humanistic impulse was strongly tied to the Reformation, the Protestant struggle against the Catholic Church in the 1500s. The humanists' new translations of the scriptures led to areas of disagreement with the Church's traditional teachings. Many of the humanists were very antagonistic toward the Church, and some (those convinced that the Church had strayed from the early Christian teachings) began to break away and form new churches. Because they protested the actions of the Catholic Church, those humanists were called Protestants. Martin Luther, the founder of today's Lutheran Church, was a major leader of the movement in Germany.

The Protestants often were more supportive of physical activities than the Catholic Church. The Protestants believed that physical activities might help to prevent corruption of the body in word and deed, and therefore were of moral value. The Protestant belief that everyone had the right to read and interpret the scriptures, which required some degree of literacy, increased the interest in education for the general public. Most education under the Catholic Church had been limited to its leaders and scholars. The idea that each individual should have a say in personal beliefs and actions was a new concept for the time. Previously, the Church told people what to believe and what to do. The Protestants were interested in education for both sexes, though women were not considered equal. Women's status had been raised somewhat in the Catholic Church by the emphasis on the Virgin Mary, but that emphasis was on the woman in the home setting, rather than as a partner and equal to man.

As the struggles over religion spread across Europe, some rulers used them as one more way to consolidate their powers. Henry VIII, for example, made himself head of the Anglican Church, the English national church that replaced the Catholic Church. As the nations gradually became modern states, similar to the nations of today, the stage was being set across Europe for the gradual move into the modern era.

Renaissance Sport

As we move from the Middle Ages through the Renaissance period, we find no radical changes in sport. Because the classics of the ancient Greeks were imitated, many of the Greek theories of physical education and sport also were copied. Apparently the sport dichotomy (the distinction between the upper classes and the common people in sporting activities) continued in Italy, where the Renaissance originated.[15]

The Renaissance was also the period of university expansion, many of which were founded at the height of the Middle Ages. University sports may have been just as popular in the Middle Ages and Renaissance as they are today. However, sport was an area of student activity that the schools often tried to suppress or limit because physical activities were believed to interfere with academic studies. The student sports of the Renaissance were similar to today's intramurals, rather than varsity athletics.

The Renaissance concept of the all-around person, developed intellectually and physically, helped to contribute to physical training and sport. Sporting skills were considered as important as intellectual skills for the well-rounded person. Team games were developed, and individual competitive activities (such as those in the military skills) were popular.

Like education, sport was for the elite, the aristocrats. Many activities were enjoyed, such as swimming, running, horseback riding, acrobatics, archery, swordsmanship, and wrestling. At the same time, more activities were learned for use in court and social functions, such as dancing, ball games, recreational hunting, singing, and playing musical instruments. Castiglione's *Book of the Courtier* (1528), followed by Thomas Elyot's *Book of the Governour* (1541), included chapters on physical education, promoting the classical Greek and Roman physical activities (along with fencing, archery, tennis, and dancing) as good exercises. By 1600, physical education was widely accepted as part of the education of young aristocrats at school.

As we move closer to the modern era, sport was still in a low-level, informal state. Games had general forms and rules, but they were not standardized. Many variations of the same basic game could be found across Europe. Although the concept of nationalism was growing, national or international sport had not yet emerged. No sporting contests on the scope of the early Greek Olympics had appeared in any nation. It is only in relatively recent times that sport as we know it today arose: a more formal activity with set, standardized rules, and competition both within and among nations.

Seventeenth-Century European Physical Education and Sport

Education and Physical Education in the 1600s

The seventeenth and eighteenth centuries saw more progress toward our current educational practices than at any previous time, except perhaps ancient Greece. To follow this progress, we must look not at the different nations at that time, because there were still no national programs of education, but at the people who were the most prominent educational theorists.

The seventeenth century saw the rise of the realists, whose goal was to tie education to reality, or life as it really was. They questioned the humanists' total reliance on ancient languages and teachings in the contemporary educational process. They believed that education should teach more useful things to prepare students for life. They also encouraged teaching in the students' native language, rather than in the classical languages, such as Greek and Latin. They wanted to get away from imitating the past.

Three slightly different groups of realists can be defined according to the degree to which they wanted to break away from the theories of the humanists.[16] The first group, the *humanist realists*, wanted to retain classical education as the foundation for all education. Although very similar to the humanists, this group wanted to modify the process of the classical studies by emphasizing the content, but no longer copying the style, of the ancient writers. The humanist realists' ideas were heavily classical.

The second group, the *social realists*, wanted more modification of the classical tradition. This group believed that the goal of education should be preparation for a career, rather than the humanist aim of simply training scholars. The social realists wanted education to develop closer ties to contemporary needs and problems.

The third group, the *sense realists*, believed that knowledge was best obtained through the senses, that is, by observation and experience. This group wanted the schools not only to teach in the vernacular, the language that the students spoke every day (rather than in the classical languages), but also to teach useful arts and sciences. The sense realists tried to base their educational methods on scientifically proven principles.

These groups included many different people. Their ideas are examples of the progress in educational thought and practice that appeared during this time. Education was still limited primarily to the upper classes and to males, but theorists were beginning to suggest that such a concept of education was far too limited. Physical education was still a minor part of the educational process, but as educational theory developed, so did the idea that physical education could be a valuable part of the curriculum. More theorists were beginning to call for the use of physical activities in education, although their primary reason was for improved health.

One of the earliest of the humanist realists was the Frenchman François Rabelais (1495–1553).[17] He wrote of the education of a boy named Gargantua, who studied the classics for their content but was not concerned with their style. His education included practical training and physical education activities as well. Physical activities were used to prepare him for war because he was being trained to become a scholar and a knight. In earlier times he would have been trained for one or the other, but never for both. The physical activities were to strengthen his body and to serve as recreation. Objects in nature were used in the educational process.

Another prominent humanist realist and also a forerunner of the Enlightenment period of the eighteenth century was John Milton (1608–1674), the English writer. Milton believed that a classical education was useful, but he thought that 8 years of study could be condensed into a single year. He wanted to include physical exercises in the studies and divide each day's activities into three parts: study, exercise, and meals. His exercises were basically war oriented. The humanist realists thought that play and games were good training for skill and alertness, but they had little interest in the potential of such activities for developing social or recreational skills.

One of the great theorists of the social realists was the Frenchman Michel de Montaigne (1533–1592). His theories concerned the education of aristocratic boys. He believed that experience and reason were the roads to knowledge. He expressed strong opposition to rote memorization by saying "To know by heart is not to know."[18] His use of physical activities to further a pupil's experiences was very similar in manner to John Dewey's later theories of "learn by doing." Montaigne stressed the education of the mind and the body at the same time, but he was not interested in providing learning experiences through games. Much of modern educational theory can be traced to Montaigne's ideas.

An English social realist, John Locke (1632–1704) used the now-popular phrase of physical educators, "a sound mind in a sound body,"[19] which was originated by Juvenal, a Roman writer. Locke believed that mind and body were separate entities and all ideas came from personal experiences, which might be better described as the experiences of the senses combined with mental reflection or thought based on the experiences. He stressed physical exercise as a way to health and also believed that dancing helped to develop grace. He thought of recreation as a useful and beneficial break in the normal pattern of activity. This view is similar to Jay Nash's twentieth-century statement of recreation as the "re-creation" of the person through a change in the pattern of the individual's activities. Locke's ideas were a major factor in the development not only of contemporary educational theory but also of other educational theories during his time.

Despite such forward-looking ideas, education under the social realists remained oriented toward the aristocracy, rather than the common people. For this reason, many of the ideas of physical activity were an attempt to overcome the tendency of the aristocrats to pamper their children, who usually became overweight, unhealthy students.

A leading sense realist was Richard Mulcaster (1531–1611) of England. He believed that students should be taught at a school with other students, rather than individually by a tutor at home. Mulcaster also was convinced that teachers should be trained professionally. He suggested that both men and women should receive some education, rather than only the males, and he was one of the first to suggest coeducational activities among children.[20] He was interested in physical and moral training through exercise and thought that mass education, unlike the more common tutorial system, could lead to the development of social values through the use of physical activities. Mulcaster, who was one of the strongest early proponents of physical education, urged its use far more than any other person of his time. Although he did not have much immediate influence, his works were rediscovered during the late 1800s.

Wolfgang Ratke (1571–1635) of Germany was another great theoretician of educational reform, although, like many of the other theorists, he was unable to successfully translate his theories into action.[21] The major points in his attempt to develop education as a science included following nature in its teaching methods (teach the students what they need to learn, and teach it at an age when they are ready to learn it); going only one step at a time with new information and utilizing repetition to assist learning; not forcing learning or stressing memorization; learning through experience; and educating all children, without exception. Although Ratke was unable to translate his formulas into personal success, he is considered the father of modern educational theory.

John Comenius (1592–1670), a Czechoslovakian, became a Moravian minister in Bohemia. For religious reasons, he was forced to move frequently. He lived at times in Poland, England, Sweden, Hungary, and finally Holland, where he died. He wrote education books that included illustrations to improve the teaching process. He wanted children to exercise to develop and preserve their health, but he also believed that they could learn much through recreational activities, which was not a widespread idea at the time. Comenius believed in the importance of play in educating young children, and he believed that all children should be educated.[22]

Sport and the Puritans

The Renaissance was combined with the Reformation in northern Europe and England, as its influence spread like ripples on a pond outward from Italy. Partly because of this mixing, and because the Reformation showed a stronger, more strictly moralistic side in the northern areas, there was less interest in balanced physical and mental development. Instead, with the strong influence of the severe views of John Calvin, the tendency was toward asceticism: "Puritanism was an intensely controlled channeling of human energies which had two sides. It was repressive . . . [but it] was also liberating . . . it favored the growth of self-reliance, self-control and a sense of personal worth that made democracy possible and necessary."[23]

In essence, the Puritans of the 1600s believed that the nature of mankind was sinful and vile; they wanted to put as many restrictions as possible on what people were allowed to do in their public and private lives. Consequently, they changed sports and recreations from simple leisure activities to political questions. Many sporting activities included informal gambling, which the Puritans opposed. They also were very concerned about the wasting of time. They considered work more important than anything else except worship. In its most extreme form, under John Calvin:

the Council of Geneva arranged yearly visits to every home to question the members on whether they had engaged in any forbidden activities: gambling, card-playing, profanity, drunkenness, dancing; whether they had sung irreligious or indecent songs, or been excessive in their dress or entertainment; whether they had worn colors of clothes prohibited by law, used more than the legal limit of dishes at a meal, worn jewelry or lace, or piled their hair too high. They were not questioned about their habits at the theater, because eventually even religious plays were forbidden.[24]

The Puritans were very strict in many ways, but most were not opposed to recreation. Instead, they were opposed to idleness and wasting time, and many of the popular recreations of the day went hand in hand with drunkenness and gambling. Puritans were not opposed to drinking, but they opposed drunkenness. They were not opposed to singing, art, or beauty. Their concerns were based on the grounds of wasted time or money.

There were many positive aspects to their beliefs. They were good at cooperative activities, generally well educated, active readers and writers, and supporters of scientific research. Their attitudes about sex came largely from their belief that "the family was almost as sacred as the scriptures and they would tolerate nothing that would disrupt it." They placed a high value on time and work, but not in today's profit-focused sense: They were opposed to taking advantage of another person's need. Indeed, as Goodale and Godbey state, "to the puritans we owe much of our sense of human and personal responsibility."[25]

One can still find reflections of the Puritans' beliefs in our everyday life. For example, if one looks at attitudes toward work and salvation from the Middle Ages, to the Puritans, and on to today's world, one can find these common traits:

Since the early monastic period, hard, back-breaking strenuous, physical work was useful in this respect: since man was basically evil and work hard and strenuous, working was a way of performing penance, recognizing and admitting sinfulness and trying to make amends. Even in a more secular sense, work was and sometimes still is thought of as useful and necessary discipline.[26]

Great social changes were occurring during the sixteenth and seventeenth centuries. In England, people had to move into the towns or to new villages because farmland was being enclosed by large estates, upsetting the stability of social life and limiting the places available for recreation.

One village event that became famous during the early 1600s was the Cotswold Olimpick Games, revived by Robert Dover in the hills west of Oxford, along the flat top of a ridge overlooking the village of Chipping Campden. The games included wrestling, the quintain, fighting with cudgels (the quarterstaff) and pikestaffs, leaping, foot races, handball, pitching the bar and the hammer, and women's smock races.

To respond to Puritan complaints about people's recreation, James I (known for his support of the Bible translation known as the King James Version) issued his *Declaration on Lawful Sports*, known as *The King's Book of Sports*, in 1618. The declaration ordered that legal recreations should not be interfered with or discouraged, even on Sundays, so long as they did not infringe on or cause the neglect of Sunday church services.

The declaration was reissued by his son, Charles I, in 1633, but by 1641 the Puritans had gained enough strength to put the king to flight, eventually executing him. William Baker sums up the period:

> *Even the public pastimes proved to be remarkably resilient. Although the Puritans controlled the government and the laws of the land, they were a minority whose rigorous views remained unacceptable to the bulk of the population. Rural laborers continued to live their lives in terms of seasonal cycles, with periodic festivals and games compensating for times of intense labor. Puritanism was too urban in character, too austere, ever to be fully acceptable to that preindustrial society. Puritan prohibitions against sports and games were doomed to fail. In the end, only the Puritan Sunday established itself firmly in the lives of Englishmen, to become sacrosanct, free of sports and public amusements, until the 20th century.*[27]

Eighteenth-Century European Physical Education and Sport

Education and Physical Education in the 1700s

The realism of the 1600s was followed by the Enlightenment of the 1700s, a movement that attempted to spread rationalism and knowledge to all people. The concurrent trend toward the belief in the essential equality of all men still did not necessarily apply to women. The educational theorists were beginning to move away from the idea that only the aristocracy should be educated. Those theorists of the Enlightenment helped to reinforce the work begun in the seventeenth century; they used many of the realists' theories as the starting point for many of their own theories. John Locke is considered the founder of the English Enlightenment because his focus on educating people through rational, natural means led to the later theories of Rousseau.

Jean-Jacques Rousseau (1712–1788) of France was one of the most important theorists of the Enlightenment. He published two extremely influential books, *Emile* (1762) and *The Social Contract* (1767). *The Social Contract* expanded on his views that all humans are free and equal by nature and that inequality appeared only after they had gotten away from nature and developed governments. Rousseau considered people good by nature but corrupted by so-called civilization.

In *Emile*, Rousseau wrote that the task of education was to develop all of a child's capabilities freely, as nature intended, and to avoid anything that would hamper this natural development. His book was considered a revolt against the education and society of the day and was at first banned by the Catholic Church, then condemned by governments.

Rousseau's plan of education for the imaginary Emile required a tutor, for the child was educated alone. Nature was the primary teacher, and the tutor was the guiding force. Rousseau believed that the child could not be taught by logic, as Locke had suggested, because as a youth the child would not yet have developed common sense. Rousseau wanted to let children progress naturally—learning what they wanted to learn, when they were interested in learning it.

Children were given tasks that were geared toward learning from nature and experience and were considered to be age appropriate. When they became young adults, they would be introduced to languages and to classical authors, who were thought to be closer to nature than the contemporary writers were.

Rousseau also discussed the education of Sophie, Emile's future wife. Sophie was educated in her parents' home in the manner that was traditional for girls. She was taught the skills needed to be a wife and to make her husband's life pleasant. Rousseau had many liberal ideas in his theories, but he was not liberal where women were concerned. He said that all *men* are born equal before nature, and he *did* mean *men*.

Rousseau regarded play as both healthful and educational, but he did not think it should be forced. He was opposed to compulsion in any area of education, believing it to be contrary to the ways of nature. Although Rousseau stressed equality of men in his educational theories, his idea of a tutorial educational process required a one-to-one pupil–teacher ratio and thus was beyond the reach of all but the wealthy.

Rousseau's theories combining the education of the mind and of the body were very similar to contemporary educational thought, but the influence of his works cannot be estimated. The most visible immediate influence was on the Germans, who followed rapidly in developing his theories of naturalism into actual educational practice.

Johann Basedow (1724–1790), a German educator, had experimented with an educational system that was based on the theories of Locke and others and involved physical activity. His discovery of Rousseau's work *Emile* was the basis for the development of his own version of an educational system. In 1774, with the help of a number of financial supporters, Basedow was able to start a coeducational school called the *Philanthropinum*, later known as the Dessau Educational Institute. He tried to educate the children without the influence of any particular church, and he preferred to treat the children as children, rather than as small adults. Basedow published several illustrated books that explained his educational theories and gave examples of the methods and content to be used when teaching children.[28]

He placed a heavy stress on physical activities. The 10-hour day in his school included 5 hours of classes, 3 hours of recreation (including fencing, riding, dancing, and music), and 2 hours of manual labor that taught a craft to the student.

He also planned a camping experience that shared some similarities with today's concept of outdoor education.

The school hired Johann Simon as its teacher of physical education. Simon can be thought of as the first modern physical education teacher. He taught fencing, dancing, games, and some crude gymnastics activities that he developed. He held a contest similar to the ancient Greek Olympics. In 1778, Simon was succeeded by Johann Du Toit, who expanded the gymnastic activities. The exercises were performed outdoors with apparatus built from natural materials.

Basedow, who was unable to make the school work under his direction, left in 1778, but the school (which reached its peak in the early 1780s) continued until 1793. Although the school did not survive, its experimental program, which recognized the importance of physical activities to the child, was very influential throughout Europe.

It had a strong influence on Christian Salzmann (1744–1811), who founded the Schnepfenthal Educational Institute in 1785 near Gotha in eastern Germany. His institute was a good copy of the *Philanthropinum*, only his version succeeded. One year after the founding of the school, Salzmann hired a new, young teacher, Johann GutsMuths (1759–1839), who taught there for 50 years and became one of the most eminent of German physical educators.[29]

Strongly influenced by the writings of Basedow, GutsMuths developed an outdoor gymnastics program that included many activities, with exercises in tumbling, climbing, jumping, vaulting, the horizontal bar, balance beam, and rope ladders. He organized his activities by age level and difficulty and kept careful records of each student's progress. His book *Gymnastics for the Young* was published in 1793 and was reprinted in many countries, including the United States in 1802 (with Salzmann listed as the author). The text "laid the basis of a scientific and evidence-based physical education."[30] GutsMuths's work set the pattern for German gymnastics, which was introduced to the United States around 1825 and was a less formal system than the one that developed later in Germany.

GutsMuths's influence was widespread across two continents because of both his writing skill and the interest of many prominent theorists and practitioners of the day. Friedrich Jahn, Adolph Spiess, and Immanuel Kant were among those who visited Schnepfenthal to study the work carried out at the school until Guts-Muths's retirement in 1835. Many of his practices are similar to those suggested and followed in today's schools.

Johann Pestalozzi (1746–1827) was a Swiss teacher who was also extremely influential among the educational reformers of the early 1800s. He taught at his school at Yverdon in Germany from 1804 to 1825 and wrote a number of books on his theories. His most important book, *How Gertrude Teaches Her Children*, was an expansion of the educational ideas he had introduced in an earlier novel, *Leonard and Gertrude*.[31]

Pestalozzi stressed early education in the family by writing of humans as social creatures. He tried to connect education with life and make it useful. He believed that the learner had to be stimulated to *want* to learn and that the teacher should act as a guide, rather than force the child to learn. He wanted learning to follow

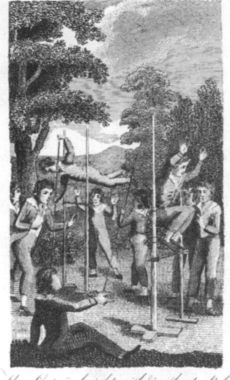

The Leap in height with & without a pole

An example of the outdoor gymnastic popularized by Guts Muths in Germany.
Source: Reproduced from G. Muths, J.C. Friedrich. *Gymnastics for youth: or A practical guide to healthful and amusing exercises for the use of schools.* Printed for P. Byrne, 1803. Courtesy of the Harvard Medical Library in the Francis A. Countway Library of Medicine [HOLLIS number 003017820].

the natural process from easy to difficult activities according to a child's level of development. He saw education as having three aspects: intellectual, practical, and, most important, moral. Physical education also was important to bring the mind and body into full harmony.

His school offered many physical activities, including a daily hour of gymnastics 5 days each week. The gymnastics program gradually became structured as the influence of the formal German system spread. Though it was not advanced, it provided a great impetus for the development of physical education activities on the part of people from many nations who visited the famous school.

Philipp von Fellenberg (1771–1844) based many of his ideas on Pestalozzi's writings and began one of the first European schools for vocational education, sometimes referred to as schools of manual labor. There was one essential difference between Fellenberg and most of the educational theorists: His ideas worked.

Fellenberg's activities were a practical success throughout his life; his school, started in 1804 at Hofwyl, was an immediate success.[32]

Fellenberg believed in the value of physical activity, although he felt that his vocational students received enough activity without having a planned program. He considered their manual work sufficient exercise. It also kept them outdoors, which was important. He encouraged outdoor activity and allowed his students a free choice of activities in their leisure time.

Friedrich Froebel (1782–1852) developed a theory of play based on his experiences studying and teaching at Pestalozzi's school at Yverdon from 1808 to 1810. He stressed that play was essential to the education and development of children. He developed a philosophy of play that went far beyond previous ideas. He expressed some of his ideas in a book titled *Education of Man*.[33]

In 1837, his interest in the education of children and play activities led him to found a school, which he called a kindergarten, for young children in Germany. His ideas on education, which, along with those on the kindergarten, were carried out by his disciples, became a major influence on early childhood education.

During the last part of the Enlightenment period, the ideas of the European theorists were beginning to influence the development of education in the United States. From about 1800 onward, educational theories in Europe moved rapidly to the United States as immigrants brought many of the new ideas with them to the huge, growing land. Many educational developments were concurrent on both continents by 1850, but the developing American educational practices were strongly based on the work of the nineteenth-century European theorists.

The Seeds of Modern Sport

The transition to modern sport began during the 1700s, as some sporting activities started to develop higher-level organization and standardized rules. In horse racing, the Jockey Club was formed circa 1750 as an organization of rich owners and horse breeders. Club members began to write rules for racing, appointed officials, and assessed penalties for breaking the rules. Around 1770, the club published the rules and the annual racing schedules in a new publication called the *Racing Calendar*.

During roughly the same time, the Marylebone Cricket Club (MCC) was founded (perhaps in 1787), soon to play its important matches at Lord's Cricket Ground in northwest London. The MCC proposed and refined formal rules for cricket, quickly standardizing the play in that sport.

The Royal and Ancient Golf Club, founded in 1754 at St. Andrews, Scotland, published rules for golf, standardizing the game at 18 holes in 1764. Even the rough sport of pugilism (boxing) became more standardized with the appearance of written rules, first with Broughton's Rules in 1741. These became the basis of the London Prize Ring Rules of 1838 and the Queensbury Rules of 1867.

Dennis Brailsford suggests that spectator sports had developed enough during the 1700s to be a significant part of popular recreation. Such events were planned to be convenient to the working week, with most events held in the early part of the week, such as Monday or Tuesday. No events were held on Sunday because of attempts to make sports more respectable.[34]

The tempo of work increased as the week progressed. Brailsford refers to

the phenomenon of St. Monday and of a weekend which covered Sunday and Monday. . . . Monday was the nearest day to the last wage and the work day furthest from the wage yet to come. It was the day on which freedom from work was easiest to envisage and one which, for large groups of workers, was regarded as a more or less regular holiday.[35]

During the 1700s and on into the 1800s, England was

a nation rapidly changing from rural to urban, a shift of far-reaching consequences. The rural sporting ethos was passing away as the villages dwindled and the economic importance of the landed gentry decreased; the traditional sporting activities were coming to be more nostalgic than consequential in local life. Religious and civil influences were changing accepted practices from the old "bloody sports" to a taste for less cruel activities more fitting to the sensitivities of city-dwellers affected by growing straitlaced ideals. A new urban sporting ethos was developing, leading gradually to mass spectator sports and highly organized activities. A shift came about from taking the people to the event, as in the early seat of English sporting activities in the villages and fields, to taking the event to the people, moving the activities to large urban centers for the convenience of masses of paying customers.[36]

Nineteenth-Century European Physical Education and Sport

We cannot really draw a line separating the eighteenth century from the nineteenth century when we study the development of physical education because the philosophies and experimental schools of the late 1700s in Europe produced the progress of the 1800s. We have already mentioned several of the educators who were more a part of the nineteenth century; others who were equally influential during the nineteenth century had their ideas rooted in the events of the eighteenth century.

During the late 1700s, revolution was in the wind. The young United States had rebelled against Great Britain, and Rousseau's ideas still had much of Europe in shock. The educational theories that leaned toward Rousseau's views on the equality of men were given a popular boost by the French Revolution. As the year 1800 passed, Napoleon had gained power in France and was trying to gain control of Europe. As nations allied to block him, the feelings of national consciousness rose to an all-time high.

After Napoleon was put to rest and the Congress of Vienna had tried to dance its way to reestablishing the old Europe, many differences became obvious. The people were less content, and there were numerous rebellions between 1815 and 1850. People also were beginning to clamor for national systems of education. At the same time, they were fleeing the Old World in large numbers, taking a chance on finding a better life in the United States. Those who remained behind sought systems of education that would strengthen their nations and have a positive effect on national pride.

Friedrich Ludwig Jahn (1778–1852), a German educator, is often considered the father of gymnastics. Jahn was an ardent Prussian patriot who was opposed to the provincialism that kept Germany separated into a multitude of small kingdoms. He began teaching in a Pestalozzian school, where he tried to use GutsMuths's ideas in an outdoor gymnasium setting.

In 1810, he began using an open area, which he named the *turnplatz*, or exercise group, which was basically a playground with apparatus for exercises. The formal organization of his program gradually became the Turner movement (for *turnverein*). Some people have considered Jahn's system too formal. However, he did oppose artificial activities in the early development of his system and sought to use natural activities instead. A book written in 1816 by one of his followers described Jahn's work; the same year Jahn wrote *German Gymnastics* to explain his system.

Jahn's emphasis on German nationalism eventually put him in prison. The rulers of the different German states considered his views on a unified Germany a threat to their rule, and he was out of favor until the 1840s, when the political climate changed. During that interval, the success of the Turner movement depended on other men.

Adolf Spiess (1810–1858) was the man who had the greatest impact on educational gymnastics in Germany. Having met both GutsMuths and Jahn, he experimented with gymnastics as a teacher by applying the movement to the formal classroom situation. He also worked with Froebel in Switzerland, where he was strongly influenced by Froebel's views on the function of play in education. Spiess's later writings, especially his *Gymnastics Manual for Schools*, classified exercises by difficulty and by appropriate age and sex, which strongly influenced the schools.[37]

Spiess devised a system of free exercises that required almost no apparatus. He also used musical accompaniment for those activities. He stressed the idea of having professionally trained specialists to teach the gymnastics classes. He wanted indoor exercise areas in addition to the traditional outdoor areas, so that the winter weather would not limit the program. He also stressed gymnastics for girls. His free exercises were a great benefit for girls because those exercises required less strength than the apparatus activities. Although Spiess considered the existing formal systems of gymnastics inappropriate for the schools, his own system also included much marching and required discipline and obedience.

Traces of his system, which served as a model for the later German system of school gymnastics, can still be seen in use today.

Franz Nachtegall (1777–1847) is identified as the father of physical education in Denmark. Inspired by the writings of GutsMuths, he gradually became known as a leader in Danish gymnastics and physical training. In 1804, he was made director of the newly established Military Gymnastic Institute, which prepared teachers of gymnastics first for the military and later for the schools.[38] Today the Military Gymnastic Institute is the oldest training institution for gymnastics instructors in Europe. Although Nachtegall did not design his own system, he was very instrumental in the development of school gymnastics and physical programs in Denmark. He was also an influential factor in the development of Per Henrik Ling's Swedish system of gymnastics.

Per Henrik Ling (1776–1839) was the founder of Swedish gymnastics, though he also was well known for his literary works. While living in Denmark, Ling was influenced by the work of Franz Nachtegall. He later decided to train teachers of fencing and gymnastics to strengthen Sweden's army. A fierce Swedish nationalist, he became the director of the new Royal Central Institute of Gymnastics (RCGI) in 1814, where he later developed his program of gymnastics, called either the Swedish system or Ling gymnastics. His emphasis on simple, fundamental movements and exercises was a change from Jahn's complicated exercises.[39]

Although the Ling exercises were developed for both educational and military purposes, they worked better as military training. While Per Henrik Ling's medical and military gymnastics were successful, his son, Hjalmar Ling, really did the major work in developing the educational aspect of the Swedish system.

Archibald MacLaren (c. 1820–1884) was a major early influence on physical education in England. Asked to design a physical training program for the military, he developed a gymnastics program similar to Jahn's that made heavy use of apparatus activities. Above all, MacLaren stressed a balance between recreational activities (physical play) and educational physical activities, which he wanted to use in a regular class (in addition to the non-educational play time) as a part of the educational process. Although MacLaren's ideas on gymnastics never really took hold in England, his writings were a major influence on the development of physical education in England in the late 1800s. His military system of physical education also spread across England as the instructors whom he had trained for the military left military service but continued to teach as civilians.[40]

During the first half of the nineteenth century, the European theorists and their systems were a powerful influence on the development of physical education in the United States. After the Civil War in the United States, the European influence declined rapidly. American physical educators were passing beyond the point where they needed the European ideas as an impetus for developing their own programs and systems. By the end of the century, leaders in the United States were calling on their fellow teachers to work together to develop an American system instead of continuing their reliance on the European systems, which were (after all) designed for Europeans. The turn of the century saw the beginnings of that distinctly American system.

Summary

During the Middle Ages, education was primarily for the nobility or people training for the Church. Most young noblemen were trained to be knights. Physical education was the core of their training; the goals were acquiring military prowess and developing social graces and sports skills. Sport was primarily seen in the upper classes, where it was influenced by the tradition of chivalry. The other social classes gradually developed their own sporting traditions, some of which copied those of the upper classes.

The Catholic Church had mixed ideas on physical education at this time. Many leaders opposed it, in part because of their belief in the evil nature of the body. Better educated churchmen, such as Saint Thomas Aquinas, tended to view the body as a unity of parts, stating "in order to achieve happiness, perfection in both the soul and body are necessary [because] happiness completed and entire requires the well-being of the body."

The Renaissance brought a rebirth of the educational ideas of the Greeks and the ideal of an all-around person with a balanced education. This concept helped to contribute to physical training and sport. Sporting skills were considered as important as intellectual skills for the well-rounded person. The Protestants were more supportive of physical activities that they believed were of moral value. By the 1600s, the Reformation had produced the Puritans, who often opposed sport and leisure as wasteful of time, though they were agreeable to its use for healthful purposes.

The seventeenth and eighteenth centuries saw more progress toward our current educational practices, including a slowly rising emphasis on the value of physical activities first for health, then for other developmental purposes, along with a growth of the idea of universal education. Sport, however, was still primarily informal.

During the eighteenth and early nineteenth centuries, the European theorists and their systems were a powerful influence on the development of physical education in the United States. The gymnastics programs of the Germans became a major influence on the development of physical education across Europe and in the United States, although after the American Civil War the European influence declined rapidly in favor of an American system.

Further Readings

Baily, Steve. 1995. Permission to play: Education for recreation and distinction at Winchester College, 1382–1680. *International Journal of the History of Sport* 12: 1–17.

Brailsford, Dennis. 1969. *Sport and society: Elizabeth to Anne*. London: Routledge/Kegan Paul.

_____. 1999. *A taste for diversions: Sport in Georgian England*. Cambridge: Butterworth.

Carter, John Marshall. 1988. *Sports and pastimes of the Middle Ages*. New York: Univ. Press of America.

_____. 2004. The study of medieval sports, games and pastimes: A fifteen-year reflection. *Sport History Review* 35: 159–169.

Carter, John Marshall, and Arnd Krüger, eds. 1990. *Ritual and record: Sports records and quantification in pre-modern societies*. Westport, CT: Greenwood.

Clarke, Simone. 1997. Olympus in the Cotswolds: The Cotswold Games and continuity in popular culture, 1612–1880. *International Journal of the History of Sport* 14 (2): 40–66.

Cummins, John. 1988. *Hound and the hawk: The practice and meaning of medieval hunting*. New York: St. Martin's.

Gerber, Ellen W. 1971. *Innovations and institutions in physical education*. Philadelphia: Lea and Febiger.

Griffin, Emma. 2005. *England's revelry: A history of popular sports and pastimes, 1660–1830*. New York: Oxford Univ. Press.

Guttmann, Allen. 2004. *Sports: The first five millennia*. Amherst: Univ. of Massachusetts Press.

Huggins, Mike. 2008. Sport and the upper classes c1500–2000: A historiographic review. *Sport in History* 28: 364–388.

_____. 2004. *The Victorians and sport*. New York: Hambledon and London.

Krzemienski, Edward D. 2004. Fulcrum of change: Boxing and society at a crossroads. *International Journal of the History of Sport* 21: 161–180.

Malcolmson, Robert W. 1973. *Popular recreations in English society, 1700–1850*. London: Cambridge Univ. Press.

Martin, Dennis W. 1983. "A Biblical doctrine of physical education." EdD diss., University of North Carolina at Greensboro.

Muhlberger, Steven. 2003. *Jousts and tournaments: Charny and chivalric sport in fourteenth century France*. Highland, TX: Chivalric Bookshelf.

Ottosson, Anders. 2010. The first historical movements of kinesiology: Scientification in the borderline between physical culture and medicine around 1850. *International Journal of the History of Sport* 27: 1892–1919.

Park, Roberta J. 1994. From "genteel diversions" to "bruising peg": Active pastimes, exercise, and sports for females in late 17th- and 18th-century Europe. In *Women and sport: Interdisciplinary perspectives*, ed. D. Margaret Costa and Sharon R. Guthrie, 27–43. Champaign, IL: Human Kinetics.

Semenza, Gregory M. Colon. 2003. *Sport, politics, and literature in the English Renaissance*. Newark: Univ. of Delaware Press.

Strutt, Joseph. 1968. *Sports and pastimes of the people of England*. Detroit: Omnigraphics. (Orig. pub. 1801.)

Twigg, John. 1996. Student sports, and their context, in seventeenth-century Cambridge. *International Journal of the History of Sport* 13 (2): 80–95.

Vale, Marcia. 1977. *The gentleman's recreations: Accomplishments and pastimes of the English gentleman, 1580–1630*. Totowa, NJ: Rowman and Littlefield.

Wigglesworth, Nigel. 1996. *The evolution of English sport*. London: Cass.

Wilkins, Sally. 2002. *Sports and games of medieval culture*. Westport, CT: Greenwood.

Williams, Jean. 2009. The curious mystery of the Cotswold "Olimpick" Games: Did Shakespeare know Dover . . . and does it matter? *Sport in History* 29: 150–170.

Zeigler, Earle F. 2006. *Sport and physical education in the Middle Ages*. Victoria, BC: Trafford.

Discussion Questions

1. Compare and contrast education for knighthood to the educational process in ancient Athens.

2. Discuss the role of the Christian church in education during the Middle Ages. How did the Church's view affect the use of physical education? Contrast the ideas of Saint Thomas Aquinas to those of Saint Augustine regarding the human body.

3. Describe the views of the Protestants on education and physical education during the Reformation.

4. Discuss the attitudes of the Puritans toward physical education and sport. What beliefs created those attitudes?

5. Briefly define humanism, and explain its rise and effect upon education during the Renaissance.

6. Discuss the educational theories and views of physical education of two of the following people:

   a. Vittorino da Feltre   **i.** Jean-Jacques Rousseau

   b. François Rabelais   **j.** Johann Basedow

   c. John Milton   **k.** Johann Pestalozzi

   d. Michel de Montaigne   **l.** Philipp von Fellenberg

   e. John Locke   **m.** Friedrich Froebel

   f. Richard Mulcaster   **n.** Adolf Spiess

   g. Wolfgang Ratke   **o.** Per Henrik Ling

   h. John Comenius

References

1. Mechikoff, Robert A., and Steven G. Estes. 1993. *A history and philosophy of sport and physical education.* Madison, WI: Brown and Benchmark, 61.

2. Goodale, Thomas, and Geoffrey Godbey. 1988. *The evolution of leisure: Historical and philosophical perspectives.* State College, PA: Venture, 31–35.

3. Ibid., 36.

4. Gardiner, E. Norman. 1910. *Greek athletic sports and festivals.* London: Macmillan, 25.

5. Broekhoff, Jan. 1968. Chivalric education in the Middle Ages. *Quest* 11 (December): 24–31.

6. Moolenijzer, Nicholas J. 1968. Our legacy from the Middle Ages. *Quest* 11 (December): 32–43.

7. Gillmeister, Heiner. 1988. Medieval sport: Modern methods of research—recent results and perspectives. *International Journal of the History of Sport* 5: 53–68.

8. Carter, John Marshall. 1985. The Bayeux Tapestry, Bishop Odo of Bayeux, and the pastimes of the medieval silent majority. *Canadian Journal of History of Sport* 16: 14–26; and Carter, John Marshall. 1981. Perspectives on medieval sport in twelfth and thirteenth century England. *Canadian Journal of History of Sport* 12: 12.

9. Carter, John Marshall. 1984. Muscular Christianity and its makers: Sporting monks and churchmen in Anglo-Norman society, 1000–1300. *British Journal of Sports History* 1: 109–124; and Hendricks, Thomas S. 1982. Sport and social hierarchy in medieval England. *Journal of Sport History* 9: 20–37.

10. Baker, William J. 1988. *Sports in the Western world*. Rev. ed. Urbana, IL Univ. of Illinois Press, 42–45.

11. Freeman, William H. 1982. Henry VIII and Francis I at the Field of Cloth of Gold: The last gasp of chivalric sports? In *Proceedings: 5th Canadian Symposium on the History of Sport and Physical Education*, ed. Bruce Kidd, 94–103. Toronto: Univ. of Toronto.

12. Goodale and Godbey, *Evolution of leisure*, 40.

13. Todd, Terry. 2005. Quoted in "Fitness Collection receives oldest known book on physical culture and sports medicine." Press release by the Office of Public Affairs, Univ. of Texas at Austin, March 22.

14. Weimer, Herman. 1962. *Concise history of education*. New York: Philosophical Library, 38–42.

15. McIntosh, Peter C. 1973. Physical education in Renaissance Italy and Tudor England. In *A history of sport and physical education to 1900*, 249–266. Champaign, IL: Stipes.

16. Hackensmith, C. W. 1966. *History of physical education*. New York: Harper and Row, 98–107.

17. Gerber, Ellen W. 1971. *Innovations and institutions in physical education*. Philadelphia: Lea and Febiger, 54–56.

18. Ibid., 57.

19. Ibid., 70.

20. Ibid., 61–64.

21. Weimer, *Concise history*, 73–77.

22. Gerber, *Innovations*, 65–69.

23. Calhoun, Don W. 1987. *Sport, culture, and personality*. 2nd ed. Champaign, IL: Human Kinetics, 86.

24. Ibid., 88.

25. Goodale and Godbey, *Evolution of leisure*, 46–47.

26. Ibid., 42–43.

27. Baker, *Sports in the Western world*, 81–82.

28. Gerber, *Innovations*, 83–86.

29. Ibid., 115–121.

30. Renson, Roland, and Pieter Ameye. 2011. Lost in translation: Johann Christoph Friedrich GutsMuths (1759–1839) and his reception in international literature. *2011 NASSH Proceedings*, 75–76.

31. Ibid., 87–92.

32. Hackensmith, *History*, 124–126.

33. Gerber, *Innovations*, 93–99.

34. Brailsford, Dennis. 1982. Sporting days in eighteenth century England. *Journal of Sport History* 9 (Winter): 41–54.

35. Ibid., 52.
36. Freeman, William H. 1982. Book review. *Journal of Sport History* 9 (Winter): 81–82.
37. Gerber, *Innovations*, 139–144.
38. Ibid., 177–180.
39. Hackensmith, *History*, 142–144.
40. Ibid., 215–219.

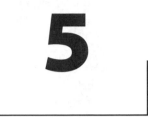
The Development of American Physical Education to 1941

We have discussed the evolution of physical education in the Western world to the mid-1800s. We now turn our attention to the developments in colonial America and the United States before the Civil War. To understand the development of physical education in the United States, one also must look at the developmental period of the nation itself and the ways in which it was influenced by the European ideas of the time. After the mid-1800s, Europe began to lose its influence on the United States. It is important to see how that period of declining influence affected the later directions that American physical education took.

Physical Education in Colonial America (1607–1783)

In colonial America, there was no physical education as we think of it. The colonies made attempts to start schools, but their primary concern was to provide the rudiments of a practical education: learning to read, write, and handle basic mathematics. Physical education activities (such as those being developed in Europe) would have been considered a frill at that time. The colonies of the New World were expanding into wilderness areas, and the pioneers, who frequently faced the threat of attack by Native Americans, usually got more outdoor exercise than a European would receive in the most educationally advanced school of the day. During this period, the non-work physical activities of the people were primarily recreational activities.

The developing colonies were a diverse culture, a mixture of many nationalities and religious groups. The Puritans in New England were opposed to many activities that might be viewed as pleasurable. They considered such activities to be either distractions from more serious concerns or questionable because they might eventually lead to sin. The Puritans were the most negative group of the colonial settlers regarding the pursuit of physical pleasures, but the Quakers, who settled in Pennsylvania, were also strict in their outlook. The Virginia colony, predominantly Anglican, was officially opposed to many recreational activities in its early days. Other groups in the New World, such as the Dutch in today's

New York City and Hudson River valley areas, were more inclined to allow such activities. However, official policy and public practice rarely agreed with each other. People still participated as they pleased.

The colonies, which were widely separated in their early days, might be compared to the ancient Greek city-states: All were of the same nation, but they were more competitive than cooperative. The spirit of cooperation among the states was noticeably thin even during the Revolutionary War. After the revolution, the nation was still largely rural and widespread, so there was little spirit of nationalism. People were from Massachusetts, or Virginia, or Pennsylvania, rather than from the United States.

The hard nature of the life of the settlers led to the gradual development of a society far more tolerant of differences among people than had been the case in their native European countries. Ancestors had little to do with a settler's ultimate survival or value to colonial society. As the political development of the colonies proceeded, strong regional antagonism developed among three groups of people that were established in many states.

In colonial society, the new elite were the residents of the coastal areas that had been settled earliest. Many of these people were well-to-do traders. They were better educated than the other groups, and they had regular contact with Europe. The second social group included the people of the piedmont and foothill areas, who were primarily farmers. They lived in less settled areas than the coastal dwellers and had little in common with them, either in wealth or in politics. The third group, the settlers of the still-unopened areas, was gradually moving into the mountains and beyond. They were almost as out of touch with the coast as they were with Europe. They had some ties with the piedmont farmers because often they were farmers themselves, but they had nothing in common with the coastal people. The result of the differences among these three groups of people was a long period of political struggle in the state legislatures between the people in the East, who had the power, and those in the West, who did not.

The schools in the colonies were copies of the European schools of the time. The first were Latin grammar schools, which proved to be of little value and were gradually replaced by academies that focused primarily on basic instruction. Advanced educational institutions, also modeled after European schools, were primarily for men who were going into the ministry. An example is Harvard University, which was founded in Massachusetts in 1636.

Physical activities served almost no official function in colonial education, but many unorganized recreational games and sports were a form of entertainment. The daily activities of the pioneers involved the survival skills used in hunting, fishing, and swimming and required physical activities such as running, jumping, lifting heavy objects, and fighting. Dance gradually became more acceptable as the Puritans became more affluent.

Although no real physical education existed in colonial times, the idea was supported by some prominent men. Thomas Jefferson wrote in support of physical education, and Benjamin Franklin was a swimming enthusiast, although swimming was considered a quaint but questionable custom in his time. One of the few educators who supported physical activities in the schools was Samuel Moody, headmaster of one of the first private boarding schools in America.[1] He promoted physical activities as vital to the health of the students, but most activities were the strictly traditional ones inherited from European backgrounds.

There was little nationalistic spirit in the United States until after the War of 1812. Americans shared a basic reluctance to submit to any centralized form of government. Thus, nationalism was not the strong force in promoting physical education that it was in the European nations in the late 1700s and early 1800s. The second impetus in Europe, pursuing physical training to serve the military needs of the country, was also weaker in the United States. The Americans were concerned with the strength and fitness of the military only in times of war, so physical training was of no concern during the rapid expansion across the Appalachian Mountains and on toward the great American Midwest. Although some military schools were being formed during the early 1800s, the idea of military instruction did not become popular until the time of the Civil War in the 1860s.

Physical Education in the Early National Period (1783–1820)

Colonial America and the early national period were not times when educational theory was of great interest. The major concerns before 1800 were survival and politics, in that order. As the nation became more settled and the larger population centers became more stable in their lifestyles, the interest in education beyond the lowest level grew. The first real attempts to put physical education into the educational curriculum were in the 1820s and 1830s. Experimental schools and academies began to open under the direction of men and women who had been influenced by the growing interest in physical education within the new European schools.

Much of the impetus for the improvement of physical activity programs before the Civil War came from Europe. However, three movements in the United States enhanced the effects of the European influence. The first was the women's education movement, seen particularly in the growth of female seminaries. The second was the move of religious groups into education and later physical education. The third was the growth of sport in the United States during the years before 1860.

The European theories popular in the United States at this time were the ideas of Johann Pestalozzi, Joseph Lancaster, Philipp von Fellenberg, and the German gymnastics system. His internationally famous school was visited by people from many nations. One of his guests from the United States was William McClure (1763–1840), who also visited Fellenberg's school. McClure, who wanted to open a Philadelphia school that would follow Pestalozzi's methods, hired Joseph Neef (1770–1854), an instructor at Pestalozzi's school. The Philadelphia school, which opened in 1809 and offered many physical activities and military exercises, was among the early American schools that were beginning to follow Pestalozzi's example in the 1820s.

Joseph Lancaster (1778–1838), an Englishman, developed a system of instruction that used student assistants to share the teachers' duties, similar to contemporary teachers' aides or paraprofessionals. Lancaster's assistants were called monitors. After they had learned a lesson, they would teach the same lesson to another group of students.

His ideas, published in 1803, included a recommendation for the use of playgrounds and play activities as part of the educational process. Most of the American schools of this type were established in New England and followed Lancaster's teaching handbook, which was reprinted in Philadelphia in 1820. As free public education gradually evolved, the Lancastrian schools dwindled in number.

Fellenberg, whose methods and views on physical activity have already been discussed, also influenced the development of American schools. His model was considered to be a well-balanced combination of the academic and the useful and included physical activity as an important part of the process. Schools using Fellenberg's ideas became popular in the 1830s, although many teachers thought the manual labor requirements removed the need for any other physical activities. The manual labor schools gradually lost popularity about the time of the Civil War. After the war, their basic plan reappeared in the manual arts schools.

The German gymnastics system, which was based on the work of a number of men (notably Friedrich Jahn), was brought to the United States during the early years of the nineteenth century by German immigrants. Three prominent leaders appeared in the United States to do much of the work toward making German gymnastics popular in this country. Two of them were Charles Beck (1798–1866), who taught at Round Hill School in Massachusetts, and Charles Follen (1796–1840), who taught at Harvard University. Both arrived in the United States from Germany in 1824. Francis Lieber (1800–1872), who also taught at Harvard, came from Germany in 1827. All three generally followed Jahn's teachings in their programs and helped to spread his system, which played a role in the development of American physical education programs prior to 1900.[2]

During the late 1700s and early 1800s, women's education grew in popularity, though the growth was not rapid. First supported strongly by Dr. Benjamin Rush (1745–1813), female seminaries or academies were founded in many communities. Tuition was required at the private institutions because providing free public education to women was not yet considered worth the expense. Attempts to open public high schools for women in Boston and New York City in the 1820s were failures because too many women wanted to attend, and the taxpayers thought the cost was too high.

Antebellum Physical Education in the United States (1820–1860)

Many new developments in both education and physical education took place between 1820 and 1860. As Rebecca Noel writes,

> *Educators and reformers from 1830 to 1860 became increasingly convinced of the need for designated play spaces and times, and even formal athletic activities, often for girls as well as boys. Boarding schools put special emphasis on exercise, but all schools were urged to provide for frequent outdoor recreation. German and Swedish gymnastics and calisthenics, long walks and ball games, domestic chores (for girls) and manual training (for boys) all figured as solutions.*[3]

The Round Hill School was opened in Northampton, Massachusetts, in 1823 by Joseph Cogswell (1786–1871) and George Bancroft (1800–1891).[4] This college preparatory school was the only American school that advocated the idea of individualized instruction. It also recognized the importance of physical activity as part of the education program. The founders had observed the programs of the German gymnasiums and of Fellenberg and had decided to try an experimental school based on those ideas.

The Round Hill School provided a classical education, but it also included dancing, riding, and gymnastics. The classes were small, usually about six persons each, and the instruction was individualized for each student's level. Cogswell, who ran the school, tried to be like a father to the students. He abolished most systems of punishment and rewards and, because he especially liked long hikes and running, led much of the exercise himself.

Charles Beck taught Latin and gymnastics at the Round Hill School from 1825 to 1830. Beck had translated a gymnastics book of Friedrich Jahn's into English, and following Jahn's system, he started the first outdoor school gymnasium as well as the first school gymnastics program in the United States at Round Hill. His program served as the introduction of German gymnastics into the United States. As Roxanne Albertson noted: "During the late 1820s many academies and colleges provided German gymnastic apparatus for students to use during recess or idle time. A small number of academies followed the example of Round Hill and included gymnastics in their regular curriculum."[5]

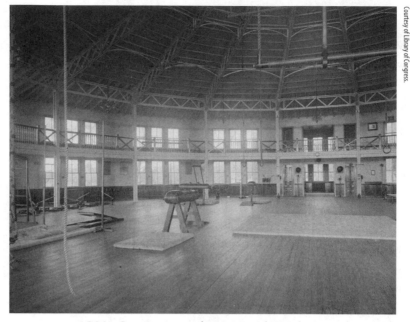

1890s Gymnasium of U.S. Naval Academy.

The Round Hill School closed in 1834. Although the school had some financial problems, the primary reason for its closing was its uniqueness compared to other American schools. The educational work had been superior, and the school's graduates were ready for the last year of work at most colleges. However, many colleges required their students to pay for the full 4 years of college work even if they entered the college as advanced students. This practice made the Round Hill School a financial hardship for many of its graduates.

In the years prior to the Civil War, there was a gradual increase in school gymnastics programs and in the construction of gymnasiums. The first college gymnasium, which was furnished with the types of equipment commonly used in German gymnasiums, opened at Harvard in 1820. By the 1850s, many colleges had begun providing gymnasiums for their students, and the gymnasium construction boom was under way.

This period also saw an increased interest in swimming and a boom in the construction of swimming pools. Benjamin Franklin, who had long been a disciple of swimming, was quoted liberally in William Turner's *The Art of Swimming* in 1821. In 1827, Francis Lieber opened the first public swimming pool under the control of the Boston gymnasium. The first college to construct a swimming pool was Girard College in 1848. The college's four indoor pools in its dormitory basements, as well as its outdoor pool, were all planned by Lieber.

Public education also began to develop during this time. Although many public schools for elementary education were being opened, most opportunities for secondary education remained in the private academies—schools that charged tuition. The academies, which were frequently coeducational, stressed terminal education. That is, they were not college preparatory, and they were more practical than classical in their curricula. Because of the large number of private academies, the first public schools often were ridiculed as schools for the poor.

Early academies in the United States were modeled on the British public schools. They were influenced both by the early developments in American physical education, copying Dr. Edward Hitchcock's Amherst College physical education programs, and by the British school sports. They utilized the boys' interest in sports as a way to develop character and purpose, but they also valued it for the health benefits.[6]

The first public high school for boys opened in Boston in 1818. In 1852, Massachusetts became the first state to pass legislation requiring all children to attend school. The problems of public education for girls have already been mentioned, but the similar disinterest in forming colleges for women was overcome in 1853 when the first 4-year college for women, Elmira (New York) College, was established.

By the 1830s, aristocratic tendencies were beginning to disappear from the rapidly growing nation and its educational system. Following the example of President Andrew Jackson, more democratic feelings began to emerge. The people wanted a more useful education than was offered at the classically oriented private schools. By the middle 1800s, people were pressing for free education for both sexes.

In 1832, John Warren (1778–1856), a Harvard professor of anatomy, published a book supporting physical education in education. This work, *The Importance of Physical Education*, is the first theoretical book on physical education because it was philosophical in nature. However, most colleges were not very interested in physical education. Although they had begun to provide gymnasiums and other facilities for physical activities, the improvements were primarily the result of student agitation for the facilities, rather than any administrative or scholarly interest in the value of exercise for students. In short, they were a tool for student recruitment. The outdoor gymnasiums that developed in many schools in New England followed the leadership of the German gymnastics model set up by Charles Follen at Harvard in 1826. Those gymnasiums were not recognized as a part of the official school programs, however.

A prominent leader in physical education for women in the antebellum period was Catharine Beecher (1800–1878). She was conservative in most of her ideas concerning women because she believed that a woman's place was in the home (which was a popular idea with the men). Unlike other women of her time, Beecher felt that women should be educated as homemakers. She viewed the mother as the core of the family and believed that mothers needed guidance if they hoped to do a good job at their difficult task. Beecher objected to the clothing styles of her time as too restrictive and heavy to permit good health. She emphasized the idea of exercising to improve health. For her students, both women and children, she prescribed exercises similar to Per Henrik Ling's Swedish gymnastics, which were not widely used in the United States until the 1860s.[7]

Although Beecher was in favor of sports and games as good exercises and considered them useful in promoting family unity, she was very puritanical in her opposition to other activities. She considered hunting for recreational purposes to be sinful, and she was suspicious of the directions in which dance might lead people. She was more interested in women's role in the home than in their intellectual role. Because women were beginning to struggle for their civil rights at this time, Beecher's ideas were not extremely popular with some women. Even so, they were refined and spread by Dio Lewis after the Civil War.

During the 1830s and 1840s, a developing trend in the heavily populated cities concerned public health.[8] Doctors began to notice the large number of unhealthy citizens, particularly children, and assessed the problem as one caused primarily by a lack of exercise. There was no place in most cities for people to get any country-type exercise away from the city's crowded, dirty environs. Boston was fortunate in having its large common, which had been used as a pasture, but it was an exception among cities. Gradually, other cities in the United States began to try to provide public parks for their citizens' exercise. European parks were studied by people who began to develop the architecture of public parks. This civic concern for low-level recreation was the start of a long period of gradual growth toward the important field of recreation.

The United States was gradually becoming a land of large cities complete with slums, and it was beginning to face for the first time some of the problems that the European cities had faced for centuries. Fortunately, most American cities were young enough or small enough to be able to set aside land for parks in their interior, which was impossible for most European cities. This period of interest in public health and public parks continued until the Civil War, and it progressed with increased vigor after the war.

Religious groups also began to get involved in physical education and recreational activities during this period. The recreational life of many people centered about the church, which was a common gathering point in rural areas.

In 1844, in London George Williams founded the Young Men's Christian Association (YMCA) to help young men to lead moral lives. It came to the United States in 1851. The YMCA programs in the United States added physical education when interest grew in gymnastics and other health-oriented activities after the Civil War. The Young Women's Christian Association (YWCA) was organized in Boston in 1866. Meanwhile a Young Men's Hebrew Association (YMHA), which had been founded in 1854 as a literary society, also began adding physical education activities.

The number of colleges began to grow rapidly before the Civil War. The government set aside land in each state to be used to provide money for education for the people. That impetus led to the founding of many state colleges, sometimes called land grant colleges. The earlier colleges had been formed by religious groups, except for Benjamin Franklin's school, which later became the University of Pennsylvania.

Perhaps the most influential factor in the development of physical education in the United States in the last decade or so before the Civil War was the example of the turnvereins, or German gymnastic societies. The *turnverein*, or Turner movement, grew in the United States as the unsettled political situation in the many states that later became Germany caused increasing numbers of Germans to immigrate to the United States. Those immigrants brought many of their customs with them, and by 1848 the Turners had established their first group in the United States, probably in Louisville, Kentucky, followed quickly by Cincinnati, Ohio, and New York City.[9] The first national Turnfest, a large, organized, outdoor gymnastics meeting, was held in Philadelphia in 1851.

The popular Turner groups were much like family physical and social clubs because they were as much social organizations (including entire families) as they were physical activity-oriented groups. The goals of the Turners in this country were to promote physical education, to improve the individual's intellect, and to provide opportunities for socializing with other members.

The demarcation point in the nineteenth-century development of physical education can be set at 1861. In that year, Dr. Edward Hitchcock (1828–1911), who had recently graduated from Harvard's medical school, was hired by Amherst College as a professor of hygiene and physical education, the first such recognized position in the United States. He was asked to develop a program to contribute to the health of the students at Amherst. Hitchcock's program began as heavy gymnastics, using large, fixed apparatus in the German manner. Later, he modified it to light gymnastics, using light hand apparatus and exercising to music, which he felt was more beneficial to the students. He began to record measures of the students' body dimensions and gradually developed a large pool of anthropometric measurements that were useful to later physical educators. He also started one of the nation's first intramural school sports programs.

Hitchcock headed the Amherst physical education program for 50 years, until his death in 1911. His hiring represented a turning point in the evolution of U.S. physical education because it was the first recognition by a college of the value of physical education in its students' educational program. The Amherst program served as a major example to other U.S. schools for many decades.

Another major factor in the development of physical education in the year 1861 was the start of the Civil War, which marked the beginning of a period of drastic change in the United States. The country was changing from a primarily agricultural nation into a highly industrialized one. Over the next half-century, radical changes in the complexion of the nation led to an increased demand for physical education activities and gymnastics.

The Professionalization of American Physical Education (1860–1900)

At the close of the Civil War, many changes were taking place in the country. The teaching of physical education was expanding rapidly. Dio Lewis (1823–1886) was a major influence on the development of American physical education at this time.[10] Although Lewis's only degrees were honorary, he practiced medicine. He had some academic learning and practical experience in the medical field, and he was an enthusiastic supporter of health-related activities, particularly physical education pursuits and temperance campaigns against the use of alcohol.

Lewis developed his own system of gymnastics, which he referred to as the New Gymnastics.[11] He was especially concerned with the development of the upper body, and he tried to develop a system of exercises that would be applicable to men, women, and children. He used no large or fixed equipment, preferring free exercises and activities using wands, Indian clubs, rings, and even bean bags. In his program the students performed the activities to music.

Lewis started the Normal Institute for Physical Education in Boston in 1861 to instruct teachers in his system of gymnastics. The course was a 10-week training session with classes in anatomy, physiology, hygiene, and gymnastics. This first teacher-training institution for physical education in the United States remained open until 1868 and graduated between 250 and 400 teachers during its existence.

Lewis was something of a charlatan–salesman. Although he practiced medicine without a degree, gave many lectures based on little experience, and made many unscientific claims that could not be supported, he was an excellent salesman of physical education. He did more to popularize gymnastics than anyone in his time. His system became a major influence in the use of gymnastics in the schools because it required minimal equipment and expense. His book of instructions for the system, first published in 1862, went through 10 editions in 6 years. Lewis also devoted much of his life to the work of the Woman's Christian Temperance Union (WCTU), which he founded, and the organization became an avid supporter of physical education in the schools.

The Turner School

The German Turners also formed a school to train teachers of their system, though their school had many early difficulties.[12] The school, which opened in New York City in 1866, was called the Normal School of the North American Gymnastic Union. (The Turners had been split by politics before the Civil War, but they dropped all political concerns afterward and changed their name to the North American Gymnastic Union.) Their primary objective of physical training was evident in the new school. The 1-year course included the history and aims of physical education, anatomy, first aid, dancing, and gymnastics instruction, combined with work in teaching methods. The classes met during the evenings, so the students could hold jobs during the day. The first class began with 19 students, 5 of whom graduated.

In the years that followed, the teacher's course varied in length from 4 to 10 months, and the site of the school shifted from New York to Chicago and back, then to Milwaukee (for 13 years), to Indianapolis, and back to Milwaukee, where the course was a 2-year program from 1895 to 1899. The curriculum gradually became diversified and similar to a junior or senior college program as the Turners discovered that they needed to broaden their program if they wanted their influence to reach beyond the German community. By 1907, the school was moved to Indianapolis to stay. It offered a 4-year degree program, granted a Bachelor of Science in Gymnastics (BSG) degree, and later became affiliated with Indiana University.

Development of Other Schools and Systems

Dr. Dudley Sargent (1849–1924) was named director of the Hemenway Gymnasium at Harvard University in 1879. He received a Doctor of Medicine (MD) degree at Yale and taught there and at Bowdoin College. He developed a gymnastics program based on the German and Swedish systems, constructed many types of apparatus to be used in his program, and also experimented in anthropometric measurements. He referred to his system as the Sargent System, an eclectic system that drew from all other systems. He required a thorough medical examination as the basic preliminary to any program of physical activity.

The school that Sargent founded in 1881 to prepare physical education teachers was originally called the Sanatory Gymnasium. It later became the Sargent School for Physical Education, which eventually merged with Boston University. In 1887, Sargent introduced a summer session (which met at Harvard) to train physical education teachers. Sargent became a key figure in the development of modern American physical education, along with Dr. Edward Hitchcock of Amherst and Dr. Edward Hartwell of Johns Hopkins University, who also directed influential American programs of gymnastics and physical education.

Other plans and systems of physical education that were introduced into the United States in the 1880s included the Swedish system of gymnastics based on Ling's work. This system was first taught by Hartwig Nissen (1855–1924) in Washington, DC, then at Johns Hopkins University, and later in Boston. Nils Posse (1862–1895) also taught the Swedish system in Boston. A graduate of Sweden's Royal Central Institute of Gymnastics, Posse came to Boston in 1885.[13] He was hired by Mary Hemenway to teach the Swedish system to 25 women teachers. Later he became director of the Boston Normal School of Gymnastics when it was founded in 1889.

The Swedish system, which began to replace the German system in popularity, used no apparatus and was more free and less rigid than the German system. Flexibility was the strength of the Swedish system because it allowed the program to adapt more easily to local conditions than the German system could. Posse added exercises with Indian clubs and other objects because they were popular in America. His goal was to achieve the desired health benefits rather than to maintain the purity of the Swedish gymnastics.

Before his death at the age of 33 years, Posse wrote three popular books on his version of the Swedish system and published a journal that rapidly spread word of the system throughout the United States. He had formed his own school of teacher training in 1890, and he was succeeded as its director by Nissen. Posse was very influential in developing the popularity of Swedish gymnastics.

The system of François Delsarte (1811–1871) of France also enjoyed some popularity in the late 1800s. Delsarte had worked with the use of body movements to express feelings. His exercises were aimed at training actors, singers, and public speakers, but because he left no writings about his ideas, his followers developed his work into a program of physical exercise that they called the *Delsartean system of physical culture*. His system of expressive exercises was used as a counter to the German and Swedish systems, although its influence was much smaller. The system was later absorbed by dance, to which it was more applicable.

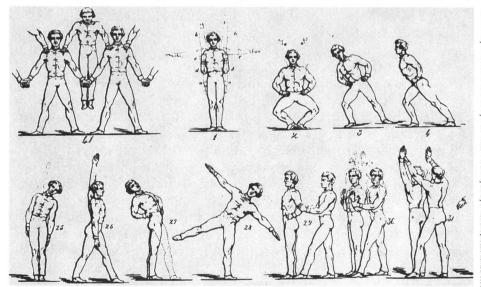

These examples of the Swedish system, or Ling gymnastics, show the simple, fundamental movements involved.

The Physical Education Requirement

After the Civil War the first steps were taken toward requiring physical education activities and instruction in the public schools. In 1866, under the leadership of John Swett, the superintendent of public instruction, the California state legislature passed the first law requiring physical education in the public schools.[14] This first state law did not lead to a dramatic surge in the number of such laws, however. The second state law was not passed until 1892, by Ohio, but it required physical education only in the larger schools in the state. Much of the work leading to the passage of such state laws around the turn of the century was done by the Turners and the WCTU. The WCTU, in seeking to gain more public recognition of the place of physical education in the educational process, was also instrumental in having a physical education division organized within the National Education Association (NEA) in 1895.

The Move Toward Professional Organization

A focal point in the history of physical education in the United States was the 1885 formation of the Association for the Advancement of Physical Education (AAPE). Most teachers of physical education were then called gymnasium teachers or directors of gymnasiums. There were not many leaders in physical education, and few of the better-known teachers had received formal training in the work they were doing. Most teachers had learned more by trial and error (and reading) than they had through teacher-training programs.

William Anderson, MD, a teacher of physical training at Adelphi College in Brooklyn, wanted to learn what other teachers were doing, so he called for a meeting of people interested in gymnastics. The group met in Brooklyn on November 27, 1885, and 60 people attended. Dr. Edward Hitchcock was appointed chairman and later elected the first president as 49 people joined the new AAPE. Most of the leaders in the new organization held MD degrees and were interested in physical education for the health benefits that they believed it provided.

The group met in the same place during the following year but changed its name to the American Association for the Advancement of Physical Education (AAAPE). Members stated that their objectives were "to disseminate knowledge concerning physical education, to improve the methods, and by meetings of the members to bring those interested in the subject into closer relation to each other." A new member was Edward Hartwell, MD, PhD, who had helped to define the field of physical education and show the extent of its practice with the publication of his 1885 report to the government called *Physical Training in American Colleges and Universities*.

The Boston Conference of 1889 might be considered an outgrowth of the AAAPE. Whether or not this is true, the AAAPE did cancel its convention that year so its members could go to the Boston meeting. The meeting was called by Mary Hemenway, assisted by Amy Morris Homans. The two women were advocates of the Swedish system, but the conference was designed to discuss all of the systems. Although many prominent leaders of physical education spoke on the German, Swedish, and Sargent systems, it is interesting to note that no speaker addressed games and sports, probably because those activities were not included in the curriculum of the schools and colleges at that time. The 1889 conference was significant because it was the first meeting that brought together American physical education leaders specifically to discuss the various systems of physical education and which program might provide the best help to the American people:

> *Physical training was associated with some form of systematic exercise regimen . . . influenced by the European style of calisthenics, primarily German or Swedish. These systems reflected contemporary thinking, which sought to develop bodily symmetry through disciplined, well-ordered, and progressively graded exercises. . . . The most notable feature of the German system was the use of heavy apparatus, including jumping [vaulting] horses and horizontal bars, and light equipment such as dumbbells and wands. . . . It was not unusual to see devotees of German gymnastics marching in formation or doing calisthenics or other similar drills by command. . . . The Swedish system used light equipment such as dumbbells and chest weights, but to a lesser extent than the German program.*[15]

By this time, the *Battle of the Systems* between the German and Swedish systems of gymnastics was growing to fever pitch. During the 1892 convention of the AAAPE, many arguments were presented on both sides. Nils Posse, a champion of the Swedish system, suggested that the greatest need was to develop an American system based on the needs of the American people, rather than to adopt totally either the German or Swedish system.

Another speaker at the 1892 convention was George Fitz (1860–1934), who called for physiological research into the benefits of physical activity. He hoped that research would provide proof of the benefits and, at the same time, help to determine which activities were actually beneficial to the body.[16] An MD who taught physical education in Harvard's short-lived (1891–1899) bachelor's degree program in physical education, Fitz was the impetus behind the formation of the *American Physical Education Review*, as well as its first editor. He also founded the first American physical education research laboratory at Harvard in 1892.

George Fitz's brief career in physical education is notable for several reasons. First, it echoed the science and health focus of the developing profession. Second, it shows that even in the earliest stages of the profession, there was a strong interest in the medical side of physical education. Many of the most prominent early leaders were from the medical profession. The earliest professional training was moving in the direction of today's science and kinesiology focus. However, as the new century dawned, American physical education was drawing away from its scientific health and medical foundations and allying itself with the growing teacher education movement. As it did so, its preparation focus shifted from the sciences to educational methods and their application.

The Rise of Scientific Research on Human Performance

During the early years of organized American physical education in the late 1800s, many of the leaders were holders of MD degrees. As such, they were exposed to the developments in both medical and academic doctoral programs that were influenced by the new focus on scientific research in the German universities of their day. Unlike most other universities, whose research might be limited to a subjective examination of evidence, the Germans were attempting to create a science of research, using objective and experimental methods, so the results would be unquestionably correct. Those practices were even found outside the sciences, such as attempts to do scientific historical research.

When it came to the human body and performance, research of any nature was rare, and the objective use of measurement data was almost unheard of. In physical education, with its concern for improving the physical health and vitality of students, one of the first concerns was to find a way to describe their goals. But how can they have goals if they had no idea what is normal?

Roberta Park writes that "Christian Friedrich Jampert's 1754 publication of heights and weights taken at the Royal Orphanage of Berlin is thought to have been the first study involving children."[17] She continues:

> In A Treatise on Man and the Development of His Faculties *(1835)*, *[Adolphe] Quetelet wrote: "If the average man were completely determined, we might consider him as the type of perfection; and everything differing from his proportions would constitute deformity and disease." His conception of "l'homme moyen"—"average man"—would have considerable influence on early American physical educators who devoted a great deal of time to measuring students.*[18]

During the late 1800s, anthropometric measurement of students was a common research subject for college physical educators. These measurements of a wide range of physical dimensions (height, weight, length, and circumference of parts of the body, and distance from one marker to another) were attempts to determine the norms for their students. Eventually they settled on top athletes as having the ideal proportions, which at that time was long and lean or wiry with muscle tone and strength.

Dr. Edward Hitchcock was measuring Amherst students by the early 1860s. By the 1890s, many studies of children's norms and rates of growth were being used by cities to determine community health and by physical education teachers to determine student progress. In 1893, Thomas Denison Wood called for more scientific research to deal with the many issues in physical education. However, a weakness of the use of anthropometric data was that teachers tended to use it mostly to decide which students needed remedial exercise to bring their measurements up to the local norm. Gradually, anthropometric measurement began to be replaced by the newer measures of motor ability and motor efficiency.

American Physical Education at the Turn of the Century (1900)

By 1900, there were 1076 members of the AAAPE, although no members came from west of Nebraska.[19] As physical education continued to spread and evolve, the association played an increasingly important role in providing channels of communication among teachers. At the turn of the century, the Battle of the Systems was being decided in favor of the Swedish system, but that issue was becoming less important. As the new century dawned, the influence of sports, including games and play activities, moved irresistibly into programs of physical education, to the point of almost replacing the gymnastic activities.

Thus, at the close of the nineteenth century, physical education was becoming recognized for its value in the educational process. States were beginning to require its inclusion in the public school programs (though most states did not do so until after 1900), and in turn, the schools were beginning to require more physical education teachers.

Although no regular 4-year degree programs were designed to prepare teachers of physical education, several institutions had begun training them. The list of those schools begins with Dio Lewis's school and includes the Turner school, Sargent's regular school and his Harvard summer session, the Boston Normal School of Gymnastics, the Posse–Nissen School, and the newly expanding International YMCA School (later Springfield College) at Springfield, Massachusetts. The first graduates of such programs appeared at the close of the century. Apparently, Harvard awarded the first baccalaureate degree in physical education, earned by James F. Jones in June 1893.[20] That fall he became an instructor at Marietta (Ohio) College, which was the first college in the United States to hire a college-trained physical educator.[21]

Stanford University offered another early 4-year degree program. It awarded a degree to Walter Davis in 1897 and a degree to the first female physical education graduate in the United States, Stella Rose, in 1899.[22] The first state university degree was awarded by the University of Nebraska to a woman, Alberta Spurk, in 1900. By 1900, four colleges offered a 4-year degree in physical education: Harvard, Stanford, and the Universities of California and Nebraska.[23] The big boom in 4-year physical education degree programs was to follow over the next 30 years, from 1900 to 1930.

The Uneasy Joining of Physical Education and Sport (1900–1941)

From about 1900 to 1930, sports were gradually included in the school curriculum, partly in response to the problems that non-school sports had created for the schools and partly because of a very strong student interest in sports. This student interest showed itself not only in changes in the physical education curriculum but also in the rapid growth of intramural sports as many colleges began responding to student desire for sports participation.

The first real mixing of sport and physical education occurred in the early twentieth century, particularly from 1900 to 1930. Two aspects of this growing relationship (and conflict) are noticeable: (1) the gradual addition of competitive athletics, including intramurals, to the school programs, followed by a boom in popularity after World War I; and (2) the addition of sports and games to the school physical education curricula, the *American System*, or the *New Physical Education*.

Those two developments were separate during the early years of the century; yet they were gradually drawing the areas of athletics and physical education closer together. The resulting conflict between athletics and physical education is visible even today. There was the fear that athletics would be overemphasized, which happened many times, in addition to the physical educators' fear that athletics might gain control of the entire program and subvert its goals and objectives. One can see those fears reflected in the conflicts related to women's sports in the 1930s and again in the 1960s and 1970s.

Today physical educators have to work out philosophical differences in school programs that combine physical education and sport programs. As they work to solve the problems and smooth the relationships, they need to understand how the shaky relationship between physical education and athletics developed.

There are roughly three phases of development in the history of American school sport between 1880 and 1930. The first phase was a time of student control of the sports programs in the schools. It lasted until about 1905, when the National Collegiate Athletic Association (NCAA) was formed. The second phase saw increasing control of sports by the schools, peaking in 1922 when a national federation was formed for high school sports. The third stage, the New Physical Education, lasted from 1922 to 1930 and was the time of greatest change in moving sports into the physical education program.

From 1905 to 1922, six trends were visible in physical education and sport.[24] The first three were in sports: (1) the gradual assumption of control over intercollegiate sport by the NCAA and by college athletic conferences, (2) the effort of high schools to control their sports programs, and (3) the rapid growth in women's athletics.

A fourth trend was the boom in intramural sports, or sports involving only the students within a single school. The school intramural program was an offshoot of the earlier student-run sports programs. Intramurals became popular in the colleges, and in 1913 the University of Michigan became the first university to form a department of intramurals (led by Elmer Mitchell) to run programs for the student body. The great boom in intramural sports that followed World War I is evident in a slogan of the times: "A sport for every student and every student in a sport." The emphasis was on the number of participants, rather than on how much they participated, which created a temporary sidetracking of the intramural program goals.[25] Intramurals were to become an important part of the total physical education program as it evolved toward its present state.

A fifth trend was the addition of games and sports to the physical education curriculum. Though the change was gradually accomplished over 3 decades, the new programs were a radical change from the formal systems of gymnastics that had been at the heart of American physical education for almost a century. Games and sports were more popular with the students, and the acceptance and enthusiasm for physical education improved considerably as a result.

A sixth trend was also visible during this time. The emphasis of physical education gradually shifted from a health focus to a general education focus. It signaled the acceptance of a much broader concept of physical education—one that was consistent with the developing philosophy of the American school system—and permitted the use of games and sports in the curriculum. This further increased student acceptance of the physical education requirement. It also caused a major change in teacher training. Rather than being products of medical schools and formal gymnastics training courses, teachers became graduates of regular college training programs in education and physical education. The eventual results were a more widely accepted physical education program as well as more and better trained teachers of physical education.

The Move Toward a Unified American System

Before 1900, American physical education was more narrowly defined than it is today. To most teachers it meant gymnastics, or physical training, or physical culture. The goal was to develop good health for the student, rather than have a total educational program. A dualistic philosophy existed—educating the mind and training the body. Educators viewed them as two separate processes, related but not very similar. Thus, most of the ideas for unified programs of instruction came from abroad, instead of the United States.

At the 1892 AAAPE convention, Nils Posse argued that American leaders should stop using foreign systems of training and develop an American system based on the characteristics and needs of the American people. Such efforts began around the turn of the century as new leaders became prominent in education and physical education.

A major leader in the progressive movement in education was John Dewey (1859–1952), who was teaching at the University of Chicago when his ideas on education first became known.[26] Later a professor of philosophy at Columbia University, Dewey sought social changes through an experimental form of education that centered on the child. He was best known for a work on education called *Democracy and Education*, published in 1916.

Dewey, who strongly believed in the unity of mind and body, suggested that the Greek education system succeeded because the Greeks never tried to separate the mind from the body in the educational process. His teachings included the concept of the whole child, combining the mental and the physical as areas that cannot be separated in education. This concept led to a gradual shift in the aim of physical education in the United States from a health-centered concern for the student's body to a concern for all educational values; that is, to a unified view of the child and of education.

Because Dewey considered the school a social institution, he believed that education had social goals and outcomes. He included physical education in this role and followed a philosophy sometimes called the "learn by doing" method of education. He was convinced that play was very important in education because children are interested in play activities. If children enjoyed an activity, they would become more involved, which would result in greater accomplishments. This was a pragmatic approach that allowed the teacher to take useful things from many activities to form a better activity or group of activities. Dewey's theories were used in producing the New Physical Education in the 1920s.

The New Physical Education (1922–1930)

John Dewey's theories of education were applied to physical education by Thomas D. Wood, Clark Hetherington, and Luther Gulick. Hetherington called for a particularly American form of physical education, and Jesse Feiring Williams popularized a broader concept of it. Sports activities were creeping into the curriculum until the writings of Wood popularized their use in a well-planned program of physical education activities. His New Physical Education was simply the acceptance of games and sports activities as a legitimate part of the school physical education curriculum. He referred to it as "a program of naturalized activities for education toward citizenship."[27] He included games and sports, as well as activities other than gymnastics, in his program aimed at meeting the needs and interests of his students. Hetherington emphasized that the physical education program must be a product of American society if it is to contribute to the total education of the American child. Gulick's work in recreational activities included camping and outdoor education and stressed the social values of education.

Although the trend away from the older, more rigid systems of physical education was beginning, the move toward the New Physical Education was delayed by a lack of teachers of physical education who were trained to teach the new program. After World War I, however, the new system began to catch on in the schools. Wood and Cassidy's textbook promoted the New Physical Education,[28] as did the efforts of Williams, in the philosophy and principles of physical education, and Jay B. Nash, whose major work was in recreation.

The physical education program was caught in a cross-current of three conflicting philosophies, and it tried to apply all three together. C. H. McCloy believed that the function of physical education was physical training and development, but Jesse Feiring Williams argued for education *through* (rather than simply *of*) the physical, even as Jay Nash focused on education for leisure activities.[29] As Ellen Gerber puts it, "Physical education projected itself into the anomalous situation of holding classes in accord with McCloy's suggestion, of advocating the activities urged by Nash, and of committing itself to accomplishing the social goals delineated by Williams."[30]

Physical education and sport were beginning to be forced together by the schools. One sign of this growing integration was the founding of the nation's first School of Physical Education at the University of Oregon in 1920. Led by Dean John F. Bovard, the school organized a unit of four departments that previously had been separate: the Department of Men's Physical Education, the Department of Women's Physical Education, the University Health Service, and the Department of Intercollegiate Athletics. The interest in this unified organization of different departments related to physical education spread across the country and was adopted by many other schools.

The period from 1922 to 1930 can be summarized from the viewpoint of either physical education or sport. For physical education advocates, it was the time of the New Physical Education, and for sports-minded people, it was the Golden Age of Sport. Athletics experienced a great boom in the United States for a decade after World War I. Postwar prosperity strongly affected the country: The standard of living was higher, the cities were growing, and the people had more leisure time available.

Expanding Program Options (1900–1930)

At the same time that popular sports were entering the school program, another activity was moving into the program with equal vigor: dancing. Dance, particularly folk dancing, was presented in depth at the 1905 convention of the renamed American Physical Education Association (APEA, formerly the AAAPE). This meeting might be called the Dancing Convention, for the bulk of the program was devoted to explanations and demonstrations of various dancing programs and their educational benefits. Some educators feared that the rapid growth in popularity of dancing programs would push gymnastics from the school curriculum.

From 1900 through the 1920s, many new programs of professional preparation were developed, first at the undergraduate level, then at the graduate level. Trained teachers of physical education were needed because many schools began to require that their teachers have bachelor's degrees. Few such programs were available in physical education. Many state normal schools (colleges for teacher training) were built at this time, and existing state schools expanded their programs. Universities added physical education majors to their programs. Teachers College of Columbia University in New York City awarded the first master's degree in physical education in 1910, and (along with New York University) offered the first doctoral program in physical education in 1924.[31]

The recreation movement was growing, led by people such as Luther Gulick. Larger cities in the United States began to expand their recreational facilities, and programs of recreation and play received more attention from the federal government. After World War I, great interest in recreation was evident, and during the Depression the government provided jobs for out-of-work citizens to construct public recreational facilities.

The National Park Service, formed in 1911, increased public interest in parks and recreational opportunities, and camping and outdoor education became part of a large movement. Many schools began camp programs, the most prominent of which was in New York City. Other interested groups, especially the new youth groups such as the Boy Scouts, the Girl Scouts, and the Camp Fire Girls, moved into the area of camping.

The American Melting Pot and Better Babies Through Eugenics: Social Prejudices in Action

Despite the idea that the United States was a great melting pot of people from foreign lands, attitudes of social and racial prejudice were common. One reflection of this was the eugenics movement, which began in the late 1800s and reached a peak in the 1920s and 1930s. It was based on the ideal of racial purity, generally for people of white, English, and western European descent.

The eugenics movement evolved from anthropometrics, Social Darwinism, and the development of the science of genetics. This confluence of scientific developments led eugenists to espouse the "perfectibility of man and society" through "good breeding." Eugenists sought to improve the species by promoting the reproduction of the best members while reducing the reproduction of less desirable members.[32]

The eugenics movement affected physical education in part because the field was focused on improving student health and, in a sense, perfecting the bodies of the students. The primary research area in the early years of the profession was anthropometric measurement. Thousands of students had many of their physical measures taken, then treated statistically to determine their group norms.

These data gave educators an idea of the physical proportions found in the average college student of that time, a group that generally represented a privileged part of society. The researchers also focused their research on the best athletes of their time; from those measures they calculated what they considered to be the ideal physique.

They then focused part of the training in physical education classes on trying to develop students physically in a way that would move their personal physical measures closer to a match with the ideal measures. In a sense, this preoccupation with perfection of the human body was an early step toward today's obsession with reshaping the human body to meet artificial ideals, as in the sport of bodybuilding and many types of personal fitness programs.[33]

As Lynn Couturier writes,

Physical education was in its infancy in the last quarter of the nineteenth century. Proponents of the new field sought to define their profession as "it ha[d] not yet crystallized." Initially, the backgrounds of physical educators were quite heterogeneous: professional training had not yet been standardized. Comprised of physicians and other individuals with varied, specialized training, physical educators were strongly influenced by the changes in American life and new scientific developments. The field began as systems of gymnastics and calisthenics but quickly evolved to include physical training, corrective exercises, anthropometrics, and hygiene as important aspects of the curriculum. Given the interests and backgrounds of early physical educators, it is not difficult to imagine possible connections with the themes of the eugenics movement.[34]

Eugenics found its way into physical education because it was concerned with what it called "improving the race," moving toward perfection not only of the individual, but also of the larger group of which the individual was a member. The result was research that identified supposed physical and psychological traits by racial and national groups, with the white English and German groups inevitably being deemed superior; this was hardly a shock because the researchers were from those same groups.

Effects of the Great Depression (1930–1941)

The Depression, which took several years to fully develop and affect the entire country, lasted from 1929 into the start of World War II (1941). The lack of money in communities hit physical education and sports very hard. Many physical education programs were dropped from the school curriculum, based on the claim that it was an expensive frill that wasted money. This attack on the position of physical education in the school program came as a surprise to physical educators. For the first time they became aware of the need for a good public relations program; they realized that people simply did not understand the purposes of physical education and how it contributed to the education of the students. The move to drop physical education as a requirement in many states forced physical educators to defend their programs vigorously.

The onset of the Great Depression created great social changes. The United States gradually shifted from its old idea of rugged individualism to a new concern for the group (society) and for equality of opportunity. The trend toward social and recreational goals in physical education programs continued through the Depression but began to slow down in the years just prior to World War II. The Depression forced both physical education and athletics to give up ground in terms of both the scope of their programs and their public acceptance.

The 1940s brought a radical reversal of that trend. War demonstrated the need for physical education and athletics in the school program. New programs in many European nations, which showed their aims to be fitness for war and the development of a stronger sense of nationalism, resulted in a gradual shift of the American programs back to emphasis on physical fitness.

Summary

Physical activities had a limited place in colonial education, but many recreational games and sports were used for entertainment: hunting, fishing, swimming, and the necessary activities such as running, jumping, lifting heavy objects, and fighting. Organized sport was still in its early stages by 1860 and was primarily a creature of the larger cities.

The idea of physical education was supported by early civic leaders such as Thomas Jefferson and Benjamin Franklin. Samuel Moody was one of the first American educators to promote physical activities as vital to the health of students. The first real attempts to put physical education into the educational curriculum were made in the 1820s and 1830s and were led by schools such as the Round Hill School. Before 1860, the major instructional ideas came from Europe. These were influenced in the United States by the women's education movement, the move of religious groups into education, and the early growth of sport.

The major American physical education programs of the 1800s were based on German and Swedish gymnastics, leading to the Battle of the Systems. Programs were also affected by college students' interest in gymnasiums and swimming pools, which were appearing by the 1850s. A trend in the cities was a concern for public health, which led to the parks movement.

By the 1860s, some colleges were beginning to provide for formal physical education, a movement led by Amherst College's hiring of Edward Hitchcock. In the same era, the earliest professional preparation programs were appearing, led by the German Turners, the YMCA, and programs started by a small number of prominent leaders, such as Dio Lewis, Dudley Sargent, and Nils Posse. By 1900, physical education was appearing as a state requirement for public schools, thus increasing the need for professional education and organization. The early national leaders were primarily medical doctors, reflecting their interest in student health. Though a few early programs followed a scientific orientation, by the early 1900s the field had shifted from a scientific educational program to an applied teacher education focus. Eugenics, with the ideal of producing a stronger race, was a growing area of interest for society.

From 1900 to 1941, six trends were visible in physical education and sport: (1) the gradual assumption of control over intercollegiate sport by the colleges, the NCAA, and the college athletic conferences; (2) the effort of high schools to control their sports programs; (3) rapid growth in women's athletics, followed by a period of abolishing it; (4) a boom in intramural sports; (5) the addition of games and sports to the physical education curriculum (the New Physical Education); and (6) a shifting of the emphasis of physical education from a health focus to a general education focus.

The Depression of the 1930s hit physical education and sports very hard because of the lack of community money. Physical education programs were dropped as expensive frills, and few people could afford tickets for sports events. The big boom was in recreation.

Further Readings

Adelman, Melvin L. 1986. *A sporting time: New York City and the rise of modern athletics, 1820–70.* Champaign, IL: Univ. of Illinois Press.

Block, David. 2005. *Baseball before we knew it: A search for the roots of the game.* Lincoln NE: Univ. of Nebraska Press.

Borish, Linda J. 1987. The robust woman and the muscular Christian: Catharine Beecher, Thomas Higginson, and their vision of American society, health and physical activities. *International Journal of the History of Sport* 4: 139–154.

_____. 2005. Benevolent America: Rural women, physical recreation, sport and health reform in ante-bellum New England. *International Journal of the History of Sport* 22 (6): 946–973.

Bundgaard, Axel. 2005. *Muscle and manliness: The rise of sport in American boarding schools.* Syracuse, NY: Syracuse Univ. Press.

Byrd, Ronald. 2000. The physical side of George Washington. *Physical Educator* 57: 83–87.

Cazers, Gunars, and Glenn A. Miller. 2000. The German contribution to American physical education: A historical perspective. *JOPERD (Journal of Physical Education, Recreation and Dance)* 71 (6): 44–48.

Chisholm, Ann. 2008. Nineteenth-century gymnastics for U.S. women and incorporations of buoyancy: Contouring femininity, shaping sex, and regulating middle-class consumption. *Journal of Women's History* 20 (3): 84–112.

Daniels, Bruce C. 1995. *Puritans at play: Leisure and recreation in colonial New England.* New York: St. Martin's.

Gerber, Ellen W. 1971. *Innovations and institutions in physical education.* Philadelphia: Lea and Febiger.

Guedes, Claudia. 2007. Physical education and physical activity: A historical perspective. *JOPERD (Journal of Physical Education, Recreation and Dance)* 78 (8): 31–32, 47–48.

Lucas, John A., and Ronald A. Smith. 1978. *Saga of American sport.* Philadelphia: Lea and Febiger.

McCullick, Bryan A., and Michael Lomax. 2000. The Boston Normal School of Gymnastics: An unheralded legacy. *Quest* 52: 49–59.

Park, Roberta J. 1992. The rise and demise of Harvard's B.S. program in anatomy, physiology, and physical training: A case of conflicts of interest and scarce resources. *Research Quarterly for Exercise and Sport* 63: 246–260.

_____. 2007. "Embodied selves": The rise and development of concern for physical education, active games and recreation for American women, 1776–1865. *International Journal of the History of Sport* 24 (12): 1508–1542.

_____. 2007. Science, service, and the professionalization of physical education: 1885–1905. *International Journal of the History of Sport* 24 (12): 1674–1700.

Pfister, Gertrud. 2009. The role of German Turners in American physical education. *International Journal of the History of Sport* 26 (13): 1893–1925.

Rader, Benjamin G. 2008. *American sports: From the age of folk games to the age of televised sports.* 6th ed. Englewood Cliffs, NJ: Prentice Hall.

Struna, Nancy L. 1994. The recreational experiences of early American women. In *Women and sport: Interdisciplinary perspectives,* ed. D. Margaret Costa and Sharon R. Guthrie, 45–62. Champaign, IL: Human Kinetics.

_____. 1996. *People of prowess: Sport, leisure, and labor in early Anglo-America.* Champaign, IL: Univ. of Illinois Press.

Swanson, Richard, and Betty Spears. 1995. *History of sport and physical education in the United States.* 4th ed. Madison, WI: Brown and Benchmark.

Todd, Jan. 1998. *Physical culture and the body beautiful: Purposive exercise in the lives of American women, 1800–1875.* Macon, GA: Mercer Univ. Press.

Welch, Paula D. 2004. *History of American physical education and sport.* 3rd ed. Springfield, IL: Charles C Thomas.

Wrynn, Alison M. 2010. Eliza Maria Mosher: Pioneering woman physician and advocate for physical education. *International Journal of the History of Sport* 27: 1173–1190.

Discussion Questions

1. Discuss the effect of European plans of education and physical education upon the development of American education during the early 1800s (1800 to 1850).

2. Discuss the part played by two of the following in the early development of American physical education:

   a. Charles Beck, Charles Follen, and Francis Lieber (one choice)
   b. Round Hill School
   c. Catharine Beecher
   d. YMCA
   e. Turnverein movement
   f. Dio Lewis
   g. Edward Hitchcock
   h. John Swett
   i. Dudley Sargent
   j. Mary Hemenway
   k. Nils Posse
   l. AAPE
   m. Boston Conference of 1889
   n. Battle of the Systems
   o. George Fitz

3. Discuss the start of public education in the United States, including the education of women.

4. Discuss the development of teacher education in American physical education from 1860 to 1900.

5. Discuss why the early profession of physical education gradually changed from its early focus on scientific health and medical foundation to a focus on educational theory.

6. How did the teachings of John Dewey and Thomas Woods's and Rosalind Cassidy's New Physical Education change physical education in the early 1900s?

7. The physical education philosophies of C. H. McCloy, Jesse Feiring Williams, and Jay Nash are in conflict. What are their philosophical differences, and how might those differences affect a physical education program?

8. Discuss the theory of eugenics. What were the strengths and dangers of the idea for society?

9. Discuss the changes in programs of sport and physical education that were a result of the Great Depression.

References

1. Rice, Emmet A., John L. Hutchinson, and Mabel Lee. 1969. *A brief history of physical education*. 5th ed. New York: Ronald Press, 146.

2. Gerber, Ellen W. 1971. *Innovations and institutions in physical education*. Philadelphia: Lea and Febiger, 245–251.

3. Noel, Rebecca R. 1997. Antebellum school exercise in the United States: Consumption and Ned Wright's dilemma. In *1997 North American Society for Sport History Proceedings*, ed. Catriona M. Parratt, 71. Iowa City, IA: North American Society for Sport History.

4. Gerber, *Innovations and institutions*, 245–251.

5. Albertson, Roxanne. 1974. *Physical education in New England schools and academies from 1789 to 1860: Concepts and practices*. Eugene, OR: Univ. of Oregon, 90–91. Microfiche.

6. Bundgaard, Axel. 2005. *Muscle and manliness: The rise of sport in American boarding schools*. Syracuse, NY: Syracuse Univ. Press.

7. Gerber, *Innovations and institutions*, 252–258.

8. Betts, John Rickards. 1972. Public recreation, public parks, and public health before the Civil War. In *Proceedings of the Big Ten Symposium on the History of Physical Education and Sport*, ed. Bruce L. Bennett, 33–52. Chicago: Athletic Institute.

9. Barney, Robert K. 1984. America's first turnverein: Commentary in favor of Louisville, Kentucky. *Journal of Sport History* 11: 134–137.

10. Leonard, Fred E. 1922. *Pioneers of modern physical training*. 2nd ed. New York: Associated Press, 83–88.

11. Gerber, *Innovations and institutions*, 260.

12. Ibid., 267–275.

13. Ibid., 314–318.

14. Ibid., 100–105.

15. Mechikoff, Robert A., and Steven G. Estes. 1993. *A history and philosophy of sport and physical education*. Madison, WI: Brown and Benchmark, 219–220.

16. Gerber, *Innovations and institutions*, 302–307.

17. Park, Roberta J. 2006. "Taking their measure" in play, games, and physical training: The American scene, 1870s to World War I. *Journal of Sport History* 33:194.

18. Ibid., 194–195.

19. Lee, Mabel, and Bruce L. Bennett. 1960. A time of gymnastics and measurement. *JOHPER (Journal of Health, Physical Education and Recreation)* (April): 33.

20. Park, Roberta J. 1992. The rise and demise of Harvard's B.S. program in anatomy, physiology, and physical training: A case of conflicts of interest and scarce resources. *Research Quarterly for Exercise and Sport* 63: 246–260.

21. Kroll, Walter. 1982. *Graduate study and research in physical education*. Champaign, IL: Human Kinetics, 58–59.

22. Lee, Mabel. 1973. Further discussion of the first academic degree in physical education. *JOHPER (Journal of Health, Physical Education and Recreation)* (April): 89.

23. Swanson, Richard, and Betty Spears. 1995. *History of sport and physical education in the United States*. 4th ed. Madison, WI: Brown and Benchmark, 183.

24. Bucher, Charles A., and Ralph K. Dupee Jr. 1965. *Athletics in schools and colleges*. New York: Center for Applied Research in Education, 8.

25. Van Dalen, Deobold B., and Bruce L. Bennett. 1971. *A world history of physical education*. 2nd ed. Englewood Cliffs, NJ: Prentice Hall, 441–443.

26. Gerber, Ellen W. 1974. *The American woman in sport*. Reading, MA: Addison-Wesley, 106–111.

27. Swanson and Spears, *History of sport*, 185; and Wood, Thomas D., and Rosalind F. Cassidy. 1972. *The new physical education*. New York: Macmillan.

28. Wood and Cassidy, *The new physical education*.

29. Swanson and Spears, *History of sport*, 228–229.

30. Gerber, Ellen W. 1972. The ideas and influences of McCloy, Nash, and Williams. In *Proceedings of the Big Ten Symposium on the History of Physical Education and Sport*, ed. Bruce L. Bennett, 98–99. Chicago: Athletic Institute.

31. Van Dalen and Bennett, *World history*, 441–443.

32. Couturier, Lynn E. 2005. The influence of the eugenics movement on physical education in the United States. *Sport History Review* 36 (May): 21.

33. Wrynn, Alison M. 2005. Less than perfect: Physical education and the pursuit of the perfect human body. In *North American Society for Sport History Proceedings*, 61–62; and Huskins, Heather A., and Jan Todd. 2000. From a strongman comes forth a new woman: The influences of Eugen Sandow on women's body ideology, 1900–1925. In *North American Society for Sport History Proceedings*, 29–30.

34. Couturier, Influence of the eugenics movement, 24.

The Rise of Modern Sport in the United States and England to 1941

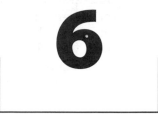

Social Sport in Colonial and Early National America (1607–1860)

This period of sport was premodern by the characteristics discussed later in this chapter. Sport in colonial and early national America was essentially recreational in nature and not very highly organized. The primary emphasis of sport at this time was social. Life was not easy for the early settlers, who had few chances to relax and enjoy themselves. On the frontier, people often were widely separated and had few opportunities to meet each other. They welcomed the chance to get together socially on such occasions as holidays, militia training days, election days, court meeting days, and church meetings and revivals.

The religiously oriented colonies usually were opposed to recreational activities as wasteful idleness. They passed *blue laws* designed to prevent any irreligious activities on Sundays. They passed other laws against many sporting activities, but they were not very successful in preventing the activities. Though we think of the Puritans in New England as being stern people opposed to any sport or recreation, it is an incorrect belief. The Puritans came to America seeking religious freedom, as they interpreted it. They interpreted it to mean that, instead of someone else telling them how to worship, the Puritans would tell everyone else how to worship. They believed in a hardworking, serious life, yet it was not one that ruled out laughter or sport.

The Puritans held to a strong work ethic, and they passed laws to see that the citizens worked hard and observed the Puritan religious beliefs. They observed no religious holidays (not even Christmas) other than the Sabbath. They objected to anyone either feasting or fasting on the Sabbath, and their rules against Sunday sport were intended to see that the religious nature of the Sabbath was observed. Their rules were not against sport, but against anyone forgetting that Sunday was primarily a day with religious meaning.

Indeed, early accounts note the streets of Boston "full of Girls and Boys sporting up and down."[1] For the most part, the Puritans recognized a value for recreational and sporting activities in the sense of recreation or change-of-pace activities that refreshed people and permitted them to work with renewed energy and zeal.[2] At the same time, as their colony grew in size, stability, and wealth, they were fighting a losing battle against the outside world's influence. People with a stable, prosperous life were less interested in a relatively ascetic life when it was no longer necessary for survival. As Don Calhoun notes:

> *Puritanism was strongest on the rural frontier and among the Anglo-Saxon population, and began to weaken with the development of towns and cities and their settlement by non-WASP immigrants (like the Germans, with their tradition of Sunday picnicking and beer-drinking).*[3]

Nancy Struna divides colonial sport into three phases.[4] The first phase (1607 to 1670) involved a relatively narrow range of activities that generally were not a transfer of English customs to the New World. The second phase (1670 to 1730) saw a wider range of activities and extensive imitation or adaptation of British practices. The third phase (1730 to 1790) saw the emergence of two distinct sporting styles, those of the vernacular (ordinary citizens) and the gentry. The vernacular style showed many regional or local variations in accepted rules and practices, while the gentry style was more elaborate and less regional. The gentry style also dominated, although the two styles also interacted considerably.

By the 1790s one can see

> *a shift within popular culture. Partly because of their numbers and their enterprise, as well as by the "unbecoming" of the gentry among some early national successors to the provincial squirearchy, America's middle ranks assumed this new standard of conduct. They resolved [Governor] Winthrop's [Puritan idleness] dilemma by establishing work as the precursor to play, and play as something at which one worked.*[5]

As the colonies became more solidly based and the citizens had more free time, more recreational activities appeared. Sports were not very highly organized at that time; people played games they had learned as children, or they followed the directions for games given in the English sporting magazines and game books. Because most of the early settlers were English, most of the early games were of English origin. English publications, which became widely spread in America during the late 1700s and early 1800s, helped to make the development of English sport a major influence on the later organization of sport in the United States.

As the settlers moved westward, life again became difficult, and the sporting activities also became much tougher. The most popular competitive activities during early national times were contests such as horse racing, cockfighting (matches between specially trained fighting roosters), gambling, rowing, and baseball. Indeed, one of the major objections of religious groups to many sporting activities, if not the very idea of sport, was the heavy use of such activities as an excuse for gambling. For the colonial aristocracy, just as for the English aristocrats, gambling lay at the heart of most sporting activities.[6] Horse racing, with both open races and match races, was always popular throughout the colonies. Aspects of modern organization appear in other activities, but Melvin Adelman argues that harness racing was the first modern sport in the United States.[7] Cockfighting also was popular, particularly in the southern states. Rowing developed in the mid-1800s as one of the first collegiate sports.

Baseball gradually evolved from English ball games, until it was considered a native American game. Documented references to the game go back to the 1740s as a game played by schoolboys.[8] One reason baseball was popular was because it was one of the few sporting activities that showed no distinction between the social classes.

Although many sporting activities were popular in early times, the real growth of sport in the United States came only after the nation had become more settled and urbanized. Some stability and a certain level of wealth and leisure time are needed before sport can become highly organized in a society. Those conditions were not very noticeable until after the mid-1800s. As the young nation moved into the mid nineteenth century, there was a growth of sporting events that were more commercial, planned for urban areas to attract a large audience of paying customers. Reflecting similar developments in England, races were popular early mass leisure events. Horse races were popular, and foot races or *pedestrianism* was quite popular for a time. Boat races also were in favor, ranging from sculls similar to today's Olympic races to larger manned boats to yachts. The rise of improved transportation, such as steamboats and railways, resulted in attempts to organize large spectator sporting events that would draw passengers traveling to the heavily promoted events.

Despite the popular English influence toward Muscular Christianity, inspired by writings such as *Tom Brown's Schooldays* and the diligent work of exercise and health enthusiasts such as Oliver Wendell Holmes and Thomas Wentworth Higginson, Americans were not very physically vigorous or healthy, nor were they as inclined to take part in strenuous sports as Europeans were.[9] In part, this was the effect of the growth of an urban, industrial nation because city dwellers had only limited opportunities for recreational exercise. At the same time, Americans still showed little interest in devoting themselves to exercising and spending their money, as wealthier Europeans did. Yet another generation was required for that development.

During the first half of the nineteenth century, interest in sports began to grow rapidly. Most of the Puritan-based objections to games and sports had gradually disappeared as the nation grew larger and more stable. Groups of various nationalities had brought their own favorite games to the United States, and the melting pot of peoples became a melting pot of sports. The time when sports would begin to organize had not yet come, however.

By the time of the Civil War, the stage was set for the United States to develop a modern system of sport. It was rapidly becoming a wealthy nation with an advanced technology, particularly in transportation and communications.[10] Once the bloody bitterness of the Civil War had passed, the United States shifted from a nation on the move to one on the run. Sport was part of its leap toward the future.

The Characteristics of Modern Sport

Although we defined *sport* in the first chapter, the term *modern sport* must be explained. Many scholars have proposed definitions or characteristics of modern sport, but Allen Guttmann's work can serve as a model.[11] He suggests seven characteristics that distinguish modern sport:

1. Secularism
2. Equality
3. Specialization
4. Rationalization
5. Bureaucracy
6. Quantification
7. Records

Secularism

Secularism indicates that sport lost any religious meaning that it may have had in earlier times. Early sporting activities had religious overtones, if not actual religious functions. Even during the Middle Ages, some of those meanings lay close beneath the surface.

Guttmann notes that modern sports are more like Roman sport than Greek sport, and the new secular nature of sport was a factor that caused opposition by religious leaders from the 1600s to the 1800s. He writes that "modern sports are activities partly pursued for their own sake, partly for other ends that are equally secular. We do not run in order that the earth be more fertile. We till the earth, or work in our factories and offices, so that we can have time to play."[12]

Equality

Equality refers to two types: Any person may compete, and the conditions under which that person competes will be the same. Equality may be the most difficult characteristic to achieve because it is as difficult to define in sport as it is in education and in law. It means that each person is treated the same under the rules and that each person has an equal opportunity to participate. It does not mean that each person is guaranteed the right to perform regardless of ability, nor does it mean that the results are equal.

Sport is competitive, and the less skilled performers will lose. People are created equal before the law, but that does not mean that their talents, abilities, or skills are equal. They are not. Just as in other areas of life, the people with greater inherited and developed talents will rise higher than those who are less talented. Equality of access and competitive conditions do not give a person of limited ability the right to compete in an Olympic contest. As Guttmann notes,

> *equality of opportunity is not the same as equality of results. . . . The more equal the chance to participate, the more unequal the results will be. For men and for women, the distance between the ordinary athlete and the international champion is greater every year. . . . Inequality of results is an essential characteristic of modern sports.*[13]

At the same time, sport, even in modern times, has fallen short in the area of equal access to competition. Guttmann points to the code of amateurism, developed during the 1800s and based on medieval ideas of separating social classes. The old rules defining the amateur evolved from Victorian and Edwardian England, where sport was controlled by an upper class that was as concerned with keeping the classes separated as with providing competition at a high level. Indeed, under the early rules, certain occupations (such as laborers) were declared automatically professional. Social inferiors were not to compete against (and perhaps defeat) their social "betters."

One can understand the amateurism controversy by looking closely at the people who form the rule-making bodies. The International Olympic Committee (IOC) members are primarily wealthy (and often titled) white males. They have very little sympathy for athletes who have to earn a living while training on the side.

Guttmann describes the code of amateurism as "an instrument of class warfare . . . [designed] to limit sports to gentlemen of means."[14] The basis of the rules often is difficult to understand. In part, the amateur code was an attempt to protect people who only participated for the enjoyment of sport from having to compete against people who considered sport a way of life or an occupation. We still face that difficulty today. How does an athlete working 40 hours a week compete to make an Olympic team against an athlete who makes a living at the sport and thus has no other task in life except to train?

Other rules have equally complicated bases. The objection to women athletes was the result of the Victorian view of women—weak creatures who needed to be protected against harm. Objections were as much for their protection (the rule makers believed) as from any objection to the idea of women competing. This protective attitude, coupled with a profound ignorance about the capabilities of women, severely limited women's sporting opportunities until the 1970s. Only in the 1980s did the IOC decide that women were physically capable of competing in endurance events, such as running a marathon, without doing themselves severe harm.

The equality of the competitive conditions is reflected in the development of standardized rules and sport settings. Instead of a site that varies according to local geography and terrain, we now have modern stadiums and competition sites that exhibit what Edward Relph called "placelessness"; that is, every site is essentially the same.[15] No site is distinctive of its locale, a characteristic feature of today's sport.

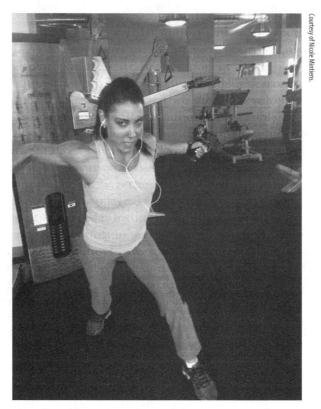

Courtesy of Nicole Minters.

Equality of opportunity is a characteristic of modern sport.

Specialization

Specialization grew out of an emphasis on success. Years ago, a dozen men who formed a football team would play both offense and defense. Today, nearly 100 athletes are on a team. Some of them may have no function other than that of substitute kicker or opposition player for practice sessions.

There are specialists who handle the off-the-field details, such as field maintenance, equipment upkeep, business details, scouting, recruiting, and coaching. Guttmann suggests that specialization is an inevitable development, along with professionalism: "To an extent, they are the same thing. . . . The plain fact is that world-class competition is usually incompatible with an ordinary vocation."[16]

Rationalization

The development of standard rules of conditions and procedures of competition is called rationalization. Greek sports are an example of earlier developments, because even if the discoi at Olympia were all the same size, their size differed from those at Nemea or Delphi. There was some rationalization, but it was not complete.

At the same time, the Greeks apparently were the first to study sports performance and how it could be improved. The distinction is important, as Guttmann says,

> *The Greeks did more than practice. They trained. The distinction is important. Training implies a rationalization of the whole enterprise, a willingness to experiment, a constant testing of results achieved. . . . There was a whole way of life concentrated on the single goal of athletic excellence.*[17]

Bureaucracy

A bureaucracy is needed to write and apply the rules that are developed for a sport. Modern sport began in England with the rise of organizations devoted to a single sport. An organization would write the rules, standardizing the equipment, the site, and the procedures for competitions. The first organizations were usually local clubs. Real progress came with the appearance of national bodies, which provided widely standardized rules and national championships, followed by international groups that started world championships.

The bureaucratic structure is seen today in the Olympic movement. The IOC oversees the Olympic Games, but subgroups set the rules for individual Olympic sports. Each nation has its own national body for each sport, as well as a national Olympic Committee below the IOC. As Guttmann says:

> *One of the most important functions of the bureaucracy is to see that the rules and regulations are universal. Another is to facilitate a network of competitions that usually progress from local contests through national to world championships . . . [and] another function of sports associations [is] . . . the ratification of records.*[18]

Quantification

Quantification (measuring and keeping performance records) is a critical characteristic of modern sport. Almost every modern sport is viewed in terms of some measurable standard of perfection. A bowler wants a 300-pin game; a baseball player wants more hits, more home runs, or a higher batting average; and a team wants more victories. Some people believe the stopwatch is a symbol of modern sport because it was invented 250 years ago to time horse races.

Guttmann notes that "at least one theorist suggests that sport be defined as that physical activity which can be measured in points or in the c–g–s system (centimeter–gram–second)." Even sports in which performance cannot be easily measured are changed to make performances measurable. In gymnastics and in diving, for example, points are subjectively awarded against a perfect performance and its degree of difficulty, leading Guttmann to refer to the modern person as *Homo mensor,* or "measuring man." This quantification is linked to the industrial age, when precise measurement first became a common feature.[19]

Records

The concept of the record is modern and is based on the idea of progress, a belief that we will always be able to improve, that performances can always become greater or faster. It requires quantification because measuring and recording are combined with the desire to win. The result is the desire to be the best ever: the record holder. Guttmann states that the Greeks had no word meaning record. In fact, the use of that term in English dates only from the 1880s. He speculates that, with the secularization of society, people no longer run "to appease [the gods] or to save our souls, but we can set a new record. It is a uniquely modern form of immortality."[20]

Guttmann summarizes the development of modern sport by citing Hans Lenk, who said that "achievement sport, i.e., sport whose achievements are extended beyond the here and now through measured comparisons, is closely connected to the scientific-experimental attitudes of the modern West." Guttmann expands the explanation by noting that

> *the mathematical discoveries of the seventeenth century were popularized in the eighteenth century, at which time we can observe the beginnings of our modern obsession with quantification in sport. . . . The emergence of modern sports represents neither the triumph of capitalism nor the rise of Protestantism but rather the slow development of an empirical, experimental, mathematical [worldview]. England's early leadership had less to do with the Protestant ethic and the spirit of capitalism than with the intellectual revolution symbolized by the names of Isaac Newton and John Locke and institutionalized in the Royal Society, founded during the Restoration, in 1662, for the advancement of science.*[21]

Melvin Adelman has taken Guttmann's model and modified it to show the difference between what he calls premodern sport and modern sport.[22] It provides a simpler model for deciding how far sporting activity has progressed toward what we call modern.

In defining premodern sport, that is, sport as it makes the transition from its early forms to the modern form, Adelman suggests six characteristics:

1. Organization
2. Rules
3. Competition

4. Role differentiation
5. Public information
6. Statistics and records

All six of these characteristics either exist at a simple or local level or do not exist at all. Organization is very limited and is usually done by local people of limited expertise. The rules are still unwritten and vary from one place to another. The competitors are limited to the local or regional area. National reputations do not yet exist. Role differentiation is limited; that is, there is little difference in the role played by any team member. In fact, spectators may occasionally take part in the competition. Public information is limited; it is usually oral and passed along locally. Finally, there are no records or statistics kept.

The appearance of these characteristics quite clearly forms modern sport. However, we must remember that the premodern period of sport was not brief: Adelman's study of New York City covered half a century (1820 to 1870). George Kirsch narrows the focal period of development toward modern sport in the United States to 1840 to 1860. Other arguments are possible, as it happened at different times in different parts of the nation. Henrik Sandblad suggests that the 1860s and 1870s were the focal time of the shift toward organized sports in a Europe that was greatly influenced by the British sporting practices of the time.[23]

The Birth of Modern Sport in England and Europe

Most of what we have come to know as modern sport developed from the growth of sport in the nineteenth century, primarily in Europe. From 1850 to 1900, there were three particular trends or developments of interest: the continuation of the class dichotomy in sport; the origins of organized competitive sport, as opposed to informal or folk sports; and the revival of the Olympic Games under Baron Pierre de Coubertin in 1896.

The Sport Dichotomy Continues

Our best example of the sport dichotomy comes from the British public schools, which are actually private, because they preserved their traditional educational patterns for centuries. The British public schools had a strong tradition of sport as an activity for the leisured gentleman. The school system that promoted sports was also strongly class conscious. England had very clearly defined social classes, and the upper classes were very hesitant to associate with the other classes.

The educational system in Victorian England upheld the class structure, even in "the type of play it allowed and promoted." The public schools tried to develop "such qualities as manliness, strength, loyalty, discipline and powers of leadership, and arrived at a convinced philosophy that games, especially team games, were an ideal medium through which to achieve these character-molding goals."[24] In the United States, these views were extended until "athletics and, in particular, team sports were regarded as symbols of democracy and as integrative mechanisms which taught traditional small-town values to urban youths."[25]

The graduates of the British public schools were a major influence on the development of organized sport. Not only were they the primary leaders in organizing sport, but it was organized within the framework of the public school philosophy: Sport was purely for the sake of competition and pleasure. Winning was, at best, a secondary interest. This philosophical direction was probably one of the most fortunate aspects of the early development of organized sport, although it created problems then and continues to create problems now.

Another notable aspect of the British public school influence was the definition of amateurism. The requirements for amateur status, which enabled the athlete to enter organized competition, made participation very difficult for the lower classes. Their jobs did not allow them time to train. The lower classes were discouraged (if not barred outright) from competing with the leisured gentlemen who made the rules. The accepted sports were still largely a domain of the upper classes. As Richard Holt puts it, the standard for amateurism was not money or profit: "It was an assertion of the class system. . . . The distinction was social rather than financial."[26]

Sport as a Moral Virtue

Dennis Brailsford asserts that "the great recreational discovery of the later Victorians was that sport could be equated with virtue."[27] Gary Cross simplifies our view of the rise of modern sport when he writes that

the key to change was in making sport respectable. Activity that the religious middle classes had associated with gambling, drunkenness, and violence gradually gained legitimacy in the 19th century when sport became an extension of moral power concretely expressed in the display of physical courage. By training the body . . . the individual disciplined the will. Morality continued to mean self-restraint, but it also increasingly implied vitality and action in the "real world," values that could be inculcated in sport.[28]

This was a complex, even a confusing, idea. By the 1850s, Charles Darwin's theory of evolution was being adapted into what was later called social Darwinism, the idea of changing people over time in deliberately planned ways. As Holt writes,

The idea of the healthy mind and body merged into a garbled Darwinism that was itself often intermingled with notions of Christian and imperial duty. All this was contained within a framework where the fierce individualism that was required for economic success had to be balanced against the need for social cohesion and political stability.[29]

Throughout society the idea was that this new sport, this "good" sport, would not allow "the old rowdiness, the drunken company, the brutality and the cruelty, the flouting of working hours, the inveterate gambling, the vice, crime and corruption in which sport had spent [its] earlier years."[30] This new sport was part of the movement called *Muscular Christianity*.

Muscular Christianity

The traditional leader in the sport movement in the British public schools was Rugby School, with its famed headmaster Thomas Arnold. Actually, Arnold is an English version of the American Abner Doubleday, for just as many people wrongly believe Doubleday invented baseball (a game that was played before his birth), others wrongly believe Arnold made public school sports a vital part of the curriculum. The reality is explained by J. A. Mangan:

> *From 1850 onwards, games were purposefully and deliberately assimilated into the formal curriculum of the public schools. . . . It must be made quite clear that the conviction that Arnold was responsible for the "athletic sports system" of the public schools . . . does not accord with the evidence and should be firmly rejected. . . . Arnold appears to have been insensitive to the possibilities of an athletic ethos with team games as the instrument of moral conditioning, as a mechanism of control, as a desirable antidote to vandalism and even as a measure of personal enjoyment. In plain fact, at no time in his life did Arnold appear to be much interested in such activities. . . . In Arnold's own contributions to educational theory there is not a single reference to physical activities.[31]*

Instead, the leadership role went to headmasters at Marlborough, Harrow, Uppingham, and other schools. They "took the then novel step of encouraging pupils and staff to consider games as part of the formal curriculum."[32] Thomas Hughes popularized the changes with his novel *Tom Brown's Schooldays*, published in 1857 for a wide British and American audience. The real influence at Rugby, and in the novel, was G. E. L. Cotton, a master who promoted sports in Arnold's time and then became an influential headmaster at Marlborough, where he continued to preach the gospel of sports.[33]

The term *Muscular Christianity* was probably coined by T. C. Sandars in 1857, though the "ideal of manliness and the association of physical prowess with moral virtue" were promoted widely by the writings of Charles Kingsley. Sports participation was encouraged as moral education, a character-building experience. The goal was not victory; indeed, "the educational value of defeat and failure . . . was a recurrent theme in Victorian England."[34] The value of sports in education lay in its encouraging youths to learn to cope with defeat, with losing or falling short, as most people will do in competition and life. The value was in taking part, in striving for victory, rather than the victory alone.

Victory was valued just as highly then as it is now. Practice time was probably as extensive as with today's athletes. Even so, the *struggle* to succeed was seen as the true virtue in education. The Victorians believed that winning was all very well but that most people will not win. They must learn to accept defeat, yet not give up.

Competition was encouraged "on the moral grounds that games were a preparation for the battle of life and that they trained moral qualities, mainly respect for others, patient endurance, unflagging courage, self-reliance and self-control, vigour and decision of character."[35] Sport helped to develop an attitude, a philosophy of striving to do better, regardless of the conditions faced. This idea, called Muscular Christianity, became very popular in both England and the United States during the second half of the nineteenth century, the formative period of modern sport. It became part of the new definition of masculinity, broadened from the old job and family identities to include character and the physical self.[36]

The Birth of Modern Organized Sport

Organized sport really dates from late in the nineteenth century. During much of the first half of the century, wars and national revolutions in Europe created unstable conditions that were not conducive to the development of sport. In the second half of the century, times became more peaceful, and nationalism continued to grow. Sporting organizations were beginning to develop, along with a consciousness of national pride.

Sports clubs developed during that period. Although there was some mixing of the classes in club memberships, the policies and practices were dominated by the public (i.e., private) school graduates. Local championships were organized, playing fields were constructed, and eventually steps were taken to form national sporting bodies.

We can see six rough stages of development during the rise of organized sport. The first stage was the growth of university sports. The second stage was the growth in popularity of sport, as people became interested first as spectators, then as participants. This popularity led to the third stage, the development of sports clubs. Participants banded together with other people interested in the sport to provide competition and playing facilities that would permit them to follow their particular sporting interests. (Some sports clubs included several sports, whereas others concentrated on a single sport.) In the fourth stage, national organizations and national championships were begun for each sport. The fifth stage, common national and international rules for each sport, was followed by the sixth stage (where it was applicable), keeping national and international records. Most of these stages were completed during the nineteenth century, when the emphasis on informal sport ended and the move toward standardized national and international sports competition began, although the majority of international organizations originated in the twentieth century.

Wray Vamplew suggests that the development of modern rules went through seven stages, beginning with rules that applied only to a single meeting between two individuals or teams, and rising through increasing numbers of affected people or teams until it reached the level of rules designed to meet international standards.[37]

An example of these developmental stages can be seen in the changes in English track and field during this period. Competition within the universities began in the 1850s, although the choice of events was highly variable from one competition to the next. The first intercollegiate meet was between Oxford and Cambridge in 1864. Numerous sports clubs formed, and the first English championship meet was held in 1866.

The time and place of the meets caused considerable conflict among sports clubs. Most nonuniversity students and citizens who lived any distance from London were unable to attend the championships. After the Amateur Athletic Association, a national track and field body, was formed in 1880, the national meet was changed to a time of year when all athletes could compete. The site of the meet was changed from year to year as well. The move to develop international rules and records came in the next century with the 1912 formation of the International Amateur Athletic Federation, whose task was to revise the international rules and to approve world records.

As the nineteenth century came to a close, many changes had taken place in European sport. Sporting organizations made the rules more consistent. National championships started for many sports. The upper classes' influence on sport was beginning to weaken as many common people became sports competitors and spectators. The last stage in the move toward organized sport was coming closer: the development of international sport. This stage appeared as the result of work by Baron Pierre de Coubertin of France and others, who worked for years to revive the ancient Olympic Games.

The Phoenix Arises: The Rebirth of the Olympic Games

The rebirth of the Olympic Games was a complex process influenced by individuals and movements in several countries. Although local communities sometimes staged competitions that they called Olympic Games, few people promoted the events as international in scope. In his detailed account of the events leading to the founding of the modern games, David Young argues that they came about because of the fortunate combined influences of a group of men.

The first was a Greek poet, Panagiotis Soutsos, who in 1833 wrote poems calling for the Greeks to renew the games as a way to reestablish Greek culture. His 1835 proposal to the government bore many points of similarity to the games that appeared so many years later. He worked for several decades to build interest in the games. Dr. William Penny Brookes held games for more than 40 years after 1850, beginning in Much Wenlock, England. Those games were visited by Baron Pierre de Coubertin in 1890. The continued efforts of Soutsos eventually encouraged Evangelis Zappas to start a series of Greek national Olympics between 1859 and 1889. Young also cites nineteenth-century Olympic Games in Sweden (1834), Greece (Elis in 1838), Canada (Montreal in 1844), and the United States (San Francisco in 1893). Though the modern Olympic Games grew from the long-term beneficial efforts of a number of people, ultimately we credit Coubertin as the primary moving force.[38]

Although the modern Games were not his original idea, Baron Pierre de Coubertin can still be called the father of the modern Olympics. The games might not have been revived or survived as an international event without his years of ceaseless promotion. Born in France in 1863, Coubertin was a well-educated nobleman.[39] He was an ardent supporter of the British public school tradition, especially of the Rugby School. Coubertin believed that the strength of England drew from this school tradition, which stressed character, intellect, and the development of the body. Organized games were required of all students, so sport was as important a part of the educational process as intellectual training.

Coubertin was motivated by a desire to help France. He believed that lack of exercise made France a weak nation, and he strongly supported physical education programs in the schools. He hoped to develop sport with an international outlook. In 1892, he called for a revival of the Olympic Games but discovered that no one was really interested. He spent the next 3 years trying to make people conscious of what he called *Olympism*.

At an 1894 congress at the Sorbonne, Coubertin formed the International Olympic Committee, with the purpose of reviving the Olympic Games in 1896. One man was elected to represent each nation on the committee. The committee members were required to value internationalism above nationalism. They also set the standards of amateurism. The committee continued, if it did not magnify, the class dichotomy in sport because only wealthy men served on the committee. The choice was intentional. They formed an independent body and were less likely to be affected by political or nationalistic influence. Unfortunately, they also were not likely to understand the views of the common people and of the athletes.

Olympism, as Coubertin called it, was a combination of religion, peace, and beauty. The strong element of character has always been a notable part of the Olympic tradition. The love of beauty, especially as expressed in the beauty of movement, is also still clear. Today we often forget the religious aspect, but the early games were held to honor the gods.

Coubertin's experiment was an attempt to blend academic training with moral and physical education. It was designed to promote peace and to contribute to international understanding. He hoped to make the competition as pure an amateur competition as possible. He did not visualize women taking part in the games for two reasons: They had not taken part in the original Olympic Games, and, in his view, it was undignified for women to compete. His beliefs (shared by most men at that time) were not an example of the Olympic ideal carried to its logical conclusion.[40]

Coubertin succeeded in reviving the Olympic Games. The first modern Olympic Games began on Easter Sunday, April 5, 1896, in Athens. The rebirth of the games was the result of Coubertin's dream, and it was one of the greatest influences on modern sport. Although sport has changed vastly from nineteenth-century Europe, most of today's practices and problems were evident even then.

The Rise of Organized Sport in the United States (1850–1905)

Steven Riess summarizes the views of American sport historians in writing that "the rise of organized sport [in the United States] was the joint product of industrialization and urbanization." He elaborates by explaining why he considers the city and urbanization to be critical factors in the rise of modern sport:

> *The evolution of the city, more than any other single factor, influenced the development of organized sport and recreational athletic pastimes in America. Nearly all contemporary major sports evolved, or were invented, in the city. The city was the place where sport became rationalized, specialized, organized, commercialized, and professionalized.*[41]

During the second half of the nineteenth century, two significant developments took place. Teams were being formed in the schools (beginning with colleges in the northeastern United States). At the same time, athletic clubs were being formed and were working to organize sport. Both played important roles in the organization of sport before 1900.

John Rickards Betts refers to the period from 1860 to 1890 as "the age of the athletic club." Many athletic clubs began in the larger cities. Some clubs supported specific sports, while others emphasized a number of sports. Many clubs were sponsored by college students until the colleges permitted them to have school teams. One leading track-and-field club was the New York Athletic Club, which introduced the spiked shoe, the cinder track, and standardized track-and-field rules. It also promoted the sport in general.[42]

The athletic clubs led to the growth of some professional sports, particularly baseball. Eventually national organizations formed and national championship competitions were held. An example is the Amateur Athletic Union, formed in 1888 from an earlier track-and-field group started by the New York Athletic Club.

Sport also was growing rapidly in colleges. The earliest school teams were similar to today's extramural or club sports programs. They were organized and directed by the students themselves. For the most part, the schools made no attempt to control these sporting activities, beyond occasionally banning events that were considered dangerous or were interfering with academic interests. The first competition between two colleges was a rowing match between Harvard and

Yale in 1852. By 1875, intercollegiate contests were also held in baseball, cricket, football, and track and field.[43]

Although fewer than two dozen schools had teams in 1875, they were increasing rapidly in popularity. College faculties usually permitted the sports for two reasons. Allowing students to direct some of their own activities was coming into fashion, and the school teams made student life more attractive to prospective students. They became (as they are today) a marketing tool for the colleges.

Gymnasiums were constructed by cities, by athletic clubs, and by schools in many areas. The addition of year-round athletic facilities helped to promote sports all the more because activities were less limited by the weather and seasons. Gymnasiums also were being built because of a growing acceptance of the value of physical education activities for the students. At this time, however, physical education and sport had no real connection. The 1889 conference on physical education hardly mentioned sports activities because physical education was more ritual and calisthenics at that time.

By the late 1800s, many new developments were taking place in collegiate sports. The 1864 Yale crew was the first to hire a professional coach. Secondary schools developed sports teams in imitation of the collegiate teams, often to compete against the college teams. Collegiate athletic associations and conferences also were formed to organize and regulate competition, such as the Intercollegiate Association of Amateur Athletes of America (IC4A, founded in 1875) for track-and-field competition in the eastern United States and the American Intercollegiate Football Association (founded in 1876).

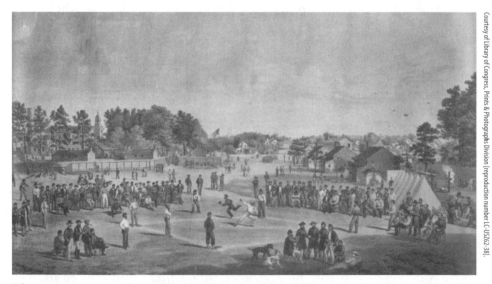

Courtesy of Library of Congress, Prints & Photographs Division [reproduction number LC-USZ62-38].

The most common theory for the growth of baseball as a national sport is that it was learned in prison camps during the Civil War, such as this game in North Carolina.

Another reason for the growing popularity of collegiate sports was the belief that sports reflected the interests and values of leading businessmen, who often gave financial support as alumni. Many of the problems common to school sports, such as professionalism and excessive outside influence, especially by alumni, date from the era when the schools did not want an official role in sports. By the late 1800s, football had become one of the most popular school sports. It was particularly influential because many of the problems it created led to a struggle in the schools to control school sports and eliminate what they considered harmful outside influences.

As Ronald Smith writes, in summarizing the rise of college athletics to 1905:

> *Twentieth-century big-time athletics became a ritual for nearly all major universities, symbolizing in physical form the intense competition for prestige existing among the various institutions. Winning athletic teams were the most visible signs of the contests for prestige taking place in all areas of university life. Nearly all universities stood for increasing undergraduate enrollment, attracting academically superior graduate students, obtaining prestigious, or "star" professors, maximizing faculty publications, accumulating university gifts and endowments, and increasing private and public research dollars. . . . With the success of Harvard and Yale as competitors in higher education and in athletics, it was not surprising that the twentieth century saw a ritualized cloning of Harvard and Yale.*[44]

American Sport at the Turn of the Century (1900)

This section examines four issues of sport in 1900: The first is the status of minorities, notably women and African Americans. The second issue is the abuses of sport at that time. The third area is the progress made toward organized sport. The fourth is the loss of student control of sports.

Women in Sport

Women's sporting activities were those that did not require the lady (that was the point of it all) to perspire or to display her body. The activities were those that could be played while fully dressed, which at that time was full indeed. Sports participation was part of respectable social encounters and usually was in individual sports, such as archery and croquet. Women's physical education was becoming accepted in the schools, and interest was also growing. Women's team sports (particularly basketball) were appearing by 1900, but they were viewed with suspicion. Women were often quite interested in sports, but the schools and the public tended to disapprove and discourage their competition as unladylike or unsafe.[45] Despite this, there were women's college teams in sports such as baseball as far back as 1866 at Vassar College and teams at Northwestern in 1869 and Smith College in 1879.[46] Collegiate physical education departments were being founded for women in the 1880s and 1890s. They soon found that many women preferred sporting activities to the traditional calisthenics and gymnastics.[47]

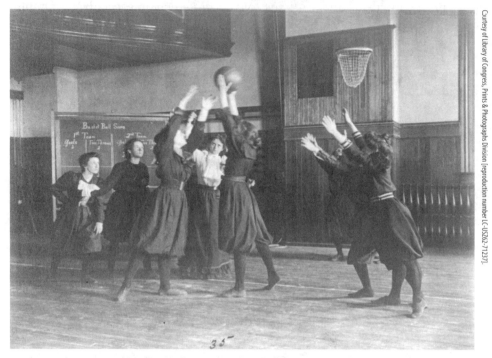

In the early years of basketball, it was more popular among girls than among boys, as shown in this 1899 photo.

African Americans in Sport

African Americans had become very involved in sport by 1900, but they were handicapped by several developments. During the slavery years, they were allowed to participate in boxing, horse racing, foot racing, and boat racing. After they were freed, they began to imitate many of the white sports, just as the middle and lower classes of the Middle Ages had imitated the sports of the nobility. Although blacks were involved in many areas of sport in the late 1800s, they were most active and successful in baseball (some were major league players in the late 1800s), horse racing (most of the top jockeys before 1900 were black), and boxing.

During the 1880s and early 1890s, a rising tide of racism in the United States resulted in the Jim Crow laws, which called for the separation of blacks and whites in many areas of life. The laws, upheld by the Supreme Court's separate but equal decision in 1896, removed blacks from many previously integrated activities. Baseball barred black players in the 1880s; white players were pressured to refuse to play if an African American was on the team. (This segregation in baseball lasted until 1946 in the major leagues.) Efforts to bar black jockeys from horse racing were largely successful by 1900. Numerous other sports were pressured to ban blacks because they were considered "uncivilized" and thus should not be allowed to compete with whites. The racism of the late 1800s was reflected most vividly in the search for the great white hope of boxing, the long-sought savior of the whites who would defeat the African American boxing champion Jack Johnson. Johnson was an object of white hatred during the years after 1900 when he was the world's best boxer.

By 1900, black athletes usually were barred from competition with whites. Black major leagues were formed in baseball, which was perhaps the most popular sport among African Americans at that time, and black college athletic conferences provided segregated competition at the college level. In 1900, few sports were integrated, though on rare occasions African American competitors participated in mixed sporting events. Some colleges (notably Harvard) had black athletes on their teams, particularly football and baseball, but those schools encountered difficulties in arranging competitions with other colleges. Many schools would not permit a black athlete to compete against their teams, which forced the integrated school team to bench the player. The breakthrough for integrated sport did not occur until the Depression, and most sports were not integrated until well after World War II.

The Organization of Modern Sport

Sport contained many abuses in its common practices by 1900, some of which have already been discussed. Other abuses involved recruiting athletes by offering them excessive inducements, recruiting athletes from one college by another college, and the lack of concern for safety procedures. Concern about the number of football deaths was growing, as were indications that a class system was present in American sport, just as it was in English sport.[48] The primary difference in American sport was that the upper class was based on wealth, much of which was recent, rather than traditional social standing and noble origins.

Considerable progress was made toward modern organization in sport, however. Colleges formed competitive conferences as well as associations to develop rules of competition and eligibility standards. They began to take control of collegiate sport, which until that time had been in the hands of the students or outsiders. The steps the colleges were taking were imitated at the high school level, as state athletic associations began to form for essentially the same purpose.

Colleges developed internal athletic associations to control sports in their schools. Because physical education had been accepted as having an educational value, the faculties added control of athletics as one more area of educational physical activity. National rules were written, and open (noncollegiate) national championships were held. By 1900, the organizational level of sport was radically different from the 1850s.

Students Lose Control of School Sport (1880–1922)

In 1880, school sport was still largely controlled by the students. The common practice was for a group of students to form a team, then choose a team captain and a manager. Selecting a manager was a critical decision because the manager was responsible for the organizational success of a team. The manager organized the schedule of contests, arranged for practice facilities and team equipment, raised money from alumni and local supporters, handled team business, and hired a coach. This arrangement was the ultimate in student administrative control. The school had no direct connection with the team, although the members were usually (but not always) its students.

School administrators gradually accepted the value of exercise as a part of the educational process. They learned that healthier students were more successful, so they added required physical education classes to the school curriculum. Faculty members learned that sport could be a valuable part of the educational experience. They worked to bring the control of sports under the protective wing of the schools, a reaction to the many abuses of sport at that time because sports were not controlled well by any organization. Football, with its yearly fatalities, was the most conspicuous example.

Basketball was rapidly becoming a popular school sport. It was invented by James Naismith at Springfield College in 1891, with the first official game played there on January 20, 1892.[49] The game spread rapidly across the country among both men and women students. Women adopted the game so enthusiastically that in some parts of the country it was considered exclusively a women's sport.

Women were becoming involved in many sports by this time, especially in colleges, and participated in basketball, baseball, rowing, golf, bicycling, aquatics, and winter sports. They were beginning to get away from the delicate flower concept of womanhood, although decades would be required to complete the change. The women were making their own basketball rules because no national organization had been formed for women's sports. As Patricia Vertinsky notes, "The development of women's sport has remained closely tied to the fortunes of the more general movements for female emancipation."[50]

Concern over abuses and serious injuries in competitive sports led to school interference in the student control of sports. Student control faded further with the December 1905 founding of the Intercollegiate Athletic Association, which changed its name to the National Collegiate Athletic Association (NCAA) in 1910. Schools had decided to take control and were trying to put sport to some educational use.

By the turn of the century, the conflict between education and sport was growing rapidly. The formation of the NCAA was the first step toward national control of school sports by the schools. The association was formed in reaction to the outcry over the growing number of deaths in college football. The NCAA originally had three basic goals: to establish high ethical standards for college sports, to develop physical education in the schools, and to promote intramural athletics.[51] Those goals were clearly those of a group of people more concerned with the broad goals of education than with narrower sporting goals.

The Stabilization of Modern Sport

Complete School Control of Sport (1905–1922)

From 1905 to 1922, six trends were visible in physical education and sport.[52] The first was the gradual assumption of control over intercollegiate sport by the NCAA and by college athletic conferences. The NCAA developed rule books to standardize rules of sports competition. Athletic conferences and associations worked to develop consistent rules, set standards of eligibility for competition, and make fairer competitive matches in sports events.

A second trend was the effort of high schools to control their sports programs. Those athletic programs imitated the collegiate programs, just as the high school academic programs were largely patterned to meet college needs and practices. State associations, followed by some regional associations, were formed to equalize competition, standardize rules, and set consistent eligibility requirements. In 1922, a national body was formed, the National Federation of State High School Athletic Associations, which later broadened its scope of extracurricular activities beyond athletics and changed its title to the National Federation of State High School Associations.[53]

A third trend was the rapid growth in women's athletics. Between 1906 and the end of World War I (1918), supervised women's athletic programs were added in many colleges because the women students wanted sports competition. Ellen Gerber notes that the magazine *Review of Reviews* had a written symposium on women's sports in 1900.[54] Although many women wanted competitive sports, their participation was controversial. During the 1920s, many arguments were expressed both for and against women's sports. Many female physical educators opposed sports.[55] The basic reason for their opposition was a combination of Victorian standards (the belief that women must be feminine and delicate) and fear that women's athletics would end up as corrupt or uneducational as men's college athletics seemed to be.[56] For those reasons, earlier rapid growth was followed by a period of abolishing competitive school sports for women.

A fourth trend was the boom in intramural sports, or sports involving only the students within a single school. The school intramural program was an offshoot of the earlier student-run sports programs. Intramurals became popular in the colleges, and in 1913 the University of Michigan became the first university to form a department of intramurals (led by Elmer Mitchell) to run programs for the student body. The great boom in intramural sports that followed World War I is evident in a slogan of the times: "A sport for every student and every student in a sport." The emphasis was on the number of participants, rather than on how much they participated, which created a temporary sidetracking of the intramural program goals.[57] Intramurals were to become an important part of the total physical education program as it evolved toward its present state.

A fifth trend was the addition of games and sports to the physical education curriculum. Though the change was gradually accomplished over 3 decades, the new programs were a radical change from the formal systems of gymnastics that had been at the heart of American physical education for almost a century. Games and sports were more popular with the students, and the acceptance and enthusiasm for physical education improved considerably as a result.

A sixth trend was also visible during this time. The emphasis of physical education gradually shifted from a health focus to a general education focus. It signaled the acceptance of a much broader concept of physical education— one that was consistent with the developing philosophy of the American school system—and permitted the use of games and sports in the curriculum. This further increased student acceptance of the physical education requirement. It also caused a major change in teacher training. Rather than being products of medical schools and formal gymnastics training courses, teachers became graduates of regular college training programs in education and physical education. The eventual results were a more widely accepted physical education program as well as more and better trained teachers of physical education.

The Golden Age of Sport (1920s)

The end of World War I provided a great impetus to sports, although we are not sure exactly why it had such an effect. Perhaps it was because sports activities had been used extensively as a part of the military training, and after the war many men continued to play the new sports that they had learned, just as with baseball after the Civil War.

The boom in sports may have been a relieved reaction to the end of the war. John Betts refers to this time as "a decade dedicated to escapism," and thus sport, which is a popular form of escapism, grew rapidly. In fact, football reached a pinnacle in popularity. Football games were followed widely at every level of competition, and the sport created much controversy. Just after this peak of football-mania, a city championship high school game in Chicago drew more than 120,000 spectators.[58]

The abuses of sport during this decade were attacked, and the colleges called for an examination of college sports by the Carnegie Foundation. In 1929, college sports took two hard blows. The economic collapse of Wall Street started the slide into the Great Depression, and the Carnegie Report on college athletics was released.[59] The report detailed the abuses of college athletics as well as the problems of professionalism, commercialism, and lack of academic integrity that affected many college athletic programs. It suggested that many colleges were losing sight of their primary purpose. It was used as a weapon to make many changes in college sports programs.

Conflicts in Depression-Era Sport

During the Depression, the school athletic programs were also hurt because the decline in the number of sports fans with spending money was a difficult blow. The programs depended heavily on gate receipts, which were dwindling. Public support had been hurt by the Carnegie Report in 1929. Interscholastic sports extended to the junior high school level by this time, but they were widely criticized. The suggestion that intramurals replace interschool competition at that level (since intramurals would involve more students, yet cost less money) led to an increased number of junior high school intramural programs.

Small colleges, which were hurt more by the Depression than the larger schools, were forced to drop sports in many cases. The small colleges became increasingly critical of the NCAA because they thought that the NCAA had been founded by and favored the larger schools. During the late 1930s and early 1940s, national organizations similar to the NCAA were formed for small senior colleges and for junior colleges.

The big boom during the Depression was in recreation, for two reasons: (1) unemployment gave many people leisure time for recreational activities; and (2) the government tried to fight unemployment by creating jobs. Many workers were hired to build recreational facilities such as playing fields, hiking trails, and park areas. This major growth also increased the options for public recreation.

Women's sports during the 1920s were held back primarily by the efforts of the leading women physical educators.[60] One reason for their opposition was an effort by the Amateur Athletic Union (AAU) to take control of women's track and field in the United States. The women educators believed that women should control and direct women's sports. They were offended as much by the administrative procedures of the AAU as by its ambition to control women's track and field. Until that time the women had made no effort to organize sport.

The women created a Women's Division of the National Amateur Athletic Federation. It was a well-organized group that not only ran the college programs for women but also trained the teachers, extending its influence from the present to the future practices in women's sport. The women leaders had several fears that limited their support for higher-level women's competitive sports. Although they kept alive the Victorian image of women as frail creatures who might suffer serious physiological and psychological harm from competition, they also had a far more legitimate concern: the fear that a fully developed program of interschool athletics would suffer from the same excesses that plagued men's athletics. The poor example set by men's sports may have done more to hold back women's athletics during the 1930s than any other factor, although this would be difficult to prove.

Some of the arguments against sports for women during the 1920s and 1930s were merely old-fashioned, and others bordered on the ridiculous. As the 1930s drew to a close, the emphasis in women's sports was moving away from the idea of interscholastic athletic competition. Their programs centered on a *playday* emphasis more like intramurals. Those playdays were low-key sporting activities. Large numbers of people were involved, and teams were formed by mixing players from the different schools. Playdays were organized with the basic concept of education for all, with the education coming through physical activities and an attempt made to reach as many people as possible.

Early Attempts to Reform College Sports

In the earliest days of collegiate sport the students who organized the competitions were concerned primarily with game rules and fairness of competition. The primary arguments were over eligibility: Who would be allowed to represent a college? In the early years of organized college sports the teams sometimes included students from the graduate or professional schools, such as law and medicine. In a few cases, professional athletes returned to play for their old college teams.

As time passed, the college faculty and administrations took control, then expanded the issues to include questions of poor use of student time, distraction from academics, and whether professional coaches should be allowed. Sports conferences were formed to standardize eligibility rules, and the NCAA was formed to attempt to control sports at the national level. As the Carnegie Report of 1929 showed, none of the attempts at reform had a significant impact on the developing college sports system.

With the failure of the Graham Plan to reform the Southern Conference in the 1930s, the NCAA realized that it would have to move into new areas of control by developing a system of investigating violations of its rules, as well as developing and enforcing a system of penalties for institutions that broke its rules.[61]

Science for Better or Worse: Measurement, Racism, Eugenics, and Striving for Perfection

Eugenics was based on the idea that the quality of the people was declining, so measures were necessary to improve the quality of the race. Some of the activities associated with eugenics were mild, such as competitions held widely at county fairs and called Better Baby contests, supposedly to determine the healthiest small child. However, as the twentieth century progressed, considerably more sinister measures appeared, sometimes as statewide practices, other times as actual state laws. Examples were forced sterilization of people deemed inferior. At first, these people were categorized as mentally handicapped, but the effect was most widely felt among people considered part of undesirable groups, such as racial minorities and other groups, such as people from some eastern European nationalities.[62]

As Lynn Couturier writes,

> *The eugenics movement provided a scientific basis for reducing these undesirable populations. At its peak, eugenics was the rationale for*

legislation prohibiting miscegenation, limiting immigration, and autho-rizing states to sterilize the feebleminded in order to prevent race degen-eration. . . . A few notable educational and scientific leaders recognized that the data used for eugenics was often manipulated in a manner that supported popular prejudices (scientific racism) or was simply bad sci-ence. . . . By the 1920's, most scientists had discarded the idea that simple genetics could explain complex human behavior, but the power of the eugenics movement lingered. . . . There was a delay between sci-entific understanding and the dissemination of that information. The highly organized eugenics movement had infiltrated social policy, the popular press, and the educational system (particularly high school and college texts). Once successfully embedded, these ideas were difficult to combat.[63]

To today's eyes, the research on athletes during the early 1900s is heavily racist. The common position had been that Nordic white people were the supe-rior race, both in body and in mind. The number of black Olympic medalists in Berlin in 1936, topped by Jesse Owens's four gold medals, was a heavy blow to the theory of Nordic superiority. Though African American anthropologist W. Montgomery Cobb's research demonstrated that anthropometric and physi-ological test results could not separate the races, the developing view after 1936 was that blacks had a superior physiology for athletic performance—but they were inferior intellectually.[64]

The new scientific paradigm would spawn a new American racial shib-boleth. Underneath black skins in this new racial mythology resided not the reservoirs of courage and will power that had connected physical to cultural prowess in older theories of athletic genius but merely "athletic genes." . . . With the backing of science, the white majority in the United States could read black athletic prowess not as "proof of equality" but as genetic accident.[65]

The final result of the eugenics movement appeared in Nazi Germany in the 1930s, when the Nazis gradually issued laws to first repress, and then bar, people such as Jews and Gypsies from ordinary society. The 1936 Berlin Olympics was used to showcase the supposed racial superiority of the Aryan German racial stock over other "inferior" races and nationalities. This is a major reason for the fame of Jesse Owens, the African American whose four gold medals van-quished Hitler's best athletes. Ultimately, the German government moved people it considered undesirable first to forced labor camps, and finally to death camps where millions were murdered. Although the Jewish people were by far the larg-est group killed, other nationalities died, as well as Germans deemed unfit, such as mentally handicapped people and homosexuals.

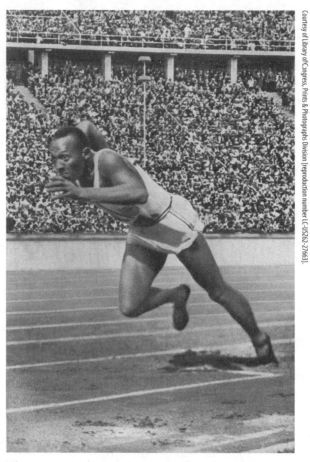

The success of Jesse Owens in the 1936 Olympic Games was a major blow to racist theories that minorities were mentally and physically inferior to whites.

The Nazi Olympics and the New World Sport Order: Politics and Promotion

Despite the focus of much writing, the Nazi Olympics were not primarily about race. Their larger impact on modern sport is as the first Olympics to represent the use of international sport for state promotion and politics.

In the first stage of the revived Olympic Games the real focus was simply the success and survival of the Games as a regular sporting event. The earlier Games took advantage of the popularity of world's fairs, staging their events at the same time and in the same location as a means of ensuring a large pool of prospective spectators.

The next stage came after World War I, when the Games were becoming stable, growing in size, and assured of returning every 4 years. By this point, the United States was staging Olympic Trials to pick teams, and those competitions were becoming more open to minorities. The 1932 Games were the largest yet, held in the massive stadium in Los Angeles and gaining worldwide publicity through the young movie newsreels.

However, it was Adolf Hitler's Nazi regime that decided to use their 1936 Berlin Olympic Games to promote the might of modern Germany, while showcasing what they expected to be a dominance of the competition by their pure Aryan athletes. The Games were awarded before the Nazis came to power, and the initial concern of the organizers was that they would lose the Games—not because of Nazi policies, but because the Nazis were not supportive of the type of sports used in the Games.[66] Despite many protest movements based on the increasingly abusive racial policies of the Nazis, the International Olympic Committee refused to move the Games to another country.[67]

The Nazi regime put a great emphasis on using psychology to sell their policies and gain support, and they soon realized that the Games would be a great marketing tool for their government. They moved quickly to take over the planning for the Games, developing extensive and spectacular facilities for the Games. In another first, Leni Riefenstahl was appointed to create a documentary of the Berlin Olympics, the classic film *Olympia*.[68] As Arnd Krüger writes:

> *Nowhere is the image of the Nazi Olympics better encapsulated than in the classic film of the event by Leni Riefenstahl. Here we can see the most perfect sport in a most perfect setting, sport in the tradition of the ancient Greeks. But this was no longer the Greece of Athens, the cradle of democracy; it was the Greece of Sparta, driven by the most barbarous of ideologies and armed with the might of modern technology.*[69]

The end result was the rise of a more modern Olympic Games, one mired in the politics of competing political philosophies. They were new Games that were used to promote the image of a nation, to advertise the success of an ideology. Although the sporting competitions received the heaviest press, the underlying message of the Games had changed. It was no longer "Look at the world's best athletes, meeting in peace and brotherhood." It had become "Look at our nation. We are successful. We have an important place in the world. Our political system is powerful, and we are now highly respected in the world's eyes." We see that side still in today's Olympic Games.

Summary

Allen Guttmann suggests seven characteristics that distinguish modern sport: (1) secularism, (2) equality, (3) specialization, (4) rationalization, (5) bureaucracy, (6) quantification, and (7) records. Melvin Adelman modified Guttmann's model to show the difference between premodern and modern sport with six characteristics: (1) organization, (2) rules, (3) competition, (4) role differentiation, (5) public information, and (6) statistics and records.

Modern sport began to develop in nineteenth-century England. From 1850 to 1900, there were three broad trends: the continuation of the class dichotomy in sport, the origins of organized competitive sport, and the revival of the Olympic Games. At the same time, there was a social trend to redefine sport as a moral virtue, thus making it more respectable. The example of the British public schools was influential in the rise of Muscular Christianity, the "ideal of manliness and the association of physical prowess with moral virtue." Sports participation was encouraged as moral education, a character-building experience. Sports encouraged youths to learn to cope with defeat; the value was in taking part, in striving for victory.

There were six rough stages of development in the rise of organized sport: (1) the growth of university sports, (2) the growth in popularity of sport, (3) the development of sports clubs, (4) the start of national organizations and national championships for each sport, (5) the writing of common national and international rules for each sport, and (6) keeping national and international records.

The rebirth of the Olympic Games was a complex process influenced by individuals and movements in several countries: Panagiotis Soutsos of Greece, Dr. William Penny Brookes of England, and Baron Pierre de Coubertin of France were the most influential. Though contests called *Olympic Games* were held in several countries during the 1800s, the extensive efforts of Coubertin resulted in the first modern Olympic Games in Athens in 1896.

A major influence on the rise of modern sport in the United States was the growth of industry and cities. They created a concentration of participants and spectators, and they provided a steady flow of money and free time that allowed participation. At the same time, colleges began to copy the sports of the British university model, though they soon replaced the English focus on amateurism with a businesslike goal of victory, which brought in elements of commercialism and professionalism. Outside the schools the athletic clubs became a widespread influence.

There are roughly three phases of development in the history of American school sport between 1880 and 1936: (1) student control of the programs, (2) increasing control by the schools, and (3) the New Physical Education, moving sports into the physical education program. From 1900 to 1936, the trends in sport were (1) the gradual assumption of control over intercollegiate sport by the colleges, the NCAA, and the college athletic conferences; (2) the effort of high schools to control their sports programs; (3) rapid growth in women's athletics, followed by a period of abolishing it; (4) a boom in intramural sports; and (5) the addition of games and sports to the physical education curriculum (the New Physical Education).

Collegiate sports became popular in part because of the belief that sports reflected the interests and values of businessmen, who then gave financial support to the colleges. As a result, the colleges gradually took control of athletics from the students, effectively recasting them as a marketing arm of the schools. Collegiate sport was finally brought under stronger university control with the 1905 founding of the NCAA.

Minority groups, including gender and racial minorities, were limited in their opportunities for sport in the 1800s. Women were limited by social custom and the medical belief that they would be harmed physically and mentally by strenuous sport. Racial minorities were limited by the legalization of racism, by enactment of the Jim Crow laws, and the Supreme Court decision that validated a separate but equal society. Despite those handicaps, women's college teams were appearing by the 1860s, while racial minorities created their own systems of school and professional sports. Real equality of opportunity did not appear until the 1960s and 1970s.

Women's sports during the 1920s were held back primarily by the efforts of the leading women physical educators, in part so women could control and direct their own sports, but also because they accepted the idea that women might suffer serious physiological and psychological harm from competition, and that women's athletics would suffer from the same excesses that plagued men's athletics. Their programs centered on a playday emphasis more like intramurals.

The eugenics movement accepted the idea that there were superior and inferior races, and it sought to improve the dominant race. It led to many abuses, including forced sterilization in some states. Nazi Germany used the idea as one excuse for later mass murder of "undesirable" people.

The Nazi Olympics of 1936 were the first Olympics to represent the use of international sport to promote a nation and its social and political beliefs. This is still a trait seen in today's Olympic Games.

Further Readings

Adelman, Melvin L. 1986. *A sporting time: New York City and the rise of modern athletics, 1820–70.* Champaign, IL: Univ. of Illinois Press.

Ashby, LeRoy. 2006. *With amusement for all: A history of American popular culture since 1830.* Lexington KY: Univ. Press of Kentucky.

Ashe, Arthur R., Jr. 1988. *A hard road to glory: A history of the African American athlete.* 3 vols. New York: Warner.

Block, David. 2005. *Baseball before we knew it: A search for the roots of the game.* Lincoln NE: Univ. of Nebraska Press.

Bonde, Hans. 2009. The time and speed ideology: 19th century industrialisation and sport. *International Journal of the History of Sport* 26 (10): 1315–1334.

Bundgaard, Axel. 2005. *Muscle and manliness: The rise of sport in American boarding schools.* Syracuse, NY: Syracuse Univ. Press.

Couturier, Lynn E. 2012. Dissenting voices: The discourse of competition in *The Sportswoman*. *Journal of Sport History* 39: 265–282.

Davies, Richard O. 2007. *Sports in American life: A history*. Oxford: Blackwell.

Dyreson, Mark. 2001. American ideas about race and Olympic races from the 1890s to the 1950s: Shattering myths or reinforcing scientific racism? *Journal of Sport History* 28: 173–215.

Erdozain, Dominic. 2010. *The problem of pleasure: Sport, recreation and the crisis of Victorian religion*. Woodbridge, England: Boydell Press.

Hoffman, Shirl J. 2010. *Good game: Christianity and the culture of sports*. Waco, TX: Baylor Univ. Press.

Huggins, Mike. 2008. Sport and the upper classes c1500–2000: A historiographic review. *Sport in History* 28: 364–388.

Hurd, Michael. 1999. *Black college football, 1882–1992*. Virginia Beach, VA: Donning.

Kirsch, George B. 2003. *Baseball in blue and gray: The national pastime during the Civil War*. Princeton, NJ: Princeton Univ. Press.

Ladd, Tony, and James A. Mathisen. 1999. *Muscular Christianity: Evangelical Protestants and the development of American sport*. Grand Rapids, MI: BridgePoint.

MacAloon, John. 1981. *This great symbol: Pierre de Coubertin and the origins of the modern Olympic Games*. Chicago: Univ. of Chicago Press.

Mangan, James A. 2001. *Athleticism in the Victorian and Edwardian public school*. Rev. ed. London: Cass.

Martin, Charles A. 2002. The color line in midwestern college sports, 1890–1960. *Indiana Magazine of History* 98 (June): 85–112.

Mewett, Peter. 2002. From horses to humans: Species crossovers in the origin of modern sports training. *Sports History Review* 33: 95–120.

Miller, Patrick B. 1998. The anatomy of scientific racism: Racialist responses to black athletic achievement. *Journal of Sport History* 25: 119–151.

Oriard, Michael. 2001. *King football: Sport and spectacle in the golden age of radio and newsreels, movies and magazines, the weekly and the daily press*. Chapel Hill, NC: Univ. of North Carolina Press.

Overman, Steven J. 2011. *The Protestant ethic and the spirit of sport: How Calvinism and capitalism shaped America's games*. Macon, GA: Mercer University Press.

Park, Roberta J. 2011. Physicians, scientists, exercise and athletics in Britain and America from the 1867 boat race to the four-minute mile. *Sport in History* 31: 1–31.

———. 2012. Contesting the norm: Women and professional sports in late nineteenth-century America. *International Journal of the History of Sport* 29: 730–749.

Pauly, Thomas H. 2012. *Game faces: Five early Americans and the sports they changed*. Lincoln NE: Univ. of Nebraska Press.

Rader, Benjamin G. 2008. *American sports: From the age of folk games to the age of televised sports*. 6th ed. Englewood Cliffs, NJ: Prentice Hall.

Radford, Peter. 2001. *The celebrated Captain Barclay: Sport, gambling and adventure in Regency times*. London: Headline.

Reel, Guy. 2006. *"The national police gazette" and the making of the modern American man, 1879–1906*. New York: Palgrave Macmillan.

Smith, Ronald A. 1989. *Sports and freedom: The rise of big-time college athletics*. New York: Oxford Univ. Press.

———. 2011. *Pay for play: A history of big-time athletic reform*. Urbana IL: Univ. of Illinois Press.

Stanley, Gregory Kent. 1996. *The rise and fall of the sportswoman: Women's health, fitness, and athletics, 1860–1940.* New York: Lang.

Todd, Jan. 1998. *Physical culture and the body beautiful: Purposive exercise in the lives of American women, 1800–1870.* Macon, GA: Mercer Univ. Press.

Vettenniemi, Erkki. 2010. Runners, rumors, and reams of representations: An inquiry into drug use by athletes in the 1920s. *Journal of Sport History* 37: 415–430.

Wrynn, Alison M. 2010. The athlete in the making: The scientific study of American athletic performance, 1930–1932. *Sport in History* 30: 121–137.

Young, David C. 1996. *The modern Olympics: A struggle for revival.* Baltimore: Johns Hopkins Univ. Press.

Discussion Questions

1. What characteristics define sport as modern? Discuss the characteristics in terms of the models of Guttmann and Adelman.

2. What effect did the issue of virtue and morals have on the development of modern sport?

3. Riess argues that the rise of modern sport was a joint product of industrialization and urbanization. Explain his argument.

4. Trace the stages in the development of organized sport to 1941, including the history of the participation of minority groups in American sport from the early 1800s to 1941.

5. Discuss Pierre de Coubertin's work and the start of the modern Olympic Games. Include factors that helped the Games, as well as those that worked against them. Who were the early influences on Coubertin?

6. Discuss the evolution of the school athletic program from its origins, and describe the stages through which it passed.

7. Discuss the formation of the NCAA and the factors that led to its founding.

8. Discuss how social class or wealth has played a part in the evolution of sport. What influence did they have on the definition of the amateur?

References

1. Struna, Nancy L. 1977. Puritans and sport: The irretrievable tide of change. *Journal of Sport History* 4: 7.

2. Guttmann, Allen. 1995. Puritans at play? Accusations and replies. In *Sport in America: From wicked amusement to national obsession*, 3–11. Champaign, IL: Human Kinetics.

3. Calhoun, Don W. 1987. *Sport, culture, and personality.* 2nd ed. Champaign, IL: Human Kinetics, 93.

4. Struna, Nancy L. 1988. Sport and society in early America. *International Journal of the History of Sport* 5: 292–311.

5. Ibid., 305.

6. Breen, T. H. 1977. Horses and gentlemen: The cultural significance of gambling among the gentry of Virginia. *William and Mary Quarterly* 34: 329–347.

7. Adelman, Melvin L. 1981. The first modern sport in America: Harness racing in New York City, 1825–1870. *Journal of Sport History* 8: 5–32.

8. Block, David. 2005. *Baseball before we knew it: A search for the roots of the game.* Lincoln, NE: Univ. of Nebraska Press, 152–162.

9. Lucas, John A., and Ronald A. Smith. 1978. *Saga of American sport.* Philadelphia: Lea and Febiger, 108–118.

10. Rader, Benjamin G. 1990. *American sports: From the age of folk games to the age of spectators.* 2nd ed. Englewood Cliffs, NJ: Prentice Hall, 42–43.

11. Guttmann, Allen. 1978. *From ritual to record: The nature of modern sports.* New York: Columbia Univ. Press, 15–55.

12. Ibid., 26.

13. Ibid., 35–36.

14. Ibid., 31.

15. Bale, John. 1993. Racing towards modernity: A one-way street? *International Journal of the History of Sport* 10: 215.

16. Guttmann, *From ritual to record*, 39.

17. Ibid., 43–44.

18. Ibid., 47.

19. Ibid., 47–48, 50–51; and Rintala, Jan. 1995. Sport and technology: Human questions in a world of machines. *Journal of Sport and Social Issues* 19: 62–75.

20. Guttmann, *From ritual to record*, 55.

21. Ibid., 85.

22. Adelman, Melvin L. 1986. *A sporting time: New York City and the rise of modern athletics, 1820–70.* Champaign, IL: Univ. of Illinois Press, 3–10.

23. Kirsch, George B., ed. 1992. *Sports in North America: A documentary history.* Vol. 3 of *The rise of modern sports, 1840–1860.* Gulf Breeze, FL: Academic International Press; and Sandblad, Henrik. 1988. Sport and ideas—aspects of the rise of the modern sports movement: An English summary of Olympia och Valhalla. *International Journal of the History of Sport* 5: 120–130.

24. Brailsford, Dennis. 1992. *British sport: A social history.* Cambridge, England: Lutterworth, 97.

25. Riess, Steven A. 1989. *City games: The evolution of American urban society and the rise of sports.* Champaign, IL: Univ. of Illinois Press, 254.

26. Holt, Richard. 1989. *Sport and the British: A modern history.* Oxford: Clarendon Press, 98.

27. Brailsford, *British sport*, 83.

28. Cross, Gary S. 1990. *A social history of leisure since 1600.* State College, PA: Venture Publishing, 143.

29. Holt, *Sport and the British*, 87.

30. Brailsford, *British sport*, 89.

31. Mangan, James A. 1981. *Athleticism in the Victorian and Edwardian public school.* Cambridge: Cambridge Univ. Press, 16–17.

32. Ibid., 18.

33. McIntosh, Peter. 1979. *Fair play: Ethics in sport and education*. London: Heinemann, 27–29.

34. Ibid., 28, 30.

35. Ibid., 29.

36. Riess, Steven A. 1991. Sport and the redefinition of American middle-class masculinity. *International Journal of the History of Sport* 8: 5–27.

37. Vamplew, Wray. 2007. Playing with the rules: Influences on the development of regulation in sport. *International Journal of the History of Sport* 24 (7): 845.

38. Young, David C. 1996. *The modern Olympics: A struggle for revival*. Baltimore: Johns Hopkins Univ. Press, 1–12, 167–169.

39. Lucas, John A. 1973. The genesis of the modern Olympic Games. In *A history of sport and physical education to 1900*, 331–340. Champaign, IL: Stipes.

40. Leigh, Mary. 1974. Pierre de Coubertin: A man of his time. *Quest* 22: 19–24.

41. Riess, *City games*, 1, 261.

42. Betts, John Rickards. 1974. *America's sporting heritage: 1850–1950*. Reading, MA: Addison-Wesley, 98; and Scott, Harry A. 1951. *Competitive sports in schools and colleges*. New York: Harper Brothers, 19.

43. Smith, Ronald A. 1989. *Sports and freedom: The rise of big-time college athletics*. New York: Oxford Univ. Press.

44. Ibid., 218.

45. Gerber, Ellen W. 1974. *The American woman in sport*. Reading, MA: Addison-Wesley, 4; Park, Roberta J. 1993. "Strong and thick-set heroines": The other side of women's sport, 1750–1900. In *North American Society for Sport History Proceedings*, 24–25; and Johnson, Scott. 1991. "Not altogether ladylike": The premature demise of girls' interscholastic basketball in Illinois. In *North American Society for Sport History Proceedings*, 54.

46. Pruter, Robert. 1999. Youth baseball in Chicago, 1868–1890: Not always sandlot ball. *Journal of Sport History* 26: 6, 25.

47. Stanley, Gregory Kent. 1996. *The rise and fall of the sportswoman: Women's health, fitness, and athletics, 1860–1940*. New York: Lang, 58–61.

48. Wettan, Richard. 1974. Sport and social stratification in the U.S., 1865–1900. In *Proceedings, North American Society for Sport History* 2: 29–30.

49. Swanson, Richard, and Betty Spears. 2001. *History of sport and physical education in the United States*. 4th ed. Madison, WI: Brown and Benchmark, 173.

50. Vertinsky, Patricia. 1994. Women, sport, and exercise in the 19th century. In *Women and sport: Interdisciplinary perspectives*, ed. D. Margaret Costa and Sharon R. Guthrie, 77. Champaign, IL: Human Kinetics.

51. Bucher, Charles A., and Ralph K. Dupee Jr. 1965. *Athletics in schools and colleges*. New York: Center for Applied Research in Education, 8.

52. Scott, *Competitive sports*, 36.

53. Betts, *America's sporting heritage*, 136; and Gerber, *The American woman in sport*, 10.

54. Gerber, *The American woman in sport*, 10.

55. Bucher and Dupee, *Athletics in schools*, 8; and Hult, Joan S. 1994. The story of women's athletics: Manipulating a dream 1890–1985. In *Women and sport: Interdisciplinary perspectives*, ed. D. Margaret Costa and Sharon R. Guthrie, 63–82. Champaign, IL: Human Kinetics.

56. Scott, *Competitive sports*, 36.

57. Bucher and Dupee, *Athletics in schools*, 6–7.

58. Betts, *America's sporting heritage*, 250, 257.

59. Savage, Howard J. 1929. *American college athletics, bulletin no. 23.* New York: Carnegie Foundation for the Advancement of Teaching.

60. Gerber, Ellen W. 1975. The controlled development of collegiate sport for women, 1923–1936. *Journal of Sport History* 2: 1–28; and Hult, Story of women's athletics, 88–93.

61. Smith, Ronald A. 2011. *Pay for play: A history of big-time college athletic reform.* Urbana, IL: Univ. of Illinois Press, 81–91.

62. Kline, Wendy. 2001. *Building a better race: Gender, sexuality, and eugenics from the turn of the century to the baby boom.* Berkeley: Univ. of California Press; and Bruinius, Harry. 2006. *Better for all the world: The secret history of forced sterilization and America's quest for racial purity.* New York: Knopf.

63. Couturier, Lynn E. 2005. The influence of the eugenics movement on physical education in the United States. *Sport History Review* 36 (May): 22–23.

64. Dyreson, Mark. 2008. American ideas about race and Olympic races in the era of Jesse Owens: Shattering myths or reinforcing scientific racism? *International Journal of the History of Sport* 25 (2): 247–267; and Dyreson, Mark. 2008. Prolegomena to Jesse Owens: American ideas about race and Olympic races from the 1890s to the 1920s. *International Journal of the History of Sport* 25 (2): 224–246.

65. Dyreson, American ideas, 249.

66. Mandell, Richard. 1987. *The Nazi Olympics.* Urbana, IL: Univ. of Illinois Press; Bachrach, Susan. 2000. *The Nazi Olympics: Berlin 1936.* Boston: Little, Brown; Large, David C. 2007. *Nazi games: The Olympics of 1936.* New York: Norton; and Guttmann, Allen. 1992. *The Olympics: A history of the modern games.* Urbana, IL: Univ. of Illinois Press, 53–71.

67. Swanson, Richard A. 2003. "Move the Olympics!" "Germany must be told!": Charles Clayton Morrison and liberal Protestant Christianity's support of the 1936 Olympic boycott. In *North American Society for Sport History Proceedings*, 85.

68. Brown, Mark. 2005. Art, sport, propaganda: The 1936 Olympic Games through the lens of Leni Riefenstahl. In *North American Society for Sport History Proceedings*, 78–79; and McFee, Graham, and Alan Tomlinson. 1999. Riefenstahl's *Olympia*: Ideology and aesthetics in the shaping of the Aryan athletic body. *International Journal of the History of Sport* 16 (2): 86–106.

69. Krüger, Arnd. 2003. Germany: The propaganda machine. In *The Nazi Olympics: Sport, politics and appeasement in the 1930s*, ed. Arnd Krüger and William Murray, 35–36. Urbana, IL: Univ. of Illinois Press.

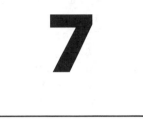

American Exercise Science and Sport from 1941 to Today

Fitness and Sport in War and Peace (1941–1963)

The coming of World War II ended the arguments over whether physical education and sport belonged in the educational program. Of the first 2 million men examined for military service, 45% were rejected for physical or mental reasons. Only part of that high failure rate could be blamed on the school programs, but extensive publicity made the public aware of the fitness problem. The government saw the need to improve the health and fitness of all citizens.

During the war, the government formed several groups to work to improve the health and fitness level of the people. The Division of Physical Fitness was formed to work first under the Office of Civilian Defense and later under the Office of Defense. An advisory board developed community fitness programs, and a sports board of celebrities and sports authorities convinced the public of the importance of fitness.

During this period, the physical education programs in the United States basically became programs of physical fitness oriented toward military needs. Sports were strongly promoted as a phase of fitness, and many prominent physical educators developed physical training programs for the armed forces.[1] They also created fitness tests to evaluate the programs and intramural sports programs for training and leisure.

Sports activities continued with few limitations. Although many young athletes were in the armed forces, and gasoline rationing hampered travel, sports were considered a positive influence on national spirit and were highly encouraged. Many sports teams on military bases competed against college teams. The armed forces encouraged intramural sports and used sports activities as a part of basic training. Unfortunately, there was a tendency to limit the objectives of school physical education to fitness for military needs.

The tendency for school physical education to adopt the physical training programs of the military and thus change from programs of physical education to physical training was the greatest problem created for physical education by World War II. The programs struggled to avoid returning to the old concept of physical training. Fitness tests, which were already available for boys, were also developed for schoolgirls. One wartime gain for physical education was that many states changed their laws from recommending to requiring physical education in the schools.

The end of the war started another sports boom similar to the one in the 1920s, as competition and sports facilities underwent great expansions. College enrollments jumped as a result of new veterans' benefits programs by the government. The American people developed a greater feeling of world unity, as seen in the formation of the United Nations, and they became more conscious of international competition with the revival of the Olympic Games in postwar London in 1948. Many international cooperative sports programs were founded to foster peaceful competitions and to help nations to meet and come to know each other on the field of sport.

The period following World War II exhibited several notable features that spread over decades. The first feature was the work done to raise the teacher preparation standards on the undergraduate and graduate levels. Major conferences on the undergraduate professional preparation curriculum were held at Jackson's Mill (1948), Washington, DC (1962), and New Orleans (1973); written reports on curriculum suggestions were published after each conference. Conferences on graduate study in physical education were held at Pere Marquette, near Chicago (1950), and in Washington, DC (1967).

Physical educators also established new professional groups according to their more specialized interests. Groups were formed for men's college physical education, women's college physical education, camping activities and recreation, and school health activities. The old American Association for the Advancement of Physical Education (AAAPE), which became the American Physical Education Association (APEA) in 1903, changed its name twice in the next 35 years, first to the American Association for Health and Physical Education (AAHPE) in 1937 and then to the American Association for Health, Physical Education, and Recreation (AAHPER) in 1938. The name was changed again in 1974 to the American *Alliance* for Health, Physical Education, and Recreation. In 1979, dance was added to the name, forming the current American Alliance for Health, Physical Education, Recreation and Dance (AAHPERD).

Physical education split into a number of separate areas of concentrated interest in the decades following World War II. Major interest groups whose concerns were health education, safety education, recreation (including park activities), and dance grew rapidly during this period. Fitness became a major concern several times after World War II, first during the Korean War and then soon afterward when the results of the widely publicized Kraus-Weber Tests implied that American elementary schoolchildren were much less fit than their counterparts in other nations.

The results of the Kraus-Weber Tests were published in the United States late in 1953. Those negative results hit the American public with explosive force.

President Eisenhower reacted to this blow to the American ego by forming the Council on Youth Fitness in 1955. The purpose of the council was to promote fitness on the local level, but it primarily served as publicity for the administration. The programs never really got off the ground.

AAHPER reacted to the study by working to develop fitness tests that could be used in the public schools. The battery of tests forming the AAHPER Youth Fitness Test was published in 1958. Despite complaints that the Kraus-Weber Test was not a genuine fitness test, the Youth Fitness Test showed essentially the same results: American children were less fit than European children.

Although the Council on Youth Fitness was allowed to fade from the public eye during the late 1950s and early 1960s, AAHPER worked to develop a program of physical fitness tests with norms for American schoolchildren. The Council on Youth Fitness was revived in 1961 by President Kennedy as the President's Council on Youth Fitness. Kennedy was an avid sports enthusiast who strongly supported more school fitness activities, a drive that was the first nonwar effort by the upper levels of the government. That action was an example of the increasing governmental concern for the state of fitness not just of children, but of all citizens.

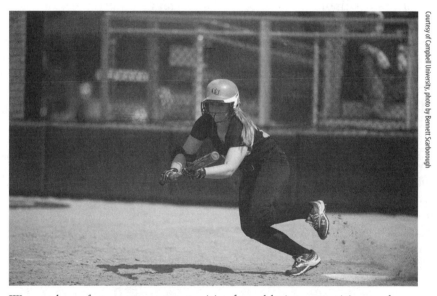

Courtesy of Campbell University, photo by Bennett Scarborough

Women have far greater opportunities for athletic competition and scholarships since the passage of Title IX.

In 1957, physical educators discovered that the required program of physical education must be defended again. When Russia orbited the first *Sputnik* satellite, the United States went into educational shock and for the first time was convinced that its schools were behind. The result was a concerted push toward the sciences and bread-and-butter education. Many educators accepted the old dualistic concept of the mind and body as separate entities. The problem of dualism reappeared in the late 1960s as an opposition to specific requirements in the educational process. The net result was to show that physical educators had neglected public relations in their dealings with the public as well as with their fellow educators.

Physical Education: From a Teaching Field to a Science

In the early 1960s, our field was essentially physical education. It was centered around the field of education, and the curriculum was largely one of applied courses once called "methods and materials," a focus on how to do the parts of the job, along with personal skill development. Since then the field has changed dramatically, with today's focus on scientific and theoretical foundations and very limited time on skill development.

The Discipline Movement

The strong relationship that physical education had developed with the field of education, rather than science, had one significant disadvantage for the field: It created the image of being a less academic field, an inferior cog in the educational machine. James Bryant Conant's 1963 book criticizing the quality of graduate programs in education struck a nerve among physical educators. The next year Franklin Henry's article called for a more scientifically focused academic discipline of physical education.

Many physical educators believe that Conant specifically criticized physical education as weak. However, as Gregg Twietmeyer notes,

> *In fact, no mention of physical education appears in the text of the* [New York Times] *articles* [describing Conant's conclusions]. *What this suggests was that the reaction of physical educators to Conant's criticism says more about what the discipline thought about itself than it does about outside pressure causing reform. Indeed, Conant's criticisms of physical education amount to only a few paragraphs out of two hundred pages. Such sensitivity on the part of physical educators implies a far deeper vein of disquiet than could have been instigated by either Conant or Henry.*[2]

The core knowledge for each area of the field, what was called the *body of knowledge* of each subdiscipline, gained new focus in the 1960s and 1970s as each subdiscipline developed its own academic structure, specialized national and international scholarly groups, and its own conventions and research journals.

As the subdisciplines developed over the years, the names of departments (and even the field itself) went through a series of name changes that represented newer views of the field's focus of study. So, too, the curriculum changed as departments reacted by requiring some new courses, by revising the approach and content to many old courses, and greatly by downsizing or removing other old courses. New major programs were added to reflect the new knowledge in the field and new career directions of students.

On the positive side, the discipline movement produced a great surge in research and the academic grounding of programs. On the negative side, the development of the individual subdisciplines (rather than a single unified interdisciplinary or cross-disciplinary field) resulted in a heavily fractured field. The question of the most appropriate title to represent the field is still not a settled question, though kinesiology is the most heavily promoted title. Most other nations use exercise science or sport science.

Changes in Teacher and Coach Education

Teacher education has changed significantly since the 1960s. At that time all programs were education-focused and application-oriented courses of study with limited scientific focus. As a result of the discipline movement the scientific bases are far more heavily emphasized today than in the past.

There was limited focus on coach education into the 1960s. Until that time the only coaches who were trained to coach were physical education teacher education students, though some undergraduates might take a coaching methods course in a particular sport.

Since that era there have been significant changes in coach education. In part, the changes were necessary because after Title IX became law in the early 1970s (resulting in a massive increase in the number of athletes on high school girls' teams) there were no longer enough licensed physical education teachers to cover all of the teams. As a result, schools began to hire part-time, external coaches.

The result of this change in the schools was a sharp increase in the number of coaches who had no actual coaching education. Often the new coaches were former athletes, but that experience rarely gave them an understanding of basic training principles or how the human body worked. In many cases the national sports organizations began to form coach education and certification programs. Many states also began to design coach education programs to deal with this influx of unprepared coaches.

Coach education and certification programs are now found in most nations, usually run by the national governing body of each sport (such as USA Track and Field for track athletics in the United States). Training and certification are done by levels, such as Level 1, which is usually aimed at coaches of youth and high school athletes. Level 2 prepares certified Level 1 coaches to work with more advanced athletes, such as college athletes. Level 3 usually prepares Level 2 coaches to work with elite or high-performance athletes, such as those who are competitive at the national level or higher.

The use of the different certification levels varies from one country to another (as does the number of levels; some sports in some nations go up to Level 5).

Although it is not the case in the United States, some nations (such as Canada) will not permit anyone to coach a national or Olympic team unless they have successful experience as a Certified Level 3 coach. This results in coaches who are more knowledgeable in preparing athletes for success at high levels of sport.

New Challenges for America's Fitness and Health

The late 1960s and early 1970s brought attacks on many traditions. American involvement in the war in Southeast Asia carried over into many areas of life in the United States. Some people felt that the country had lost its ideals, and others felt that the traditional ideals were being condemned. During this period of confrontation, many things seemed to be argued in purely political terms. Sport and physical education were attacked from numerous directions.

The opposition to the physical education requirement as a part of the curriculum was renewed at many levels. The basic argument was that, although physical activity was beneficial, the student should be allowed more freedom in deciding what activities to take, or even whether to take any. The objection to the physical education requirement was a small part of a larger educational movement of the time, which was a general attack on all course requirements in the schools. Many opponents of school structure considered physical education to be the weak link in the requirement system and thus the most logical place for an initial clash. Because of that movement, some required programs of physical education at the college level were changed to elective programs.

By the late 1970s, the resistance to school course requirements had lost most of its force. A decade of experimentation resulted in young people who were less capable of communicating and of using abstract reasoning skills. Standardized tests showed consistent drops in student scores during the time of weaker requirements. As the stress on school accountability grew, public interest in more traditional educational structures and standards increased. By 1980, schools wanted to provide more direction for students, rather than let them decide for themselves whether they would make an effort to become educated.

As course requirements were under attack, there was a concurrent trend toward a recreational emphasis in physical education activities, or what were called *lifetime sports*. That trend continued into the 1990s as more students chose electives such as racquetball, aerobic dance, and backpacking, instead of the traditional fitness and competitive sports-oriented activities. However, in 1986 national surveys showed that the fitness level of young Americans had dropped since the mid-1970s, a finding that renewed interest in traditional fitness activities.

The *wellness movement* arose in the 1990s. It indicated that many physical education programs were moving back toward the earlier strong health goal of physical educators. Physical education also increased its scope to include special populations, such as people with physical disabilities and elderly adults. Programs of recreation and fitness were expanded for elderly adults, a large group that previously received little attention from physical educators.

As during the Great Depression, the 1980s witnessed the rapid growth of school costs beyond the ability of many communities to pay. A consistent result was the threat of cutting school sports programs and limiting (if not eliminating) physical education programs as unnecessary frills. The popularity of school sports defended those programs somewhat, but a public facing the problems of inflation lost much of its sympathy for financing the programs.

By the year 2000, reports by the federal government showed unusually high levels of obesity among schoolchildren. The concern shifted somewhat away from fitness (obese children will not be fit) to the overriding health concern. With high levels of child obesity, the outlook is for adults who will have more health problems and a shorter life span. Yet despite those concerns, by 2010 little legislative action stiffened school physical education requirements or required a return to the earlier tradition of healthy lunches in the school cafeterias.

Legislation and Performance: Standards and Testing

Over the last 2 decades a major approach to improving student performance in the schools has been increased student testing. Every state now has testing requirements for high school graduation, and there are now national tests designed to measure student achievement. Testing studies three types of achievement: (1) student achievement, (2) teacher qualifications and success, and (3) school success.

For the students, there is standardized testing of achievement and progress. For the teachers, there are licensing tests and assessments ranging from the National Teacher Exam and Praxis to records of student success. For the schools, there are comparisons of individual schools through student achievement tests, such as those mandated by No Student Left Behind.

The Kinesiology Movement and the Name Game

The movement to declare that our field should be called *kinesiology* began in 1990. Although it has been influential, it has not succeeded to the degree that was expected by the research universities. Two major obstacles to the success of the term were that (1) the original description of the curriculum was too specialized to appeal to (or be easy to teach at) the other colleges and universities, and (2) over the last 2 decades the version of kinesiology taught at the research universities changed to become a health science.

The majority of traditional, exercise science, and sport-related majors are not really interested in working in the health sciences. The result is that our field still has a variety of departmental titles.

Sport Opens Its Doors

General Changes in Sport (1963–1984)

Athletics and physical education faced many problems during the late 1960s and early 1970s. As a well-publicized area of American life, athletics was an excellent target for publicity seekers. Athletics was increasingly politicized, and it created many of its own problems. Coaches claimed sports kept America a democracy, even as Russians argued that sports helped keep their nation communist. Sports leaders tried to wrap themselves in the cloaks of patriotism and religion by staging militaristic displays at football games and adding religiously oriented shows at the beginning of the festivities. The unfortunate result of those excesses was to widen the split between those who thought politics and religion should be part of athletics and those who did not. Both sides were convinced that they were morally right.

One result of those political excesses is seen in the riots and demonstrations at the 1968 Olympic Games in Mexico City and the murder of the Israeli athletes by Arab extremists at the 1972 Olympic Games in Munich. The Games have become a political symbol, and because of the intense worldwide publicity they generate, they are a perfect target for any group wanting instant, worldwide publicity. The heavily promotional aspects of the 1980 Games in Moscow and the 1984 Games in Los Angeles are cases in point because each was used to promote the home country, while their political opponents boycotted and criticized.

The Integration of School Sports: All Races Are Welcome

In the 1960s and early 1970s, the final steps were taken to promote racial integration in sports. The segregation of African American athletes was largely continued until after World War II, although there were some exceptions. The first black American competed in the Olympics shortly after 1900, and many blacks appeared in Olympic track-and-field competition after World War I. In the late 1930s, whites began to notice the abilities of the top black athletes. Even as Hitler proclaimed his doctrine of the Aryan's racial superiority, a black American, J. C. "Jesse" Owens, won four gold medals in the 1936 Berlin Olympics, and Joe Louis, the "Brown Bomber," defeated the German world champion boxer.

Finally, in 1946, Jackie Robinson became the first black athlete in professional baseball in more than 60 years as a result of Branch Rickey's deliberate attempt to integrate baseball. Robinson's obvious athletic skills, combined with his ability to withstand considerable player and fan hostility, paved the way for integration in other professional sports. Those achievements led to the integration of college sports in the 1960s, as did the early leadership of a small number of collegiate teams, such as those at Harvard that insisted on playing with integrated teams. The Supreme Court decision in 1954 that reversed the tradition of separate but equal schooling led to integrated sports in the public schools over the next 2 decades. Although there were many abuses of the African American athletes in the schools, American sports were for the most part integrated by the 1970s.

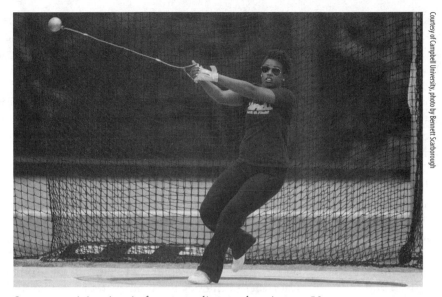

Courtesy of Campbell University, photo by Bennett Scarborough

Sports participation is far more diverse than it was 50 years ago.

Title IX and Sports: Okay, We'll Let the Women Play, Too

Starting in the 1960s, women's athletics underwent radical changes. The women's liberation movement gained strength and pushed for fairer treatment of women in all areas of life, including sport. Although women have competed in sports to some degree since at least the 1860s, women's sports programs were relatively unpopular with administrators and had only marginal educational support.[3]

In earlier years, women's school sports were controlled by the Women's Division of the National Amateur Athletic Federation (NAAF) and later by the Division of Girls and Women's Sports (DGWS) of the AAHPER, which did not accept the idea of intercollegiate sport until 1963. Control in the colleges eventually was passed to the Association of Intercollegiate Athletics for Women (AIAW), which began in 1971 to 1972.[4] The AIAW promoted sport on the national and international levels. The National Federation of State High School Associations also became more active in girls' sports and developed rule books and statewide competitions at the high school level.

The 1980s and early 1990s saw massive changes in women's athletics, both in practice and in public attitudes toward the programs. Arguments today are rarely based on whether sport is safe for women or whether they have a right to equal competition. Instead, many opponents of the programs are concerned with the cost of women's sports. When Title IX appeared in the 1970s, it led to a decade of upheaval in American school athletics. Actions in the schools, the media, and the courts resulted in a massive growth of women's teams at the high school (from 300,000 to 1.5 million girls on teams within 2 years) and college levels, a growth that began to level out only in the mid-1980s because of inflation and declining school revenues.

Unfortunately, most of the opportunities for the women were as competitors or chaperones. At the administrative and coaching levels, men continued to run the women's programs. The basic argument for this practice was that the women lacked experience, but they were given few opportunities to gain the necessary experience.

Although the increase in women's funding created financial and administrative problems, early fears did not materialize: Men's athletics did not collapse, and the colleges did not lose their sources of funding. Instead, public interest in women's athletics blossomed. Usually the schools that wanted to be powers in men's sports showed the same interest (and success) in women's sports. The challenges and benefits of the expansion have far outweighed the drawbacks. Indeed, by 1980 the success of college athletics for women was great enough that the NCAA launched an effort to take control of the programs (which they had opposed) from the AIAW.[5]

Women's athletics have continued to grow since that time. Even though there has been resistance by men's athletic programs, and even though positions for women coaches and administrators have been disappearing, women's sports have continued to improve and gain participants and fans.[6] Men's athletic departments fought the growth of women's teams with the argument that men's teams would have to be eliminated as a result of financial limitations. Although the same argument is being made today, it is not true. The only area of decrease in men's teams has been in NCAA Division I teams,[7] where in many cases the budget for football or basketball alone may exceed the cost of the entire women's program. We see this pattern of reluctance by men to share with women in the governance structure of the International Olympic Committee, where the first female member was admitted only in 1981, and even in 1996 "women comprise just 7 percent of the IOC. They hold only 3 percent of the NOC [National Olympic Committee] presidencies and 6 percent of the international sports federations' presidencies."[8]

The Death of Amateurism in Sport

Perhaps the other most noticeable development in athletics since the 1980s has been the trend toward accepting the international view of athletics in the United States. The distinctions between the amateur and the professional essentially have disappeared. Sports groups now embrace the idea of corporate support of athletes, where the athlete can receive an annual salary while training or competing. That idea was used in Europe for many years and is the Western version of the old eastern European state-supported athletics.

Youth Sport as Precollegiate and Pre-Olympic Sport

Youth sport, extremely popular in the United States, has changed radically from its original function of providing enjoyable learning experiences for children younger than high school age. Though it is not a new type of organized activity, it is far different from what it was even 50 years ago.

Sport was preached as beneficial for youths from the physical, educational, and moral vantage points. It promoted health, it taught youths to work together in a cooperative context, it taught them to strive for higher goals, and (best of all) it kept them off the streets and out of trouble. It was only natural for those suggested benefits to filter downward from college students to secondary students to primary students, until in the early 1900s organized sport was appearing in elementary schools.[9]

Physical educators eventually had second thoughts about the outcome of their well-meaning promotional efforts. By the late 1930s, physical educators were passing resolutions opposing organized sport below the high school level. The excesses of a commercialized, semiprofessional collegiate athletic scene were apparent by 1905.[10] Unfortunately, their change of heart came too late. By the late 1930s, nonschool groups were moving into children's sport, led by the organization of Little League baseball in 1939. With the addition of a Little League World Series in 1947, promoting a national championship competition for ages 8 to 12 years, the stage was set for today's model of professional, commercial sport to emerge.

The second half of the twentieth century has been a time of shifting control of youth sport from educators, to private sport groups organized along the lines of traditional amateur sport, to today's growing control of youth sport by commercial interests. Indeed, for all the criticism of the socialist sport model so prominent in the 1970s, in gymnastics the East German sport boarding schools of that era devoted only 10 hours per week to sport training for 12-year-olds, rising to 23 hours per week as 18-year-olds.[11] Contrast that to today's 12-year-old American girls who may train for 6 to 10 hours per day. Even for children, the focus in sport has turned to training and performing like a professional.[12]

There has been a continuing downward trend of the age at which youth become involved in highly organized and highly competitive sporting programs. If schools have not provided programs for the young, private clubs and competitive teams have filled the gap, especially in individual sports such as swimming, ice-skating, gymnastics, skiing, and boxing. The benefits remain to be seen, though they largely depend on the viewpoint of the individual.

There has been a rapid growth of very competitive, highly organized youth sports. However, untrained coaches' use of the approach of professional athletes with young children has caused grave concern. The impact is most noticeable in the mid- and upper-elementary school grades.

As Richard Davies notes, the growth of high-level competitive sports and sports training for youths has become "a profitable new industry in the United

States." At the same time, one of the negative aspects of this system is that "left to their own devices, children are natural cross-trainers, dabbling in many sports and related activities. But the growth of organization and adult supervision has undercut spontaneity. Many experts decry the overemphasis at an early age upon concentration on one sport."[13] As one person in the youth sports industry commented,

> We've got tennis kids who can't hop, skip or jump. . . . We've got golfers who if you threw them a ball, they'd duck—basketball players who can't swing a baseball bat. We've got some kids who are really good at their sports, but if you look closer, you'd be surprised at how unathletic they really are.[14]

High School Sport: The College Farm System

More than 3 million students per year compete in high school sports in the United States. For most of them, high school will be their last time on a competitive sports team. For the top high school athletes, however, high school is their time of seeking college athletic scholarships.

We are accustomed to the idea of farm teams in professional sports, lower-level professional and semiprofessional teams that serve as a way of preparing athletes for higher-level professional play. We fail to realize that high school sports are used by the colleges as their farm teams. At the higher levels of college sports, such as NCAA Division I, there is rarely much actual development of typical athletes. Instead, the schools recruit students who already have the needed skills to succeed. College sports will mature them, but college sports at the higher levels is not an instructional league.

I Play for Basketball Academy

Two developments of the last few decades are high school–level travel teams and the growth of small private schools that seem to exist largely to have traveling basketball teams. We could fairly call them basketball academies. Some athletes go to these small schools in part to improve their academic training because often they would not otherwise meet the academic standards to get an athletic scholarship. At the same time, they are used to allow an extra year of training, maturing, and competitive experience before college.

The traveling teams play in tournaments across the nation, with a major purpose of gaining exposure to college coaches and talent scouts. These two types of programs increasingly drain talent away from the traditional school programs, weakening them competitively, but also depriving the lost athletes of a chance to have a normal high school experience.[15] In essence, they have become professional athletes while still in high school.

Collegiate Sport and the NCAA Cartel

In the 1960s, the big-time college sports programs were attacked as an example of highly financed programs of sports for the few. Student groups worked to limit student funds allocated to athletic departments. The students preferred to have their money put into programs of intramurals, extramurals, and club sports that would reach more students. There was increasing emphasis on programs with more sports for all, rather than the existing system of limiting competition to a narrow segment of the student population.

In the long run, those protests have made no real difference. College sports today are essentially business operations, often run with budgets that are separate from those of their schools. The NCAA has worked as a cartel over the years, organizing the schools to band together in a multi-billion-dollar sports industry. Although joining the NCAA is voluntary, the reality is that a school cannot run a highly competitive athletic program unless it is a member. It will be handicapped in scheduling, in media exposure, and in potential athletic income.

This economic power wielded by the NCAA has made it a powerful and wealthy organization. Although the university presidents have the technical power to rein in overly expensive athletic programs, the reality is that they have tended to be unwilling to do so. The power of alumni contributions, combined with the high visibility of successful athletic programs, has protected college sports from many restrictions. They have become another form of big business.

Olympic Sport Becomes Professional

One of the key concepts in the revival of the Olympic Games in 1896 was that the athletes would be amateurs, just as the ancient Greeks supposedly had been. Although the ancient Greeks had little idea of amateurism and professionalism in sport, the upper-class gentlemen who revived the Games enforced it as a weapon of class distinction, designed to avoid competition with inferior people.

The code of amateurism was rigidly enforced and survived for many decades. By the 1960s and 1970s, it was becoming a shadow of its former self. International competition had become very advanced, governments were beginning to use success in sport for national prestige, and they had found many ways to skirt the boundaries of the old rules of amateurism. In totalitarian governments, such as the Soviet Union, the top athletes were supported by the government and provided everything they needed for training, from housing to meals to coaching to equipment and facilities. Officially, they were most often students or officers in the military. Leaders in American sport called this *shamateurism* and argued that they should be barred as professional athletes.

On the other hand, most of the top American athletes were students on athletic scholarships, which meant that they were receiving the same benefits as the Soviet athletes. In addition to those competing ways of supporting supposedly amateur athletes, many high-level competitions offered gifts, financial expenses, and even prize money under the table. By the late 1970s, the claim of amateurism at the international level was almost a joke.

The idea of truly amateur competition was also weakened by actions taken by the International Olympic Committee. Over a period of several decades the organization had become involved with commercial groups that pumped large amounts of money into supporting the Games (and often the members of the IOC itself). Inevitably, they received commercially valuable benefits in return. By 2000, the level of corruption on the committee was all too noticeable, with payments for votes on the awarding of Olympic Games.[16]

At the same time, the code of amateurism began to slip so that by the early 1980s athletes could set up trust funds to accept prize money. Although it supposedly could not be used until the athlete retired from competition, soon it was allowed to be used for training expenses, and within a few years the idea of separating prize money and delaying its use had disappeared. By 1988, there were professional athletes competing in the Games, and in 1992 the United States basketball team at the Olympics was staffed completely by NBA all-stars.[17]

Today's World Sport: The Name of the Game Is Money

The Impact of Media and Technology on Sport

The rapid growth of professional sports activities also had an impact on the nation. Television broadcast sporting activities as public entertainment, and the nation moved closer to becoming a society of spectators. Professional sports influenced the amateur sports to imitate the professional approach. This affected football and basketball practices most heavily. The glamour of television sports threatened grassroots amateur sports with a loss of local fans. The professional sport ethic, which reached down to the amateur level, promised many changes in sport in the years to come.

In the late 1800s and early 1900s, sport was promoted by newspaper coverage, which expanded until newspapers had a whole section devoted to sports. When commercial radio became widespread during the 1920s, live sports became available to people who lived hundreds of miles away from the actual events. This increased public interest in sports teams.

When television became widespread in the 1950s, early sports coverage was limited. The cameras were bulky, and they could not capture fast movements well. Indoor events were not easy to broadcast because they required very high light levels, which raised the temperatures in playing areas. Some of the early television events were sports like boxing, which required strong lighting for a very small area and which could be covered with just one camera.

By the early 1960s, color television was growing, and cameras and image quality were improving rapidly. The fabled Colts and Giants NFL championship game in the late 1950s was the start of a rapid growth of interest in professional football, which until that time was primarily of interest in the northeastern United States.

During the 1960s, several television events, heavily promoted by ABC network and Roone Arledge, led to great growth in the number of television sports fans. The network started a weekly Wide World of Sports program that broadcast a variety of sports events from around the world. Later in the 1960s, they initiated Monday Night Football (professional), greatly expanding the number and quality of cameras covering the games. With ABC's heavy emphasis on sports coverage, they initiated many of the improvements in coverage, such as detailed analysis of the games by experts and instant replay.

Television made fortunes from sports coverage, and in doing so hooked the NCAA and the colleges on the money that they could make by licensing their games to television networks. Because of the money involved, colleges willingly allowed television interests to override their own fans' interests. Games were played at inconvenient hours for the benefit of viewers in other time zones. Basketball tactics changed because of added TV time-outs. Insignificant tournaments and bowl games were created in the hope of an avalanche of money. In short, the focus of college sports on money became very clear.

College Sports Reform: A Century of Failure

After World War II, the NCAA set out to expand its control over college sports. It gradually gained the authority to penalize institutions that broke its rules. Almost every decade saw a new attempt to reform college athletics, from the Sanity Code of the 1940s to the Knight Commission of the 1990s. A move to put the university presidents in charge during the 1990s led to some changes, yet serious problems remain. College sports are still marked by an overemphasis on sports success, by gross commercialism, by limitations of the freedom of athletes, and by problems in the levels of academic achievement.[18]

24/7 Sports and Getting the Betting Line

By 1980, other forces had appeared that affected sports. In the early days of television, sports events were limited in time: the Friday Night Fights, the Saturday Game of the Week, and perhaps one professional football game on Sunday. Few events were shown outside those limited times. That began to change with the rise of cable and satellite television.

Today ESPN is a hugely influential and wealthy cable channel. When it began in 1979 it was a tiny cable channel covering things such as high school sports and any type of low-profile sport that it could get cheaply, preferably free. It expanded into every sport that was neglected by the major networks, moving to cover minor sports and low-level playoff games.

Midway through the 1980s it signaled its growing sophistication when it bought the rights to broadcast the America's Cup yacht races from Australia. It faced the challenge of showing events covering several miles at sea that were happening live from 1:00 to 5:00 A.M. on the East Coast of the United States.

The network used a system of dirigibles for long overhead shots, powerboats for water-level coverage, and well-placed onboard mini cameras that put the viewers onto the yachts in the middle of the crews as they discussed tactics; raised, lowered, and stowed sails; and fought for hours for tactical advantages of seconds of time. The result was an unanticipated jump in viewers staying up most of the night (during the work week) to follow the races, which were also repeated on tape the following day. The quality and innovation of their coverage showed that they were capable of covering the highest-level sports events.

During the same era, a national newspaper, *USA Today*, appeared. Sometimes called *McPaper* because of its emphasis on very short news stories, it was instantly popular in sports circles because of its detailed listing of sports results. At the same time, combined with the sports coverage range and reporting of ESPN, it was a boon to sports gamblers because it would publish the betting line on events, after which the outcome was both in the newspaper and on ESPN's *SportsCenter*.

The result is that sports coverage today is a 24/7 world, with a range of sports available through cable and satellite television day and night throughout the year. In 1992, NBC experimented with additional cable channels offering complete coverage of particular Olympic sports as pay-per-view channels. The experiment failed, and the assumption was that people were unwilling to pay for the events. A more likely reality is that NBC initially set the fees too high, while many cable systems did not offer the option to their customers, resulting in too limited a customer base for success. Even so, sports championships are starting to move from free network coverage to the pay cable and satellite systems.

The Body Dynamic: Creating the Competitive Human, or Sport, Entertainment, and the Artificial Body

Another notable development in sport is the change in the ideal of the sporting body, both male and female. Although some people believe that the focus on the sporting body is more concerned with the erotic than with performance, the image of the human body has represented a striving for perfection for thousands of years.[19]

While prehistoric representations of the human body are likely concerned with fertility, by the time of the ancient Greeks we see the depiction of the human body in art as an ideal to be attained, not simply in the erotic sense, but in the sense of its utility, its ability to perform, because many of the images are of performing athletes.

Else Trangbæk writes of four versions of the sporting body, which she calls (1) the ancient Greek ideal, (2) the modern body, (3) the post-modern body, and (4) the post-genomic body.[20] The sculpture *Discobolus* represents the Greek ideal, while Eugen Sandow in 1900 represents the modern ideal (for males).

She also terms the post-modern body the *risk-taking body*, one that is developed to an extreme by using scientific methods. An example is the underweight, even anorectic, body sometimes seen in elite female endurance runners or gymnasts. The post-genomic body is when science is taken past its limits with the use of drugs, such as steroids, and *gene doping*. In this case, we see extreme development of the body, such as heavily overbuilt muscles.

The ideal body for men and women changes over time; every generation has its mental model of that ideal.[21] Female gymnasts until the early 1970s were expected to have a relatively typical female body, fit but neither overly nor inadequately developed. The Olga Korbut and Nadia Comaneci era of the 1970s shifted that ideal to a prepubescent circus performer, doing more dangerous, athletic stunts, but having a very small, immature body. The average gymnast on the 1992 U.S. Olympic Team weighed 83 pounds, and it was not considered unusual for elite performers, who were supposedly mature females, to be 4'9" tall and weigh 75 pounds. In recent years that ideal is beginning to shift to a more mature female body, in part because of a rise in the age requirement for international competition.

Today we see human bodies that can seem like cartoons, caricatures of the real body, but heavily, sometimes grotesquely, exaggerated. Between extreme training and perhaps drug assists, sometimes with the added touch of plastic surgery to overcome reality, we see bodies that can be beyond belief. For people who have made those changes, they are seeking their view of perfection.

Are we really believers in the physical perfectability of man? Not only that he can be perfected, but that nothing should stand in the way of him being perfected? Michael Sandel has argued otherwise with his article "The Case Against Perfection." He explains:

> *I do not think the main problem with enhancement and genetic engineering is that they undermine and erode human agency. The deeper danger is that they represent a kind of hyperagency—a Promethean aspiration to remake nature, including human nature, to serve our purposes and satisfy our desires. The problem is not the drift to mechanism but the drive to mastery. And what the drive to mastery misses and may even destroy is an appreciation of the gifted character of human powers and achievements. To acknowledge the giftedness of life is to recognize that our talents and powers are not wholly our own doing, despite the effort we expend to develop and to exercise them. It is also to recognize that not everything in the world is open to whatever use we may desire or devise. Appreciating the gifted quality of life constrains the Promethean project and conduces to a certain humility. It is in part a religious sensibility. But its resonance reaches beyond religion.[22]*

Doping and Today's Sport

Drugs are widely considered the greatest problem in sport today.[23] When an athlete makes a sudden breakthrough or dramatically improves a long-standing world record, the first assumption is that drugs are involved.

The greatest concern is that drug abuse has serious short- and long-term health risks. A second concern is that it violates the concept of fair competition upon which sport competition is built because it is an attempt to gain an unfair advantage over more ethical athletes. A third concern is that young athletes will be discouraged from pursuing sport because they will believe that they cannot succeed at a high level without taking drugs.

Drug use is not a recent phenomenon. It began in ancient times with eating foods that were considered to improve performance. In the 1800s, drugs such as strychnine were used in athletic potions to give a jolt of energy. Diets were manipulated, as they are today, to give a more effective athlete's diet. From nutrition came nutritional supplements, beginning with vitamins. The 1956 U.S. Olympic Team raised questions because of its athletes' use of packages of many vitamin pills (in the days before multivitamins). The difficult question is where an athlete crosses the line in moving from diet to vitamins to other supplements to what we call *drugs*.[24]

A major problem in the struggle over the drugs issue is that at its heart sport sets no boundaries. The Olympic motto of "*citius, altius, fortius*" (faster, higher, stronger) states the basic goal of athletes. The Olympic motto and ideal create an ethical dilemma for athletes and coaches: They set no limits within the spoken goal. The primary problem is that not all races, creeds, and nations see ethical structures from the same perspective. Although fairness is a principle to which all can agree, they cannot agree on what ethical structure constitutes the practice of fair play. All sports rules are constraints formed by an ethical structure accepted by all participants.[25]

By the 1990s, Olympic sports were being heavily affected by the influence of drugs. Even today, with regular out-of-season drug testing of top athletes, drug use may be rampant. As Michael Sokolove writes:

> *Elite athletes in many different sports routinely consume cocktails of vitamins, extracts and supplements, dozens of pills a day—the only people who routinely ingest more pills are AIDS patients—in the hope that their mixes of accepted drugs will replicate the effects of the banned substances taken by the cheaters. The cheaters and noncheaters alike are science projects. They are the sum total of their innate athletic abilities and their dedication—and all the compounds and powders they ingest and inject. A narrow tunnel leads to success at the very top levels of sport.*[26]

The greatest frustration we deal with in the detection of drugs and drug usage among athletes is that there is no foreseeable solution through the detection process. It can never fully catch up with the cheaters. Regardless of the speeches and press releases of the drug testing authorities, their record is not encouraging. Any athlete or coach in high-performance sport is aware of rumors of drug usage and often has direct knowledge of its reality. Unfortunately, even dropping anti-doping rules would not make competition safe. Athletes use poor judgment in pursuing their dreams, so the number of athlete deaths would likely rise. At the same time, the use of drugs would move down to ever-lower ages and levels of sport.[27]

The Growth of the Worldwide Sporting Event

Sport is a major international concern in a world linked by communications satellites. After World War II nations were sending sports teams to other nations for friendly competitions as a sign of mutual trust and friendship and, increasingly, as a means to political cooperation. Sport was becoming a tool for political propaganda to a greater degree than ever before.

Today there are sporting events of a magnitude that they are viewed around the world. From relatively smaller events, such as the Tour de France in cycling to the Super Bowl in American football to the World Cup in soccer, there are events that are seen by hundreds of millions of spectators. But the classic world sports event is the Olympic Games, viewed by billions of people in more than 100 nations around the world. It is for this reason that we now talk of the *globalization* of sport.[28]

Events such as the Olympic Games require the host city and nation to spend billions of dollars in improving infrastructure, such as roads and transportation, in addition to the costs of building and upgrading competitive facilities. The costs have sometimes caused difficult economic problems for the host. Montreal spent 30 years repaying its debt from hosting the 1972 Games, and the cost of the Athens Olympics in 2004 may have been a factor in that nation's economic crisis a few years later. Despite those risks, cities still bid for the Games, sometimes creating scandals with their methods of winning the bid.[29]

Our Field Today

Our field has changed greatly, and significant changes are still taking place. From nearly two centuries ago it has gone from a student health focus to a concept of concern for the education and state of the whole person—mind and body unified. It has gone from a system promoted by self-taught amateurs to one supported by science and the medical profession, from one with teachers having 10 weeks (or less) of professional training to one with teachers who hold doctoral degrees. It has changed from a field interested in a small area of physical concern to a diverse body of people who might at first glance seem to have little connection with each other; they are, however, united in the broad field. Our field has become a broad and complex field, but it has become no less a satisfying field for the practitioner.

The question of the relationship of exercise science and sport has not been settled. This topic is worthy of volumes because the two areas are the same and inseparable to many people. Although there are many problems to overcome, sport and exercise science have gradually been blended together to form a broad area of interest. As they have blended, each has benefited: sport from the educational aims of physical education, and exercise science from the activity and application opportunities of sport. Both sport and exercise science are stronger as a result of the relationship, but much work is needed to realize the full benefits of the combination and to make the relationship a harmonious one.

Who has won the battle between physical education and sports? Athletics on the professional model has largely won the battle at all levels of our schools. Physical education programs are dwarfed by the focus on athletic success. School administrators at all levels seem to have adopted the Big-Time Sports emphasis on sports as a marketing device to bring attention and revenue to the school. The influence of performance-enhancing drugs that accompanies this ethic has also penetrated to the middle school level. The unfortunate reality is that physical education and exercise science are hurt by the image of sport because the public sees no difference between them.

Some people argue that physical education made an error in distancing itself from athletics in the past. They argue that we should develop a unified field that includes all areas of our interests. Part of the field's problem is a lack of communication and a failure to develop a group focus that includes every group that works in an area that is part of our broadly defined field.

In fact, the physical education versus sport conflict is disappearing in the face of newer changes in the field. Even though the conflict is still a strong force and a major problem in smaller colleges, exercise science and sport are completely separate entities at most larger institutions. At the NCAA Division I level, athletics is a major marketing arm of universities, with a significant economic impact on those schools. In those schools' exercise science programs, the concern is the consolidation toward the concept of our newly defined field, a field that meets this book's earlier definition of "the broad field of exercise science." The name changes, but the song remains the same.

Summary

The coming of World War II changed physical education programs to physical fitness oriented toward military needs. Sports were considered a positive influence on national spirit and were highly encouraged. Major conferences on the undergraduate professional preparation curriculum were held between 1948 and 1973. Fitness became a major concern in 1953 when the results of the widely publicized Kraus-Weber Tests implied that American elementary schoolchildren were much less fit than their counterparts in other nations. The AAHPER Youth Fitness Test was published in 1958.

In the early 1960s, our field was essentially physical education, while today's focus is on scientific and theoretical foundations. In 1964, Franklin Henry called for a more scientifically focused academic discipline of physical education. The core knowledge for each area of the field, what was then called the *body of knowledge* of each subdiscipline, gained new focus. New major programs were added to reflect the new knowledge in the field and new career directions of students. The movement produced a great surge in research and the academic grounding of programs, but the separate development of the individual subdisciplines resulted in a heavily fractured field. The kinesiology taught at the research universities has changed to become a health science. The best title for the field is not settled; most other nations use exercise science or sport science.

By the year 2000, reports by the federal government showed unusually high levels of obesity among schoolchildren. Yet despite those concerns, by 2010 there had been little legislative action to stiffen school physical education requirements.

The distinctions between the amateur and the professional disappeared in the 1980s and 1990s. Youth sport moved to a model of professional, commercial sport. There has been a continuing downward trend of the age at which youth become involved in highly organized and highly competitive sporting programs. In today's world of sport the name of the game is money. College sports today are essentially business operations. The NCAA has worked as a cartel over the years, organizing the schools to band together in a multi-billion-dollar sports industry. By 1988, there were professional athletes competing at the Olympic Games.

The ideal of the sporting body, both male and female, is changing as a result of media, money, drugs, and plastic surgery. The image of the human body has represented a striving for perfection for thousands of years. Today we see human bodies that can seem like cartoons, caricatures of the real body.

Drugs are widely considered the greatest problem in sport today. The greatest concern is that drug abuse has serious short- and long-term health risks. A second concern is that it violates the concept of fair competition upon which sport competition is built because it is an attempt to gain an unfair advantage over more ethical athletes. A third concern is that young athletes will be discouraged from pursuing sport because they will believe that they cannot succeed at a high level without taking drugs.

Sport is a major international concern in a world linked by communications satellites. Today there are sporting events of a magnitude that they are viewed around the world. The classic world sports event is the Olympic Games, viewed by billions of people in more than 100 nations around the world. It is for this reason that we now talk of the globalization of sport.

Our field has changed greatly, and significant changes are still taking place. It has gone from a student health focus to a concern for the education and state of the whole person—mind and body unified. It has gone from a system promoted by self-taught amateurs to one supported by science and the medical profession.

Further Readings

Barker-Ruchti, Natalie. 2009. Ballerinas and pixies: A genealogy of the changing female gymnastics body. *International Journal of the History of Sport* 26: 45–62.

Bowers, Matthew T., and Thomas M. Hunt. 2011. The President's Council on Physical Fitness and the systemisation of children's play in America. *International Journal of the History of Sport* 28: 1496–1511.

Carpenter, Linda Jean, and R. Vivian Acosta. 2005. *Title IX*. Champaign, IL: Human Kinetics.

Davies, Richard O. 2007. *Sports in American life: A history*. Oxford: Blackwell.

Dimeo, Paul. 2007. *A history of drug use in sport 1876–1976: Beyond good and evil.* New York: Routledge.

Hamzeh, Manal, and Kimberly L. Oliver. 2012. "Because I am Muslim, I cannot wear a swimsuit": Muslim girls negotiate participant opportunities for physical activity. *Research Quarterly for Exercise and Sport* 83: 330–339.

Henderson, Simon. 2009. Crossing the line: Sport and the limits of civil rights protest. *International Journal of the History of Sport* 26: 101–121.

Hoberman, John. 1992. *Mortal engines: The science of performance and the dehumanization of sport.* New York: Free Press.

Hoffman, Shirl J. 2010. *Good Game: Christianity and the culture of sports.* Waco, TX: Baylor Univ. Press.

Hogan, Lawrence D. 2006. *Shades of glory: The Negro leagues and the story of African-American baseball.* Washington, DC: National Geographic Society.

Hunt, Thomas M., and John Hoberman. 2011. *Drug games: The International Olympic Committee and the politics of doping.* Austin, TX: Univ. of Texas Press.

Kaliss, Gregory J. 2008. Un-civil discourse: Charlie Scott, the integration of college basketball, and the "progressive mystique." *Journal of Sport History* 35: 98–117.

Lamb, Chris. 1997. "I never want to take another trip like this one": Jackie Robinson's journey to integrate baseball. *Journal of Sport History* 24: 177–191.

Llewellyn, Matthew P. 2011. The curse of the Shamateurs. *International Journal of the History of Sport* 28: 796–816.

Martin, Charles H. 1999. The rise and fall of Jim Crow in southern college sports: The case of the Atlantic Coast Conference. *North Carolina Historical Review* 76: 253–284.

Overman, Steven J. 2011. *The Protestant ethic and the spirit of sport: How Calvinism and capitalism shaped America's games.* Macon, GA: Mercer Univ. Press.

Oxendine, Joseph B. 1995. *American Indian sports history.* Lincoln, NE: Univ. of Nebraska Press.

Park, Roberta J. 2010. Women as leaders: What women have attained in and through physical education. *International Journal of the History of Sport* 27: 1250–1276.

Park, Roberta J., and Patricia Vertinsky, eds. 2012. *Women, sport, society: Further reflections, reaffirming Mary Wollstonecraft.* New York: Routledge.

Pauline, Gina. 2012. Celebrating 40 years of Title IX: How far have we really come? *JOPERD (Journal of Physical Education, Recreation and Dance)* 83 (8): 4–5.

Rader, Benjamin G. 2008. *American sports: From the age of folk games to the age of televised sports.* 6th ed. Englewood Cliffs, NJ: Prentice Hall.

———. 2009. A revolutionary moment in recent American history. *Journal of Sport History* 36: 315–336.

Roche, Maurice. 2000. *Mega-events and modernity: Olympics and expos in the growth of global culture.* New York: Routledge.

Rosen, Daniel M. 2008. *Dope: A history of performance enhancement in sports from the nineteenth century to today.* Westport, CT: Praeger.

Senn, Alfred E. 1999. *Power, politics, and the Olympic Games.* Champaign, IL: Human Kinetics.

Smith, John Matthew. 2009. "It's not really my country": Lew Alcindor and the revolt of the black athlete. *Journal of Sport History* 36: 223–244.

Smith, Lisa. 1999. *Nike is a goddess: The history of women's sport.* New York: Grove /Atlantic.

Smith, Ronald A. 1998. Women's control of American college sport: The goal of those who played, or an exploitation by those who controlled? *Sport History Review* 29: 103–120.

———. 2001. *Play-by-play: Radio, television, and big-time college sport.* Baltimore: Johns Hopkins Univ. Press.

———. 2011. *Pay for play: A history of big-time athletic reform.* Urbana, IL: Univ. of Illinois Press.

Wiggins, David K. 2010. "With all deliberate speed": High school sport, race, and *Brown v. Board of Education. Journal of Sport History* 37: 329–346.

Wiggins, David K., and Brenda P. Wiggins. 2011. Striving to be in the profession and of it: The African American experience in physical education and kinesiology. *Research Quarterly for Exercise and Sport* 82: 320–333.

Wushanley, Ying. 2004. *Playing nice and losing: The struggle for control of women's intercollegiate athletics, 1960–2000.* Syracuse, NY: Syracuse Univ. Press.

Zimbalist, Andrew. 1999. *Unpaid professionals: Commercialism and conflict in big-time college sports.* Princeton, NJ: Princeton Univ. Press.

Discussion Questions

1. Discuss the changes in programs of sport and physical education that were a result of the following:

   a. World War II and the Korean War
   b. The Cold War, including Kraus-Weber and *Sputnik*
   c. The integration of school sports
   d. The opposition to requirements in the 1960s and 1970s
   e. Title IX
   f. The discipline movement
   g. The end of amateurism in Olympic sport

2. Using old college catalogs, examine the major curriculum and required courses at your school from 1960 to 1965. How does this compare to today's programs and course requirements?

3. Discuss the development of women's athletics over the past century.

4. Discuss the role of black athletes in American sports since 1941.

5. Discuss the development of youth fitness programs since the 1950s. What caused the emphasis, how has it changed over the years, and what is it like today? Has it brought about genuine change in the level of fitness of American children?

6. Discuss the discipline movement and its effect upon the field of exercise science and kinesiology over the last 50 years.

7. What is the relationship between physical education and sports today? Is the situation a good one? Explain and defend your answer.

References

1. van Oteghen, Sharon. 2009. Lest we forget the service they rendered. *JOPERD (Journal of Physical Education, Recreation and Dance)* 80 (9): 54–57, 61–65.

2. Twietmeyer, Gregg. 2007. The education of American kinesiologists: Broadening the understanding of the importance of James Bryant Conant's impact on the field. Abstract. In *North American Society for Sport History Proceedings*, 65–66.

3. Hult, Joan S. 1994. The story of women's athletics: Manipulating a dream 1890–1985. In *Women and sport: Interdisciplinary perspectives*, ed. D. Margaret Costa and Sharon R. Guthrie, 94–100. Champaign, IL: Human Kinetics.

4. Hultstrand, Bonnie J. 1993. The growth of collegiate women's sports: The 1960s. *JOPERD (Journal of Physical Education, Recreation and Dance)* (March): 41–43, 63.

5. Hult, Joan S. 1999. NAGWS and AIAW: The strange and wondrous journey to the athletic summit, 1950–1990. *JOPERD (Journal of Physical Education, Recreation and Dance)* (April): 24–31.

6. Hill, Karen L. 1993. Women in sport: Backlash or megatrend? *JOPERD (Journal of Physical Education, Recreation and Dance)* (November–December): 49–52; and Heishman, Mary Frances, Linda Bunker, and Roland W. Tutwiler. 1990. The decline of women leaders (coaches and athletic directors) in girls' interscholastic sports programs in Virginia from 1972 to 1987. *Research Quarterly for Exercise and Sport* 61: 103–107.

7. Sabo, Don. 1998. Women's athletics and the elimination of men's sports programs. *Journal of Sport and Social Issues* 22: 27–31.

8. Wilson, Wayne. 1996. The IOC and the status of women in the Olympic movement. *Research Quarterly for Exercise and Sport* 67:183–192; and Davenport, Joanna. 1996. Breaking into the rings: Women on the IOC. *JOPERD (Journal of Physical Education, Recreation and Dance)* (May–June): 26–30.

9. Berryman, Jack W. 1996. The rise of boys' sports in the United States. In *Children and youth in sport*, ed. F. L. Smoll and R. E. Smith, 4–14. Dubuque, IA: Brown and Benchmark.

10. Smith, Ronald A. 1988. *Sports and freedom: The rise of big-time college athletics*. New York: Oxford Univ. Press; and Smith, Ronald A. 1993. History of amateurism in men's intercollegiate athletics: The continuance of a 19th-century anachronism in America. *Quest* 45 (4): 430–447.

11. Hardman, Ken, and C. Fielden. 1994. The development of sporting excellence—lessons from the past. In *HPER—moving toward the 21st century*, ed. P. Duffy and L. Dugdale, 161–173. Champaign, IL: Human Kinetics.

12. Freeman, William H. 1998. The trend toward professionalism in youth sport: The implications for educational sport for all. In *Active living through quality physical education: Selected readings from the 8th European congress of ICHPERSD (Europe)*, ed. Richard Fisher, Christopher Laws, and Jackie Moses, 54–58. Strawberry Hill, England: St. Mary's Univ. College.

13. Davies, Richard O. 2007. *Sports in American life: A history*. Oxford: Blackwell, 423.

14. Ibid.

15. Jable, J. Thomas. 2006. Have skill, will travel: The impact of travel teams on high school athletics in the United States. In *North American Society for Sport History Proceedings*, 44–45.

16. Simson, Vyv, and Andrew Jennings. 1992. *Dishonored games: Corruption, money and greed at the Olympics*. New York: SPI; Jennings, Andrew. 1996. *The new Lords of the*

Rings: Olympic corruption and how to buy gold medals. London: Pocket Books; Jennings, Andrew, and Clare Sambrook. 2000. *The great Olympic swindle: When the world wanted its games back*. London: Simon and Schuster; and Barney, Robert K., Stephen Wenn, and Scott Martyn. 2002. *Selling the five rings: The I.O.C. and the rise of Olympic commercialism*. Salt Lake City, UT: Univ. of Utah Press.

17. Davies, *Sports in American life*, 343–345; and Rader, Benjamin G. 2004. *American sports: From the age of folk games to the age of televised sports*. 5th ed. Upper Saddle River, NJ: Prentice Hall, 304–306.

18. Smith, Ronald A. 2011. *Pay for play: A history of big-time college athletic reform*. Urbana IL: Univ. of Illinois Press.

19. McClelland, John. 2002. Eros and sport: A humanist's perspective. *Journal of Sport History* 29 (3): 395–406.

20. Trangbæk, Else. 2002. On the modern and the post-modern body—with a focus on elite sport. Vol. 1 of *Transformationen: Kontinuitäten und veränderungen in der sportgeschichte*, ed. Arnd Krüger and Wolfgang Buss, 65–71. Göttingen, Germany: Niedersächsisches Institut Für Sportgeschichte Hoya E.v.

21. Barker-Ruchti, Ballerinas and pixies, 45–62.

22. In Freeman, William H. 2006. The ethical paradox of *citius, altius, fortius* in a multi-cultural world. Paper presented at the International Sport Studies Conference, Melbourne, Australia.

23. Davies, *Sports in American life*, 398–409; and Polidoro, J. Richard. 2000. *Sport and physical activity in the modern world*. Boston: Allyn and Bacon, 118–122.

24. Dimeo, Paul. 2007. *A history of drug use in sport 1876–1976: Beyond good and evil*. New York: Routledge; Rosen, Daniel M. 2008. *Dope: A history of performance enhancement in sports from the nineteenth century to today*. Westport, CT: Praeger; and David, Paul. 2008. *A guide to the world anti-doping code: A fight for the spirit of sport*. New York: Cambridge Univ. Press.

25. In Freeman, Ethical paradox.

26. Sokolove, Michael. 2004. In pursuit of doped excellence. *New York Times Magazine*, January 18, 30.

27. Freeman, William H. 2006. *Citius, altius, fortius*: Motto and ethical paradox. Paper presented at the Commonwealth International Sport Conference, Melbourne, Australia; Freeman, William H. 2006. Removing drugs from sport: Is it too late? Paper presented at the European College of Sports Sciences, Lausanne, Switzerland; and Freeman, William H. 2006. If drugs didn't matter: A consideration of the potential impact of no-limits sport. Paper presented at the Commonwealth International Sport Conference, Melbourne, Australia.

28. Brookes, Rod. 2002. *Representing sport*. New York: Oxford Univ. Press; and Lafeber, Walter. 1999. *Michael Jordan and the new global capitalism*. New York: Norton.

29. Barney, Wenn, and Martyn, *Selling the five rings*; and Jennings and Sambrook, *Great Olympic swindle*.

PART 3

Our Cultural Heritage in Philosophy

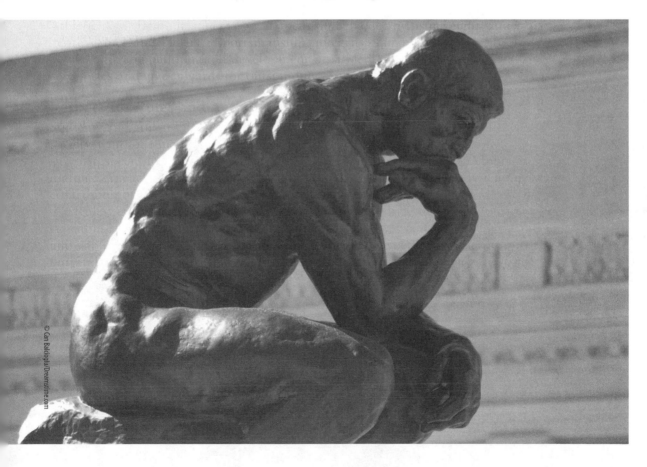

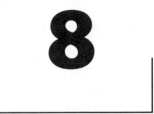

Philosophy in Exercise Science and Sport

CHAPTER

8

The study of philosophy is important to physical educators. In keeping with a whole-person concept of physical education, it helps us to develop personal philosophies that affect every area of our actions in our daily lives. An examination of four areas of interest can explain the need to understand philosophy and its uses: (1) the definition and application of philosophy in physical education and sport, (2) the newer area of sport philosophy, (3) the major philosophical teachings, and (4) how we can "do" philosophy in physical education and sport.

What Is Philosophy?

Philosophy has long been a confusing concept to students. It is difficult to define clearly because the definitions may seem to disagree. Harold Barrow, who suggests that philosophy can be viewed in several ways, presents three concepts: (1) philosophy as "a study of the truth or the principles underlying all knowledge," (2) philosophy as "a study of the most general causes and principles of the universe," and (3) philosophy as "a system for guiding life."[1] Clearly, philosophy is not a small area of interest; it is so broad that it is hard to define. Barrow views philosophy as both a process and its resulting product. The process is a method used to establish a system of values, and the product is the system of values that eventually is produced by the process.

Randolph Webster notes that the original meaning of philosophy was a "love of truth" or a "love of wisdom." It was a search for both facts and values that are studied without any bias or prejudice. As he points out:

> *Philosophy is concerned with questions of right and wrong, justice, freedom, and discretion. Though there is a distinction between philosophy and science, philosophy can be said to be a science since it organizes knowledge about man and the universe for the purpose of evaluation and comprehension. . . . Philosophy criticizes, evaluates the worth of things, and synthesizes facts; while science describes, discovers, and analyzes facts. . . . [Scientists] know how [atomic energy] works and*

how to use it, but only philosophers deliberate about where and for what purpose it should be used. Both processes are essential.[2]

In ancient times, philosophy included the physical and social sciences, but as knowledge expanded and specialized disciplines developed, philosophy was eventually left with meaning, values, appreciation, interpretation, and evaluation as its subject matter.

We might say that science is an examination of what can be proven with physical experiments and evidence, while philosophy is an examination of what cannot be proven by physical evidence. Philosophy attempts to extend meanings far beyond known facts and to provide direction for each person's life. Webster spoke of philosophy as a science, but philosophy is not a science in its common definition. Philosophy tries to go far beyond science's solid, physical facts.

Some of the relationships between philosophy and science are discussed by Elwood Davis and Donna Miller.[3] They point out that science is precise and defined by proven, concrete facts, but philosophy goes beyond the facts and into areas of speculation that probably can never be proven. Actually, the scientific method of research is very similar to the methods used to gain knowledge in philosophy. However, science requires observable data, though philosophy does not. Philosophy is concerned largely with meanings and values. The dividing line between philosophy and science is not always clear, and there is considerable overlap. Science may rely on cold, hard facts, but its directions are determined by human emotions and philosophies as much as any other area of study or life.

Religion is closely related to philosophy because religion is philosophical by nature. Religion is concerned with the idea of God and the relationship between God and people; it also includes ethics and ethical practices. Religion is often self-conscious about its lack of scientifically provable ideas, but that does not make it less valid than philosophy. Both religion and philosophy try to go beyond the known and into the unknown. Each seeks to answer questions that science can never answer.

Art is also closely related to philosophy because it does not involve scientific judgment or process. Art is an area of values where people seek to express, fulfill, and understand themselves—a complex process that goes beyond the limitations of science. Art is by its nature subjective; it is concerned with an inner self that is beyond the bounds of science. Indeed, we might argue that art and science are simply different approaches to reality.

The Branches of Philosophy

The major branches of philosophy are metaphysics, epistemology, logic, and axiology (**Figure 8.1**). When we think of philosophy, we usually think of metaphysics, or the nature of reality and being. *Metaphysics* tries to answer questions that cannot be answered scientifically about what is real and what really exists.

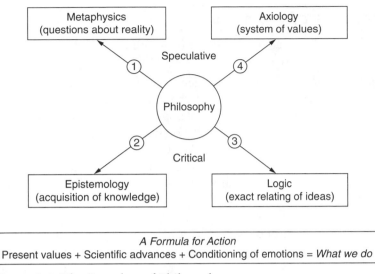

Figure 8.1 The Branches of Philosophy

Reproduced from E. F. Zeigler. Introduction to sport and physical education philosophy. Benchmark, 1990. Courtesy of Earle F. Zeigler.

Epistemology is the study of the theory of knowledge. It examines how knowledge is gained and what kinds of knowledge can be obtained, or what can be learned and how the content of knowledge can be determined. It involves the processes of perception (how we see things) and knowledge, including the process of learning, which we sometimes call the *scientific method.*

Logic is the study of the relationship of ideas to one another. Ideally, it is the method for thought and research, the steps that should be followed in relating one idea to another or in proceeding from one idea to another more advanced one. For many people, logic is the most important area of philosophy.

Axiology is the study of values in general terms; it involves the nature and kinds of values. We are most concerned with two specific subareas of axiology, ethics and aesthetics. Ethics is concerned with morals and conduct, that is, with determining proper rules of conduct. It is a study of ideal conduct and the knowledge of good and evil. It examines which actions are right and wrong, or what people should and should not do.

Aesthetics deals with the nature of beauty, which is very subjective. Earle Zeigler defines aesthetics as the "theory or philosophy of taste" because beauty is very much a matter of personal taste.[4]

By looking more precisely at the major questions philosophy tries to answer, you can develop a clearer perception of the directions that philosophical studies can take.

The Questions of Philosophy

The major questions or concerns of philosophy fall into nine areas, though this list is not necessarily exhaustive:[5]

1. *Nature of the universe.* In ancient times, philosophical discussion concerned the origin and nature of the earth and what basic materials had been used in its development. Today this issue is of little concern to philosophers because it has been largely taken over by the scientists.

2. *People's place in the universe.* Are human beings just other animals, or are they supreme creatures? Are they important or unimportant? Are they the masters of their own destinies, or are their fates controlled by higher forces?

3. *Determination of good and evil.* Are there any absolute measures for determining good and evil, right and wrong? Do such standards change depending on the situation? What constitutes the good life? These questions are still considered very important today, and in many respects they are of great concern to us in our working and daily living activities.

4. *Nature of God.* Is there a God, or do gods exist? Is there some supreme being, and if so, what are its characteristics? Where do we find God, and what is God's relationship to people? These are some of the important questions involved in the philosophy of religion.

5. *Soul and immortality.* This may be related to the previous issue, depending on the philosophy and beliefs of the person involved. Do we possess a soul, that is, some inner part that is intangible? When we die, does the soul die also, or does it continue to live on in another place or another form? This area of philosophy goes into the age-old religious questions regarding life after death: Is there life after death, and if so, what is it like?

6. *People's relationship to the state.* This area is a growing concern as the world's population rapidly expands, bringing on increased governmental regulation and monitoring of people's lives. What is the best form of government? Who should reign supreme: the people or the state? Is the answer to the question of supremacy an absolute, or can it change as circumstances change?

7. *Role of education.* What is the role of education in the social structure? What part does it play, and what should be its goals? These questions are crucial because they determine how a civilization reproduces itself or fails to do so. What should be taught in education, and how should it be taught?

8. *Relationship between mind and matter.* How do people affect, and how are they affected by, their environment and surroundings? Which is superior, mind or matter, or is one superior to the other? How do they relate to each other?

9. *Implications of philosophy for exercise science.* Though this is not a question of pure philosophy, it refers to exercise science in the broad sense, including such related areas as health and recreation. How do the answers—those we have determined for ourselves as being the best—to the questions in the first eight areas affect our programs?

As James Baley and David Field point out:

Philosophy is man's effort to see the universe in a coherent, systematic, and meaningful way. It gives our actions direction. If our objectives, principles, and methods are to be consistent, we must possess a reasonably well thought-out philosophic position. Otherwise, we are likely to be like the horseman who tried to run off in all directions at once.[6]

Most people seek to answer these questions to clarify their ideas and beliefs regarding life and how it should be lived. Philosophy can deal with both general and very specific questions. Those questions help to make our purposes and goals clearer. By doing so, they play a major role in determining how people view exercise science, physical education, and sport and their function in society; what their feelings about our field will be; and what they will try to do with them.

Issues in Sport Philosophy

A discussion of some of the issues and areas of philosophical interest will illustrate the kinds of problems studied by sport philosophers. To give a general idea of what the sport philosopher seeks to do in each area, rather than present an actual philosophical study of each area, this overview examines eight such areas of philosophical interest.

The Nature of Sport

The first question or problem that the sport philosopher faces is that of defining the field of study: What is the nature of sport? Ellen Gerber and William Morgan begin their book with a discussion and supporting readings that are concerned with this question. They suggest that "fundamental to an examination of sport in its diversified and meaningful roles is an understanding of its nature as a phenomenon." They briefly discuss four techniques that can be used to contribute to such an understanding: definition, characterization, classification, and comparison.[7]

Definition is the application of inductive reasoning to define sport in terms of those activities that are considered genuine. It provides a generalized idea of what sport is. *Characterization* uses deductive logic to determine the common elements or characteristics of sport. After the basic characteristics have been determined, the philosopher will try to discover the basic relationships. This is accomplished by *classification*, the grouping of subjects or activities according to similar elements. Finally, the philosopher will use the technique of *comparison* to see whether the theorized elements do indeed hold true when compared to other activities.

The task of defining the nature of sport is such that not all philosophers agree that it is possible. Frank McBride argues that sport is too vague and too complex to be defined in a single concept, if it can be defined accurately at all.[8] The differences seem to be semantic; there is disagreement over the exact meanings of words. Part of the problem is that many terms are used interchangeably, so the same term may have conflicting meanings. A common example is the use of the terms *sport* and *athletics*. They are often used to mean the same thing, although most philosophers agree that they are not the same, but overlap. Scholars from another nation might have less trouble in defining these terms because they probably had different meanings from the beginning. This is only one example of the problems in trying to make a generally accepted concept or definition of the nature of sport.

Sport and Metaphysical Speculation

Metaphysics is essentially a study of reality, although in sport philosophy it is similar in some respects to the study of the nature of sport. Gerber and Morgan briefly discuss metaphysical speculation in sport, raising three questions involving reality. The first question concerns the nature of the world (cosmology), though that research topic has been largely replaced by modern science. The second asks whether a divine entity or condition exists, though theological studies have largely separated from philosophy in modern times. The third question asks the nature of reality from the standpoint of human existence (ontology), which is the primary modern focus of philosophical research. This is the most common type of study in metaphysics and sport, particularly the being–status of sport.[9]

Metaphysical speculation in sport balances such themes as the mind–body relation, finiteness and infinity, time, space, and freedom. It especially notes how sport is similar or dissimilar to other human movement phenomena, such as exercise, play, dance, and games. Gerber and Morgan suggest using three approaches. The first develops the implications of major philosophical schools of thought (such as idealism) for issues that are central to sport. The second approach develops the implications of the philosophical systems of major philosophers (such as Plato) for issues of interest to sport. The third approach, which is the most difficult because it requires greater "philosophic acumen and originality," is to move into a direct philosophical examination of a major issue. Although metaphysical speculation may appear rather pointless, it does have important implications. As Gerber and Morgan point out, the ways in which people view sport are reflected in their attitudes toward it.[10] Thus, metaphysical speculation can be used by the sport philosopher to discover how people see, approach, and use sport.

The Body and Being

The area of the body and being tries to define the relationship that exists among the mind, body, and soul, including the relative values of each "dimension."[11]

The concept of a body–soul or mind–body relationship has been a matter of philosophical interest since the time of Plato. Plato viewed the body negatively and sport positively. This resulted in much interpretive argument among philosophers of physical education and sport. Monism (the oneness of mind and body) is still in conflict with dualism (the mind and body as separate, not connected).

Phenomenologists (researchers of self-awareness) delve into the philosophical interest area of the body and being. They approach their study from the unusual (in terms of tradition) point of view of the body as the primary self, rather than the mind or soul. Essentially, these philosophers examine the connection between sport and the body by studying the body experience in different sport or physical situations and by noting how it differs in nonphysical situations.

Sport as a Meaningful Experience

Sport as a meaningful experience is another complicated topic because it deals with the "mysterious relationship between subject and object."[12] Experience lies in the realm of epistemology (the gaining of knowledge) because all questions of truth or confirmation of knowledge relate to experience. Gerber cites these six universal characteristics of experience: (1) it is temporal in character; (2) it has elements of organic, physical, and cultural relatedness; (3) it involves the past, present, and future; (4) it has a space–time locus; (5) it involves some object

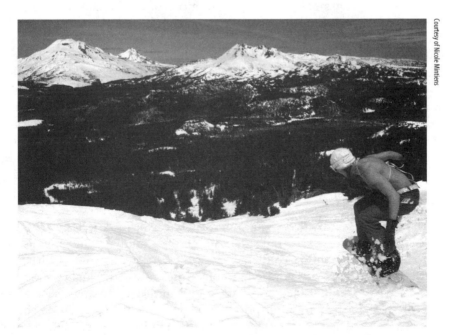

Courtesy of Nicole Mintiens

Every person experiences sport differently, which adds complexity to studying a meaningful experience.

or phenomena in the experience; and (6) it can be perceptual, imaginative, or conceptual.[13]

Each experience is different because each person perceives things differently. This factor makes philosophical studies of meaningful experience even more difficult. Sport philosophers study issues such as why people play, great moments in sport, peak experiences, and the idea of the perfect moment. A peak experience or perfect moment does not demand championship skill levels because it does not require records or other attributes of "great moments." The peak experience is "that moment when the person is totally involved, in control, and effortlessly touching that flow of personal perfection."[14] It is a time of personal fulfillment, surpassing normal potential, when everything "comes together." It is a moment crystallized and held in time to be remembered, relived, and examined. It is perhaps the essence of the sport experience.

Sport Versus Physical Education: Philosophical Conflicts

There is confusion over the difference between sport and athletics. The athletics–physical education relationship has historically been difficult. William Harper suggests that a clear understanding of the problem is complicated by the many myths that survive.[15]

One myth is the spurious continuum running from play to games to sports (represented often by intramurals) to athletics. In reality, athletes rarely come from intramural programs. Intramurals are more often the final resting place of those who are unable to compete at the interschool level. A second myth is the existence of only one viable model for the sports program. There are actually several distinct models that depend on the group setting the standards. A third myth is that certain attitudes (such as sportsmanship and fair play) are inherent in the game. A fourth myth is the preciseness of definitions used in athletics and physical education (such as those used for the terms *play*, *games*, *sport*, and *physical education*). Another myth results from disregarding the historical origins of athletics. The conflict in means and goals between athletics and physical education dates back to the ancient Greeks. We need more research in this controversial area because the problems are very real and very immediate.

Sport and Aesthetics

Aesthetics is concerned with the question of what is beautiful. Some of the most complex philosophical issues fall into this area of study. It includes issues of beauty, taste, and the nature of the aesthetic experience, as well as questions of what is art, what is beauty, and what constitutes aesthetic quality.[16] Sport has long been seen as a good subject for works of art and is increasingly seen as an art form. Moreover, participation in sport can be an aesthetic experience. This leads to the question of when a phenomenon has the quality to be considered a work of art.

The area of aesthetics is receiving more attention from sport philosophers, such as Peter J. Arnold in his "movement as a source of aesthetic experience."[17] The most extensive study is Benjamin Lowe's *The Beauty of Sport*.[18]

Sport and Values

Values represent perhaps the most critical area of concern in sport for many people because of the moral or behavioral values expressed by sports participants. Are values taught in sports settings? Are they inherent in sport or in games? These questions lie at the crux of the education–sports–athletics dilemma. One of the great all-time arguments for athletics was that it taught sportsmanship (though no evidence has ever backed up this admirable philosophy). Some of these matters will be discussed in more detail elsewhere. Two related concerns or problems that are also popular areas of study for the sport philosopher are the concept of the amateur, and fair play and sportsmanship.

The Concept of Fair Play and Sportsmanship

The place of values and moral education needs to be considered much more closely than it has been in the past, as Delbert Oberteuffer long ago suggested. We need clear ethical guidelines for sport at every level. James W. Keating has given considerable attention to competition and the competitive experience, including questions of ethics, particularly in studies such as "Sportsmanship as a Moral Category." Peter McIntosh devoted an entire book to the historical and philosophical consideration of the concept of fair play and ethics in sport and education. He argues that, although there is increasing interest in the idea of moral education, too little attention has been paid to the roles of physical education, play, and sport in moral education.[19] Justice lies at the heart of the concept of fair play, yet the ideals of sportsmanship and fair play seem to be drifting farther and farther away from the common practice in modern sport. As such, this area is of critical interest to teachers and coaches.

Contemporary Philosophies of Our Field

Five major philosophies are examined most often in relationship to physical education today: naturalism, idealism, realism, pragmatism, and existentialism. As the study of philosophy in physical education and sport develops, less emphasis is placed on the traditional schools of philosophy as a subject of study. However, a brief summary shows how educational philosophies develop.

Naturalism

Naturalism is based on its root word *nature*. It is a belief that the laws of nature govern everything in life: Because nature is unchanging, anything of value will always work. At the same time, naturalism emphasizes individualism by considering the person more important than society as a whole. Although naturalism ranks societal goals below individual goals in importance, it still accepts the need for a social system to prevent chaos. This acceptance does not make the social system good, but simply necessary.

In education, natural means are the desired method. That is, the process should be geared to the student, rather than the student to the process. The teacher is both guide and teacher. The teacher primarily helps the student see how to learn, but nature does the teaching. The student must make an active effort to learn, with punishments and rewards a part of the process. The rate of learning depends on the student because the educational process requires a physical and mental balance, rather than the promotion of one over the other.

In physical education, naturalism considers the development of the whole person, not just the physical aspect. Physical activity can be a major source of the overall development of the student (especially with younger children, as in Rousseau's *Emile*). Play is an important part of the learning process, but it can be self-directed, individual activity as well as group activity. Although competition is natural, it is not strongly emphasized, because the concentration is on the individual, even though competition is against oneself. Teaching is paced with the student's needs, using reasonably democratic, informal methods.

Earle Zeigler suggests that naturalism has one strength and one weakness, and that they are the same: The philosophical practice of naturalism is extremely simple.[20] Simplicity can be an advantage because most people find a simple education a relaxing change. On the other hand, it may be a disadvantage because the approach of naturalism may be too limited to prepare the student to cope with an increasingly complex world. A simple education may be a handicap, rather than an asset, in an advanced, scientifically oriented civilization. Naturalism was a popular philosophy during the eighteenth and nineteenth centuries, but it is no longer a major educational philosophy.

Idealism

Idealism is based on the root word *idea*, with the focus on the mind. As everything is interpreted in terms of the mind, all reality comes from the mind. People's rational (reasoning) powers help them find the truth, although they may use scientific methods to help in the discovery. According to idealism, people are more important than nature because their minds interpret everything in nature for them. Ideas are true and never change, so moral values also never change. People have the free will to choose between right and wrong.

Most of the educational process under idealism is concerned with the mind, so content is objective. Because education develops the individual personality, fostering moral and spiritual values is important, too. The teacher creates a learning environment, but the student is responsible for motivation and learning. Many teaching methods may be used, but education takes place primarily through the active effort of the student.

Although physical education can make a major contribution to the development of the intellect, idealists consider physical education less important than the more thought-oriented, educational activities. Physical education is based on known truths, principles, and ideas that do not change, so the program can be rather fixed and formal, although not without variety in activities and teaching techniques. The teacher is an important example to the students, a role model in the use of ideals and values.

Idealism is a well-developed, broad philosophy for education and physical education. It gives the student a strong place in the universe by developing a feeling of individual importance. It permits a broad physical and intellectual growth, with play and recreation making important contributions. At the same time, some people object to the idealist notion of teaching values that have been established by past experience; there is less interest today in dedication and sacrifice for older ideals. Moreover, some teachers' actions may contradict the values they seek to teach, as in the saying "actions speak louder than words." The idealist educational program may pay little attention to the body because its primary concern is to develop the mind. People's conflicting ideas of work and play can make the application of physical education under idealism difficult to explain because people may have difficulty in accepting that play can have values as great as those of work.[21]

Realism

Realism falls between naturalism and idealism. The philosophy argues that the physical world of nature is real, so people should use their senses and experiences to understand it. Experimental means, such as the scientific method, help realists discover and interpret truth. Realists believe that the physical things that happen result from the physical laws of nature. They also hold that the mind and body cannot be separated: One is not superior to the other. Although naturalism does not permit religion (it puts nature above everything) and idealism does permit religion, realism allows its adherents to go either way in determining their beliefs.

The first priority of the realist educational process is to develop the student's reasoning power because that power is considered essential to further learning. Scientific, objective standards are always part of an orderly, scientifically oriented process and curriculum. Physical education is valuable in the realist curriculum because it results in greater health and productivity. Realists believe that a healthy person can lead a fuller life. The realist physical education program is based on scientific knowledge and uses many drills to instill knowledge according to scientific progression. Social behaviors and life adjustment are important benefits of recreational and sporting activities.

Realism deals with the world as we find it because the world of cause and effect cannot be changed. It gives physical education a clear function as a healthy physical basis for life. At the same time, realism advocates a lower status for physical education because its primary function is to provide a vigorous physical basis for life. However, realism gives a more clearly defined place for physical education in the educational process than many other philosophies. The authoritarianism suggested by the realist acceptance of standardization and drill learning is not consistent with the needs of democratic societies. Societal needs and trends are negligible factors in realism.[22]

Pragmatism

Pragmatism was once called experimentalism because it is based on learning from experiences or experiments.[23] The theory argues that because change is a characteristic common to everything in life, success is the only reliable judge of any theory or truth; anything that is true can be proved. Success in social relations is important. The philosophy emphasizes societal living and preparing people to take their places in a harmonious society.

The basic pragmatic educational tenet comes from John Dewey, who advocated learning by doing or gaining knowledge through experience. At the same time, the emphasis is on the student rather than the subject area; each person is a bit different, so not all students should be forced into the same mold. Problem solving (experience) is the basic educational method, and the ultimate judgments are made in terms of a person becoming a productive member of society. The need is to develop the total person—mind, body, and soul—using a very broad process.

According to the pragmatic view of physical education, physical activities have social value because they help integrate students into society by teaching them how to act and react with other people. The curriculum is based on the needs and interests of the students and offers a variety of activities for a multitude of experiences. The problem-solving method is used even in physical education. The teacher tries to motivate the individual student, rather than rely on a standardized program.

Pragmatism is a practical approach to education that breaks down the distinctions between life in and out of school. It encourages people to cooperate by using a broad program based essentially on whatever works. Physical education has broad social uses and is important in pragmatism. However, pragmatism's experimental approach to education is difficult to apply to physical education because the end result may be an unmanageable multitude of goals. The pragmatic philosophy of education has no fixed aims or values. It does not provide the stability and direction needed by many students.[24]

Existentialism

Some people argue over whether or not existentialism is a philosophy because its basic concern is the individual. Everything is judged in terms of the individual, who interprets experiences and develops a personal system of values. The person is more important than society, and whether an individual fits into society is not an issue. Because an existentialist believes nothing can be done to change things, existentialism is often considered a negative, hopeless philosophy.

Butler maintains that no one has tried to apply existentialism formally to either education or physical education.[25] However, the implications of the philosophy on education can be surmised. From an existential viewpoint, education would be viewed as a process of learning about oneself and of developing one's own beliefs. The school would provide only a learning environment. The student would control the curriculum and methods, with the teacher acting as a stimulator. Responsibility toward oneself, rather than toward others or society, would be encouraged. Students would be made aware that they have to bear full responsibility for the consequences of their decisions.

In physical education, existentialism would allow freedom of choice within the program. This might take any form and therefore could not be planned ahead by the teacher. A wide variety of activities would result in the development of

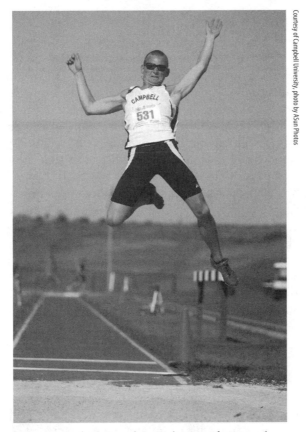

Courtesy of Campbell University, photo by ASun Photos

Many people enjoy the aesthetics of sport, the beauty of the movements, even as they enjoy the feeling of accomplishment as their skills improve.

creativity. The teacher would act as a counselor by pointing out the various available activities, and ultimately the students would be responsible for selecting the activities in which to participate.

Based on these suppositions, the philosophy would appear to have only one real strength: Individuality makes each student very important. Each person has a status not granted by any other philosophy because the existentialist educational process revolves totally around each student's personal needs and wishes. This apparent strength is also its greatest weakness because the importance each student would be accorded in the school community could never be realized in the outside society. As a result, a student would not be prepared to work within the social system. The suggestion that society is unnecessary is an approach better suited to anarchy. The overriding flaw of absolute individualism makes existentialism seem an unlikely choice as the sole basis of a successful mass education program.

Humanistic Approach to Education

Earle Zeigler defines humanism as "a position in which concern for man's welfare is central; [it] stresses the importance of man in working out his own destiny." Bucher gets closer to the heart of the educational concept of humanism, defining it as "a revolt against depersonalization and . . . the emergence of the belief that every human being is an individual and should be treated as an individual rather than as part of a larger group." Reuben Frost speaks of the necessary "humanization of education."[26] In contrast, the expansion of technology into education emphasizes the impersonal, non-humanistic direction that may be the future of mass society.

The humanistic approach to education attempts to counter the effects of the impersonal aspects of our crowded society by trying to show concern for every person. It encourages the involvement of everyone, not just some of the members of the group, in the educational process.

The humanistic approach does not try to make each person the center of everything in education. It is simply an effort to ensure that each person retains a personal identity in society. The approach tries both to maximize students' potential contributions to society and to develop maximum student self-respect. Physical education can be part of a more humanistic society because its activities include very close primary contact between individuals and groups.

Eclectic Approach to Philosophy

We have examined the major philosophies and approaches to philosophy that affect our practices in our field and our concepts of it. Each student must develop a personal philosophy of life, education, and exercise science. The last aspect for the student to consider is the eclectic approach to philosophy. Zeigler defines eclecticism as "the practice of combining a variety of theories from different philosophical schools into a body of fairly compatible beliefs."[27]

We can think of the eclectic approach as a supermarket, or pick-and-choose evolution of a personal philosophy. Each student gradually constructs a personal philosophy that has elements of several different philosophies. Zeigler suggests that the eclectic approach is an immature stage in the development of a philosophy. However, this approach is very common among educators because few of us are philosophers.

Doing Philosophy in Our Field

Why Have a Personal Philosophy?

You might wonder why you need to have a personal philosophy. What does it matter? What purposes would it serve? Elwood Davis and Donna Miller have made several observations regarding the value of having a philosophy and the functions it can serve.[28]

A Common Language

The development of a personal philosophy around common philosophical ideas helps members of a field to develop a common bond. We are facing what C. P. Snow referred to as the "two cultures"; the sciences and the arts or humanities are gradually growing farther apart and losing their former sense of a common tie.[29] A common language is needed to tie all the diverse educational areas together, and the most common bond can be found in philosophy. Further, the development of the theoretical and philosophical areas of disciplines and professions helps greatly to explain the fields to the public, in addition to increasing public acceptance.

Professions Move Beyond Isolated Concerns

We need to work more to show that our field contributes to society and its values in broad terms. Our field has traditionally been concerned with short-term, practical goals rather than the study of our contribution to culture as a whole. In essence, we are moving in this direction as we begin to expand the scope of our study of traditional physical education and sport to include fields such as philosophy, sociology, psychology, anthropology, and history. The field is undergoing a necessary diversification as it seeks to broaden its area of interest beyond its earlier narrow concern with limited aspects of exercise and hygiene.

Highlighted Professional Purpose

As we begin to develop our individual philosophies, we gradually begin to clarify our vision of the purposes of our field. People will work more to fill the needs that they see as areas where our field can make a vital contribution. Davis and Miller suggest that one reason for the low quality of many past programs designed to prepare physical educators was that no basic purpose or purposes of the programs had been developed either by the institutions or physical educators as a body. As personal philosophies develop, major purposes should clarify themselves in the minds of educators.

Examination of Basic Assumptions

Simply put, as philosophical studies are pursued and personal philosophies are developed, the basic assumptions, principles, or theories on which our professional practices have been based can be examined more closely. Often we fail to look at accepted theories and practices to see whether they still stand up before the light of current knowledge and experimentation. If ideas are no longer in line with the present state of knowledge, the pursuit of philosophical studies is likely to expose the problem. It is hoped that such an examination would result in the development of new theories or the discovery of new principles and thus lead to an improvement in the theory and practice of our field.

Self-Examination and Independent Work

As students become educated, they must learn to expand the horizons of their minds by seeking to develop their own minds and ideas rather than depending wholly on learning the ideas and theories of other people, as is common in most current systems of education. Students must learn to look inward, to look at themselves for more answers. The process of education that begins with the examination of what earlier students have learned must be carried to a logical extension as students try to go beyond what earlier students were able to learn. The desire to take part in creative, independent work throughout the professional life should be a natural outgrowth of the development of a personal philosophy.

The Levels of Discussion

One can get some idea of where philosophy fits into the search for knowledge by looking at the four levels of discussion that Harry S. Broudy uses in solving educational problems: (1) the emotional level, (2) the factual level, (3) the theoretical level, and (4) the philosophical level.[30] They are presented in order from the lowest, or least reliable, level to the highest, or most reliable, level.

The lowest level of discussion is the *emotional*, or uncritical, level. At this level, people are usually giving arguments or ideas based only on their personal experiences, which may be quite limited. The arguments are based primarily on feelings or personal prejudices, with little or no thought given to whether further study proves the views to be reasonably accurate. Only personal opinion is used at this level.

A more objective level of discussion is the *factual*, or informational, level. At this level, people seek facts to prove their arguments or make their points. Opinions cannot stand unless factual support can be provided at this level, but there are still inherent weaknesses in the factual level of discussion. Much depends on which facts are used and which are not, as well as how the facts that are used are interpreted.

A third level of discussion, a step higher than the factual level, is the *theoretical*, or explanatory, level. In this case, the facts that have been gathered are organized as proof of a more general theory that is more broadly applicable: For example, facts proved by research on teaching methods can suggest a theory on how to teach.

The fourth and highest level is the *philosophical* level of discussion; the issue has gone beyond the level of facts and theories to become concerned with questions of a more general and philosophical nature about the values, uses, and outcomes of the problem. This level is difficult to reach with satisfactory results, because philosophy goes beyond the provable and into the eternal truths of what is real and what is right.

The Hierarchy of Philosophical Ideas

It is also important to be acquainted with the hierarchy of philosophical ideas.[31] Essentially, they proceed from the lowest level of idea, which is any person's opinion, to the highest level of idea, which is that of a law.

Davis and Miller move first from the level of *anyone's opinion*, which may or may not be valid, up to the level of *authoritative opinion*, the views of people considered to be at least a little bit informed about the area being studied. One level higher is the *agreement of experts*, which is a higher form of opinion, and which is topped by the next level of *proven facts*. Facts are one step removed from the experts' agreement because we have moved from *opinions* of what is true to *proof* of what is true.

As one gets closer to the philosophical areas of concern, according to Davis and Miller, one moves toward *hypothesis*, which is a low-level generalization. Generalizing aims to take a small number of facts and explain them or show where they are leading. The hypothesis is a step beyond the fact because it tries to suggest which direction should be taken in seeking more facts or in learning more about a question.

A *theory* is one step beyond the hypothesis; it tries to determine something that is more probable or more likely to be true than the hypothesis, which is considered to be only a low probability of truth. The theory often has one or more hypotheses that have been shown to be true, but it will have others that are not yet proved. Thus, a theory is an attempt to explain some phenomenon or occurrence, but the attempted theory has not yet been completely proved true.

A *principle* is higher than a theory in philosophy; it is a fundamental, proven truth and the result of philosophical thought. A principle is a generalization based on facts and determined and proved through the philosophical process.

The highest level, however, is the *law*, which is "a generalization of wide application and high probability."[32] The law describes relationships that are always present, by saying that if certain conditions are present, such-and-such will always be the result. The laws that have been determined are the bedrock of knowledge because everything else, including the process of seeking more or higher knowledge, is built on the foundation of the laws that have been determined.

Thought and the Philosophical Process

Philosophy is often thought of as being related only to the mind, a purely mental or thought process. To see how to use philosophy, one needs to understand how to use the thinking processes. In discussing the part thinking plays in the philosophical process, Davis and Miller present five necessary aspects of the satisfactory use of the thinking processes in philosophy:[33]

1. They first refer to *intelligent striving*, that is, applying intelligent thought over time. The philosophical process is not a short one. Evaluation and reevaluation of ideas are constant necessities. The philosopher must never quit attacking a problem simply because it appears to defy analysis or understanding but must continue to make the effort to understand and clarify the questions of philosophy.

2. The philosopher must also *meet the challenge*. A challenge provides a goal or purpose for philosophical inquiry. Just as we need goals or challenges to make life meaningful and enjoyable, we need challenges in philosophy because the mind expands when faced by such challenges.

3. The *ability to discriminate* is also vitally necessary. A student of philosophy needs to be able to evaluate the relative worth of ideas and theories because they are not all of equal importance. Unless we can discriminate in judging issues and problems, we may waste much time on questions or problems of little importance and thus become slaves to the philosophical version of busywork.

4. Philosophers must be *able to draw reasonable generalizations*. They must be able to determine when they have enough information to defend their conclusions as being reasonable. Too often, one can see situations where leaders accept ideas that have not been proved and then develop ideas or programs that are of questionable value because they were based on premature assumptions.

5. Finally, *generalizations should be studied carefully*. A generalization should not be accepted as proven without considerable study by a number of people. Instead, we should consider generalizations to be tentative answers and subject to further study. Just as people may fail to draw reasonable generalizations, so they may also fail to study those generalizations enough to see whether they are really justified.

The Philosopher's Basic Questions

We can look at the *doing* of philosophy in terms of the types of questions that are asked. Scott Kretchmar suggests five questions, each dealing with a branch of philosophy:[34]

1. Questions having to do with the nature of things (metaphysics)
2. Questions having to do with what people know (epistemology)
3. Questions having to do with the value of things (axiology)

4. Questions having to do with good behavior (ethics)

5. Questions having to do with what is beautiful (aesthetics)

In asking those questions on the *doing* of philosophy, we must understand that, just as in sport training, we may gain as much from the philosophical process as from the knowledge or understanding that results from it. Kretchmar writes that "philosophy is valuable not only for the theories and propositions it produces but also for the thinking skills it requires." He goes on to explain:

> *The philosophic process is the art and science of wondering about reality, posing questions related to that wonder, and pursuing answers to those questions reflectively. It is an art and a science because the philosophic skills of wondering, posing questions, and searching for answers are grounded partly on repeatable methods that can be objectified and explained (science) and partly on intuitions, tendencies, and flashes of insight that can neither be fully predicted nor accounted for (art).*[35]

The question of method in philosophical studies is often confusing to the beginner. Ultimately, any philosophical question is subjective; empirical research is not possible because the phenomena are not observable. Indeed, Harold VanderZwaag and Thomas Sheehan state that "there is no common methodology for sport philosophers" primarily because of the highly individual nature of the process, although they do suggest that analysis and synthesis are the "two pillars of integrity" in philosophical research.[36]

Kretchmar writes of three analytical or reasoning techniques of philosophers: induction, intuition, and deduction.[37] *Inductive reasoning* is based on going from the specific to the general, that is, taking a specific situation or fact and drawing more general conclusions about it. *Intuitive reasoning* is based on being able to recognize a situation or fact and describe it without gathering further information. With intuitive reasoning, you can create and analyze situations in your mind. *Deductive reasoning* is based on going from the general to the specific; that is, taking a broad principle and trying to develop more specific information or guidelines from it.

The three basic approaches to philosophical study are *speculative* (suggesting possible answers to a question), *normative* (suggesting guidelines or norms), and *analytical* (evaluating the ideas of others). The areas or methods of philosophical study are as follows:

1. The historical background study

2. The varied interpretation method

3. The value judgment

4. Clarifying the main issues

5. Determining relationships to similar concepts

The philosophical and scientific research methods in organizing research studies are very similar. However, one needs to look at several other research methods to provide a broader exposure to the many possible approaches to philosophy. Kathleen Pearson suggests two research approaches that can be used as part of a brief self-study program.[38] The first is called the *goodness-of-fit approach* because it is similar to the statistical study that compares how closely two statistical models agree. In this case, the researcher takes a suggested paradigm or model (such as those for the relationships of play, games, sport, and athletics) and determines whether another example actually conforms to the suggested one. The second method is the *implications approach*, in which the researcher studies what something would be like if it did conform to a given model or what the implications of such a condition would be.

Robert Osterhoudt suggests that the basic method used in philosophical studies is a systematic "dialectic," or dialogue, of either of two types: speculative or critical. He believes that both types are valuable because "without the speculative, philosophy would be reduced to logic [and] without the critical, [philosophy would be reduced] to poetry. Philosophy is wholly neither."[39]

Seymour Kleinman has argued against the idea of developing a correct theory of sport.[40] He suggests that theories put structure and limits on sport that close it to anything beyond its imposed bounds, whereas sport demands openness. Kleinman discusses three methods of theorizing: formal description, logical description, and phenomenological description. *Formal description* relates the properties or characteristics of a phenomenon; *logical description* studies how a term is used in the language; and *phenomenological description* studies the experience itself. The latter method is Kleinman's preference because it concentrates on the phenomenon as it actually happens, without limits. As Osterhoudt puts it, phenomenology's method is "pure subjective consciousness." Osterhoudt also notes, however, that phenomenology does not look into many aspects of life that need to be examined, so in some respects it is not as free of "unreflective assumptions" as it supposes.[41]

How Do We Apply Philosophy in Our Field?

Philosophy is a vital part of our programs because it is a major influence on the early stages of program planning. **Figure 8.2** roughly illustrates the steps leading from what we already know (facts) through what we theorize and believe (our personal philosophy), through the various stages of development until we arrive at the actual policies and procedures that we will use in administering a physical education program.

At the lowest level are *facts*, or the base of information that has been conclusively proved. If there is no base of proven fact at the root of a physical education program, the program simply is an experimental vehicle of questionable value. With increasing demand for accountability, the program's chances of success are slight.

We next *apply our personal philosophy* to the facts at hand. In essence, we take what we know and add to it what we believe. This determines fundamental

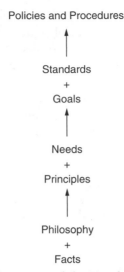

Policies and Procedures

↑

Standards

+

Goals

↑

Needs

+

Principles

↑

Philosophy

+

Facts

Figure 8.2 The Developmental Process of the Total Physical Education Program

principles on which we will base our program. Webster has defined *principle* as "a fundamental truth or cause . . . which serves as a guide for conduct and procedure . . . a guide which is used in the attainment of an aim or objective."[42] Principles are viewed as fundamental laws, although they are closer to universally accepted hypotheses or theories because principles *can* change.

When the principles have been determined, the next step is to ascertain the *needs of the program*. Blending the needs of the program with the principles that are involved produces the *goals* of the program.

The goals may include a number of closely related aims and objectives, which are simply more specific aspects of the overall program goals. They may be expressed in terms of gaining or developing knowledge (cognitive goals); attitudes, appreciations, and a sense of values (affective goals); and skills (primarily psychomotor goals in physical education).

When the goals have been determined, the *standards to evaluate the goals* must be developed. The standards are evaluative criteria that set the level of the desired outcomes. For example, how thoroughly must a skill be developed to satisfy the goals of the program?

The program is administered by the *policies and procedures* that result from the combination of desired goals and suggested standards for the program. The policies and procedures state how the actual program will be run in terms of administration, requirements, and application of the curriculum.

At the heart of the entire physical education program is its philosophy because it enters the planning process at the earliest stages and thus determines the areas that will be emphasized within a particular program. Because of the crucial part philosophy plays, the personal philosophy of each person involved should be clearly thought out. Philosophy's ultimate effect on the program is considerable.

This chapter attempts to explain the *why* of philosophy, rather than the *what*. Although it discusses briefly the process of philosophy, its primary focus is on its value to physical educators, or how it is studied. In an age of scientific advancements, we tend to forget the importance of things that cannot be tested against concrete facts.

Many scientists today have misgivings about the application of their discoveries and have become interested in philosophy. Scientists developed theories that led to the first nuclear weapons, but with it came the debate over the *morality* of such weapons. Do human beings have a moral right to develop such weapons or use them? These questions cannot be answered with simple facts.

These types of questions have shown repeatedly that although we are moving toward the two cultures of C. P. Snow, both cultures are still tied to the realm of philosophy. Unanswerable or untestable questions exist in every discipline and field of learning, and if answers to such increasingly difficult questions are to be found, all fields of learning must be familiar with the nature and uses of philosophy. The concept of the ultimate value of all learning will come to us from our studies in philosophy, not solely from those in our separate fields.

This chapter has discussed the meaning and use of philosophies, as well as their basic teachings regarding our field. Think about what your own personal philosophy of our field will be when you lead the life of a physical educator, exercise or sport scientist, or kinesiologist.

Summary

This chapter examines four areas that explain the need to understand philosophy and its uses: (1) the definition and application of philosophy in our field, (2) the area of sport philosophy, (3) the major philosophical teachings, and (4) how you can incorporate philosophy into physical education and sport. One scholar defines philosophy as (1) a study of the truth or the principles underlying all knowledge, (2) a study of the most general causes and principles of the universe, and (3) a system for guiding life.

The major branches of philosophy are metaphysics (the nature of reality and being), epistemology (the study of the theory of knowledge), logic (the study of the relationship of ideas to one another), and axiology (the study of the nature and kinds of values, including two major subareas: ethics and aesthetics).

Some of the major questions of philosophy are (1) the nature of the universe, (2) people's place in the universe, (3) the determination of good and evil, (4) the nature of God, (5) the soul and immortality, (6) people's relationship to the state, (7) the role of education, (8) the relationship between mind and matter, and (9) the implications of philosophy for physical education.

Some of the issues studied by sport philosophers include (1) the nature of sport, (2) sport and metaphysical speculation, (3) the body and being, (4) sport as a meaningful experience, (5) sport versus physical education: philosophical conflicts, (6) sport and aesthetics, (7) sport and values, and (8) the concept of fair play and sportsmanship.

The philosophies most studied in relationship to exercise science are (1) naturalism, (2) idealism, (3) realism, (4) pragmatism, (5) existentialism, and (6) humanism. Practitioners often take a less mature eclectic approach to philosophy.

The philosopher's basic questions have to do with (1) the nature of things (metaphysics), (2) what people know (epistemology), (3) the value of things (axiology), (4) good behavior (ethics), and (5) what is beautiful (aesthetics).

The three basic approaches to philosophical study are speculative (suggesting possible answers to a question), normative (suggesting guidelines or norms), and analytical (evaluating the ideas of others). The areas or methods of philosophical study are (1) the historical background study, (2) the varied interpretation method, (3) the value judgment, (4) clarifying the main issues, and (5) determining relationships to similar concepts.

Further Readings

Anderson, Doug. 2001. Recovering humanity: Movement, sport, and nature. *Journal of the Philosophy of Sport* 28: 140–150.

Arnold, Peter J. 1979. *Meaning in movement, sport and physical education*. London: Heinemann.

———. 1992. Sport as a valued human practice: A basis for the consideration of moral issues in sport. *Journal of the Philosophy of Education* 26: 237–255.

Booth, Douglas. 2009. Politics and pleasure: The philosophy of physical education revisited. *Quest* 61: 133–153.

Brown, W. Miller. 2009. The case for perfection. *Journal of the Philosophy of Sport* 36: 127–139.

Cavallini, M. Felicia. 2006. Who needs philosophy in physical education? *JOPERD (Journal of Physical Education, Recreation and Dance)* 77 (8): 28–30.

Coetzee, N. A. J. 1994. In search of a founded epistemology for human movement science. *International Journal of Physical Education* 31: 8–17.

DeSensi, Joy T. 1996. Virtue, knowledge, and wisdom: Proclaiming the personal meanings of movement. *Quest* 48: 518–530.

Estes, Steven G., and Robert A. Mechikoff. 1998. *Knowing human movement*. Boston: Allyn and Bacon.

Fahlberg, Larry L., and Lauri A. Fahlberg. 1994. A human science for the study of movement: An integration of multiple ways of knowing. *Research Quarterly for Exercise and Sport* 65: 100–109.

Fraleigh, Warren P. 1984. *Right actions in sport: Ethics for contestants*. Champaign, IL: Human Kinetics.

Gumbrecht, Hans Ulrich, 2006. *In praise of athletic beauty*. Cambridge, MA: Belknap Press of Harvard Univ. Press.

Hochstetler, Douglas R. 2003. Process and the sport experience. *Quest* 55: 231–243.

Holowchak, M. Andrew, & Heather L. Reid. 2011. *Aretism: An ancient sports philosophy for the modern sports world*. Lanham, MD: Lexington Books.

Hopsicker, Peter. 2011. In search of the "sporting genius": Exploring the benchmarks to creative behavior in sporting activity. *Journal of the Philosophy of Sport* 38: 113–127.

Kretchmar, R. Scott. 2005. *Practical philosophy of sport and physical activity*. 2nd ed. Champaign, IL: Human Kinetics.

Lodewyk, Ken, Chunlei Lu, and Jeanne Kentel. 2009. Enacting the spiritual dimension in physical education. *Physical Educator* 66: 170–179.

Loland, Sigmund. 2012. A well balanced life based on "the joy of effort": Olympic hype or meaningful ideal? *Sport, Ethics and Philosophy* 6: 155–165.

Lu, Chunlei, Johanna M. Tito, and Jeanne A. Kentel. 2009. Eastern movement disciplines and mindfulness: A new path to subjective knowledge in Western physical education. *Quest* 61: 353–370.

McFee, Graham. 2012. Olympism and sport's intrinsic value. *Sport, Ethics and Philosophy* 6: 211–231.

Mechikoff, Robert A. 2010. *A history and philosophy of sport and physical education*. 5th ed. Boston: McGraw-Hill.

Meier, Klaus V. 1991. Philosophical anorexia. *Quest* 43: 55–65.

Morgan, William J. 2006. *Why sports morally matter*. New York: Routledge.

———. 2010. Sport, wholehearted engagement and the good life. *Sport, Ethics and Philosophy* 4: 229–253.

Osterhoudt, Robert G. 2006. *Sport as form of human fulfillment: An organic philosophy of sport history*. Victoria, BC, Canada: Trafford.

Parry, Jim, Simon Robinson, Nick Watson, and Mark Nesti. 2007. *Sport and spirituality: An introduction*. London: Routledge.

Reid, Heather. 2002. *The philosophical athlete*. Durham, NC: Carolina Academic Press.

———. 2012. *Athletics and philosophy in the ancient world: Contests of virtue*. New York: Routledge.

———. 2012. *Introduction to the philosophy of sport*. Lanham, MD: Rowman and Littlefield.

Reid, Heather, and Michael W. Austin, eds. 2012. *The Olympics and philosophy*. Lexington, KY: Univ. of Kentucky Press.

Ryall, Emily. 2009. *Critical thinking for sports students*. London: Leaning Matters/Sage.

Stoll, Sharon Kay, and Allison Mathews. 2000. I play, therefore I am. *JOPERD (Journal of Physical Education, Recreation and Dance)* 71 (9): 50–55.

Thomas, Carolyn E. 1983. Thoughts on the moral relationship of intent and training in sport. *Journal of the Philosophy of Sport* 10: 84–91.

Twietmeyer, Gregg. 2010. Kinesis and the nature of the human person. *Quest* 62: 135–154.

Weiss, Paul. 1969. *Sport: A philosophic inquiry*. Carbondale, IL: Southern Illinois Univ. Press.

Zeigler, Earle F. 1994. *Critical thinking for the professions of health, sport and physical education, recreation, and dance*. Champaign, IL: Stipes.

———. 2012. *"Finding one's self" in sport and physical activity*. Victoria, BC, Canada: Trafford.

Discussion Questions

1. Discuss the value and use of a personal philosophy.

2. Discuss the following statement: Science studies what can be proven, while philosophy studies what cannot be proven.

3. Briefly define and explain three of the following branches of philosophy:
    a. Metaphysics
    b. Axiology
    c. Epistemology
    d. Logic
    e. Ethics
    f. Aesthetics

4. Give and discuss three of the questions or concerns of philosophy suggested by Baley and Field.

5. Compare and contrast the ideas on education and physical education of two of the following philosophies:
    a. Naturalism
    b. Idealism
    c. Realism
    d. Pragmatism
    e. Existentialism

6. Briefly discuss the strengths and weaknesses of two of the following philosophies:
    a. Naturalism
    b. Idealism
    c. Realism
    d. Pragmatism
    e. Existentialism

7. Briefly explain three of the following areas or methods of philosophical study:
    a. Historical background
    b. Varied interpretation
    c. Value judgments
    d. Clarifying the main issues
    e. Relationship of similar concepts

References

1. Barrow, Harold M. 1971. *Man and his movement: Principles of his physical education.* Philadelphia: Lea and Febiger, 18.

2. Webster, Randolph W. 1965. *Philosophy of physical education.* Dubuque, IA: Brown, 3–4.

3. Davis, Elwood Craig, and Donna M. Miller. 1967. *The philosophic process in physical education.* 2nd ed. Philadelphia: Lea and Febiger, 23–29.

4. Zeigler, Earle F. 1964. *Philosophical foundations for physical, health, and recreation education.* Englewood Cliffs, NJ: Prentice Hall, 22.

5. Baley, James A., and David A. Field. 1976. *Physical education and the physical educator.* 2nd ed. Boston: Allyn and Bacon, 227–232.

6. Ibid., 231.

7. Gerber, Ellen W., and William J. Morgan, eds. 1979. *Sport and the body: A philosophical symposium.* 2nd ed. Philadelphia: Lea and Febiger, 1–3.

8. McBride, Frank. 1979. Toward a non-definition of sport. In *Sport and the body: A philosophical symposium*, 2nd ed., ed. Ellen W. Gerber and William J. Morgan, 48–52. Philadelphia: Lea and Febiger.

9. Gerber and Morgan, *Sport and the body*, 69–72.

10. Ibid., 71.

11. Ibid., 145–147.

12. Ibid., 201–203.

13. Ibid., 201.

14. Ravizza, Kenneth. 1979. Raising the consciousness of the human movement experience. In *A self-study guide for the philosophy of sport and physical education*, 20. Brockport, NY: Sport Philosophy Academy.

15. Harper, William A., and Elwood Craig Davis. 1977. *The philosophic process in physical education.* 3rd ed. Philadelphia: Lea and Febiger, 250–259.

16. Gerber and Morgan, *Sport and the body*, 315–317.

17. Arnold, Peter J. 1979. *Meaning in movement, sport and physical education.* London: Heinemann, 120–161.

18. Lowe, Benjamin. 1977. *The beauty of sport: A cross-disciplinary inquiry.* Englewood Cliffs, NJ: Prentice Hall.

19. Oberteuffer, Delbert. 1963. On learning values through sport. *Quest* 1 (December): 23–29; Harper and Davis, *Philosophic process*, 231–238; Keating, James W. 1978. *Competition and playful activities.* Washington, DC: Univ. Press of America, 39–53; and McIntosh, Peter. 1979. *Fair play: Ethics in sport and education.* London: Heinemann.

20. Zeigler, *Philosophical foundations*, 65–66.

21. Ibid., 241–244.

22. Ibid., 162–164.

23. Ibid., 69.

24. Ibid., 109–110.

25. Butler, J. Donald. 1968. *Four philosophies and their practice in education and religion.* 3rd ed. New York: Harper and Row, 462.

26. Zeigler, *Philosophical foundations*, 320; Bucher, Charles A. 1979. *Foundations of physical education.* 8th ed. St. Louis, MO: Mosby, 37; and Frost, Reuben B. 1975. *Physical education: Foundations, practices, principles.* Reading, MA: Addison-Wesley, 24.

27. Zeigler, *Philosophical foundations*, 319.

28. Davis, Elwood Craig, and Donna M. Miller. 1967. *The philosophic process in physical education.* 2nd ed. Philadelphia: Lea and Febiger, 169–176.

29. Snow, C. P. 1960. *The two cultures and the scientific revolution.* Cambridge: Cambridge Univ. Press.

30. Broudy, Harry S. 1954. *Building a philosophy of education.* Englewood Cliffs, NJ: Prentice Hall, 20–24.

31. Davis and Miller, *Philosophic process*, 181–183.

32. Ibid., 182.

33. Ibid., 217–220.

34. Kretchmar, R. Scott. 1994. *Practical philosophy of sport*. Champaign, IL: Human Kinetics, 16–17.

35. Ibid., 1, 4–5.

36. VanderZwaag, Harold J., and Thomas J. Sheehan. 1978. *Introduction to sport studies: From the classroom to the ball park*. Dubuque, IA: Brown, 142.

37. Kretchmar, *Practical philosophy*, 19–25.

38. Pearson, Kathleen. 1979. A self-study guide: Two approaches to doing philosophy of sport and physical education. In *A self-study guide for the philosophy of sport and physical education*, 10–18. Brockport, NY: Sport Philosophy Academy.

39. Osterhoudt, Robert G. 1978. *An introduction to the philosophy of physical education and sport*. Champaign, IL: Stipes, 8–9.

40. Kleinman, Seymour. 1968. Toward a non-theory of sport. *Quest* 10: 29–34.

41. Osterhoudt, *Introduction to the philosophy*, 96–97.

42. Webster, *Philosophy of physical education*, 148.

Ethics and Problems in Exercise Science, Physical Education, and Sport

9

Ethics is concerned with morals and conduct; that is, with determining proper rules of behavior. It is a study of ideal conduct and of the knowledge of good and evil. It examines which actions are right and which are wrong, and what people should and should not do. It is an important concern for our field because we deal in human behavior—how it is shaped, how it shows itself, and all the shades of good and bad conduct that appear.

Because physical educators have argued that sport can develop character, one must understand what it is and why it is important. As Scott Kretchmar writes:

> *Ethics most fundamentally is about seeking and promoting the good life—about finding out what it is, celebrating it, and keeping it in focus. It is about preserving values like truth, knowledge, excellence, friendship, excitement, and any number of other good things.*
>
> > *Ethics is also about compassion and sympathy—about making sure that the good life is shared with others who inhabit this planet with us. It is about caring for others, particularly those who do not have the position or power necessary to protect themselves or have their way.*[1]

David Shields and Brenda Bredemeier describe character in terms of four virtues that a person of good character displays: compassion, fairness, sportsmanship, and integrity. With compassion, "players can be encouraged to see competitors as coparticipants, equally valuable, equally deserving of regard. . . . Fairness involves evenhandedness, equal consideration." Sportsmanship "involves an intense striving to succeed, tempered by commitment to a 'play spirit,' such that ethical standards will take precedence over strategic gain when the two conflict." Finally, "integrity enables one to act on one's convictions, even if such action is negatively received by a coach, teammates, or fans."[2]

No field is without problems, but the problems encountered in our field can be particularly difficult. In many cases, people find themselves caught in ethical dilemmas, unsure as to what is the best or most proper thing to do. As Hubert Doucet notes, "Sports and ethics have always been in a dialogue."[3] He adds that one must understand sport in the context of a technological society because the potential for abuse is much greater. Gunter Gebauer warns that we often make the mistake of interpreting ethics by ambiguous and constantly changing standards, usually in terms of the past (such as chivalry).[4] This chapter looks first at some current problems in our field, then turns to a discussion of ethics in physical education and sport, although the emphasis is on the sport setting.

Problems in Exercise Science, Physical Education, and Sport Today

Problems in sport affect our field. The public views the two areas as one, and many American coaches work in physical education departments. Sport has changed considerably over the years. Both media coverage and financial investments have risen sharply. At the highest levels of competition, athletics can become almost a full-time job. Are such requirements by coaches or colleges ethical, even with scholarships? Here is an overview of the problems and risks of one popular sport, football:

> "I wanted to be the starting quarterback and a Phi Beta Kappa at the same time. . . ." He became both [with] a double major in economics and psychology. . . . When he talks of his decision to quit football you hear tones of frustration about how college sports can practically consume the lives of the young athletes who play them.
>
> "For me it was 12 months a year. . . . You never really got to stop. . . . When you come to college, it becomes such a regimented program. It's a job."
>
> As a football player [he] had to eat breakfast every morning by 8. . . . He had to finish all his classes by 1 p.m. in order to eat lunch at 1:15 at a players' "training table." Next came meetings with coaches, film-watching sessions and scouting reports. At 3:30 his ankles were taped for practice, which lasted until 6:30. After that he had to lift weights and shower. Between 7:30 and 8:30 it was back to the training table for dinner.
>
> "For those 12 hours you haven't been able to study," [he] says. "You're starting out at 9 o'clock at night, worn out from the day you've been through. . . ."
>
> [He] frequently studied until 3 or 4 a.m. During one season he lost 15 pounds and had to have nutrients injected intravenously the day before games to have enough stamina to play.
>
> [Though he] started at quarterback for two years . . . he has decided to follow his academic interests, which he hopes will lead him to graduate studies in business and maybe a Rhodes scholarship. . . .

*"I think my potential in other areas is better than my potential
in pro football," [he] says. "The bottom line is your potential in life,
getting where you want to in life."*[5]

This example of what it is like to play football at a high level can be seen
in many other sports. Academic success and the enjoyment of college life are
not the only things at risk. A note on *the football knee* points out that 70% of
professional football players have knee surgery by age 26 years, 50% of all running backs require knee surgery, and 50,000 pieces of knee cartilage are removed
annually from football players by American surgeons.[6] This has also been a serious problem for women basketball players.

Physical risks also reach into the aftereffects of some of the more questionable training procedures in sports. Those procedures include the use of steroids
and human growth hormone, blood replacement techniques (blood doping), the
use of erythropoietin (EPO), designer drugs, so-called nutritional supplements
that mimic steroids, and even gene doping. Increased training loads add the risk
of long-term physical damage from overuse syndrome, the extreme repetition of
stressful physical movements. This can leave injuries such as carpal tunnel syndrome or back, hip, knee, and ankle damage that remain permanently when the
playing days are over. The risks reach into every modern sport; football is only
one prominent example. This chapter looks briefly at four areas of problems or
concerns in physical education and sport today.

Abuses of Sport

The first area of concern centers on the abuses in sport. Dudley Sargent lists them:
direct or indirect payments to students for athletic services, encouragement of
students to move from college to college for athletic purposes, lack of faculty
control in games and grounds, coaches of questionable morals and influence, and
bad moral effects of games when rules are broken or evaded.[7] Those abuses, inci-
dentally, were the subjects of a complaint made in 1903. Thus, while the abuses
of sport may be more intricate today, they are not new. Indeed, they were present
at Olympia 2500 years ago.

Educators need to show leadership in this area, but there has been only limited interest in a massive investigation such as the one conducted by the Carnegie
Foundation in the 1920s. The Hanford Report in the 1970s called for changes,
and the Knight Foundation Commission of the late 1980s and early 1990s acted
as an independent call for greater responsibility in school sports. A focus is growing on the long-term abuses of college sports. The mushrooming evidence of large-
scale drug abuse, ranging from narcotics to steroids to prescription medicines,
shows the need for a major study of what we are and should be doing in sports.[8]

Many Americans were shocked early in 1985 when they learned that Olympic cycling medalists from the United States admitted to blood doping before
their competition. A magazine article stated that eight cyclists blood doped either
before the U.S. Olympic Trials or before the Games themselves.[9] In addition,

86 American athletes in other sports failed drug tests given by the U.S. Olympic Committee in the 9 months before the 1984 Games.

The same magazine issue gave an account of how the sudden death (from natural causes) of a Dutch runner at an American university led to the accidental discovery of the widespread use of illegally obtained prescription drugs by college athletes, supplied by college coaches and others. Several coaches were eventually fired, but the case is only the tip of the iceberg. The 1998 Tour de France was almost destroyed by a major drug scandal among the cyclists. The response of the cyclists was that the officials were being unfair to test them.[10] Many athletes have too little faith in their ability to reach the top legally; the drugs they may take can be very dangerous. Indeed, we still know little about the long-term effects of medium and high dosages of drugs such as anabolic steroids because most research studies use only very low dosages.[11]

The overemphasis on winning and success has led to a sports world that is far from clean. Young athletes—and their teachers and coaches—need a well-developed sense of ethics, of right and wrong, to decide which course to pursue as they develop.[12]

Overemphasis on School Sports

A second concern is the overemphasis on sports in the schools.[13] If educators believe that sports make a genuine contribution to the educational process, they should expect them to be important. In many cases, though, sports are overemphasized, that is, not used for lessons, but promoted simply for the victories and fame that can be gained. This problem needs to be considered seriously because it reflects on physical education programs as well.

A prominent example is the Jan Kemp case at the University of Georgia in 1986. Kemp was a remedial English instructor in the Developmental Studies Program. The program was designed to assist students who had been admitted to the university, yet were not academically ready to do college-level work. Such students were expected to pass the remedial-level courses by a certain deadline, or they were removed from the university.

Kemp was dismissed by the university in 1983, but filed a legal suit claiming that she was fired for objecting too strongly to the favorable treatment given to athletes. In early 1986, she won her suit against the university. The jury agreed that the athletes had been treated preferentially, that Kemp was fired because of her objections to the athletes' getting passing grades when they had failed, and that teachers were pressured to give good grades to athletes.[14]

Shortly after the jury decision, the state Board of Regents delayed renewing the university president's contract and he resigned. An audit report by the Board of Regents of the University System of Georgia showed that athletes had been given preferred treatment, under pressure from the athletic department, and with the knowledge of the university's president.[15]

The Georgia case was widely publicized, but similar examples may be found at other colleges and universities in the United States. What do these practices say for the ethical standards maintained by some schools, their administrations, and their coaches, if they develop and encourage a system for using academically unqualified athletes until their eligibility expires, or if they cheat to keep them eligible?

To show that this problem is not isolated, a similar scandal erupted in 1999 when the University of Minnesota was forced to oust its winning men's basketball coach after reporters found that workers for the athletic department had written more than 400 term papers for athletes with poor grades. This scene was unfolding even as questions were raised about questionable academic scheduling to keep Ohio State University's star football player eligible.[16]

The University of North Carolina, ranked among the academic top five public universities in the United States, has been dealing with the fallout of the discovery that many of its football players were remaining eligible for taking courses that had no class meetings and set very low standards for passing, usually requiring only a lightly graded term paper.[17] This has badly hurt the school's reputation as one of the truly "clean" college sports programs.

Why did a massive system of competitive sports in the schools develop in the United States, yet not in the schools of any other country? Does the American concept of mass education have anything to do with it? Other nations have mass public education; is their concept of education different from ours? Did schools in the United States stop being regarded by the public as a place of education, becoming instead a center for youth activities? Did the school become a place for young people to stay busy and play while waiting to grow up and move out into adult society?

Indeed, recent decades have seen increased development of national high school competitions, of school teams that travel across many states for competition, and even the growth of high school basketball academies, private schools known only for their athletes who come from many states and their playing schedules that cross the entire nation.

The state of Texas was the first to try to change the direction of school sports with its no pass, no play policy in 1985. Although it resulted in many athletes losing their places on the teams, it received strong parent and court support.

Marian Kneer suggests that physical education and athletics "need a divorce," that the problems that grew from trying to teach and coach at the same time cannot be solved except by separating the jobs.[18] She argues that the teaching of physical education has been badly damaged, so new answers are needed by the profession. However, if the two are divorced, physical education cannot press for more ethical behavior in athletics.

Overemphasis on Competitive Sports in Physical Education

A third concern is whether competitive sports are overemphasized in the physical education program. Although competitive sports may be overemphasized by less skillful teachers, a good teacher will prepare a well-balanced program that exposes students to all areas of physical activity. Physical educators need to evaluate their programs constantly to ensure that they are providing physical *education*, not simply promoting physical *competition*. This is an area of great professional interest.[19] It is a factor in part because our national focus seems to shift every decade or so, moving from physical fitness to lifetime sports, to elective sports, to aerobic fitness, to wellness-oriented fitness. No consistent pattern exists over the years, other than that the pattern will eventually change.

Relationship Between Physical Education and Sport

The fourth concern is still controversial: What is the relationship between physical education and sport? In the eyes of the public, the two areas are one. The need to share facilities, equipment, and even budgets and faculty causes conflict. Each area is affected by the public reputation of the other. Whether or not physical education and athletics wish to be a single area, they are often forced together by the public. This often has unfortunate effects.[20]

Is Sportsmanship Dead?

Recent decades have shown a disturbing change in the world of sport and in society: an increasing disregard for fair play and the traditional rules of society. We have become accustomed to a sports world where we assume that the most successful athletes cheat, whether by taking illegal drugs or in other ways trying to avoid following the rules that produce fairness in competition.

We cannot be as much concerned with this development in professional athletics, as pervasive an example as it is in our society, because professional teams exist primarily for entertainment. Their only goal is to maximize profit. If the entertainment value of a sport declines, they simply change the rules to make it more entertaining. They try to avoid the development of team excellence with draft systems designed to reward incompetence and failure: The worse your team performs, the better athletes it will be assisted in signing. Again, this is not sport, but simply entertainment of a sport-like nature.

However, we see the same traits in what were once considered amateur (not-for-profit) sports, such as school sports. Increasingly, they have followed the professional model, focusing on victory and increased income. Some universities have spent hundreds of millions of dollars for facilities in an effort to attract athletes, fans, and donors and to maximize their athletic department's income. This is despite the reality that the majority of colleges and universities lose money on sports.

Because Congress and the National Collegiate Athletic Association (NCAA) have required stricter reporting standards on the academic success of athletic programs and the full cost of athletic programs, the results have embarrassed many schools. One major university was cited for having failed to graduate even one male basketball player in 7 years. The highest competitive levels of universities refuse to have a playoff system to determine a national football champion because the traditional bowl system permits many marginally successful teams to have a bowl game, generating far more money for athletic departments than a playoff system would produce. At the highest competitive levels of the NCAA, it is not about sport or character development or opportunity for students: It is all about money.

Understandably, decades of this behavior have affected our sense of ethical behavior in sport. William J. Morgan writes of his concern about the apparent changes in the ethical values of his students over a period of time. He writes:

The present sociology that informs morality in contemporary America imperils the moral life, indeed, makes it difficult for people even to think in moral terms. . . . This story of the decline of moral life is writ large in contemporary American sports. Sports . . . are no mere reflection of larger society's growing indifference to moral considerations but, in part because of their prominent standing in contemporary society, both a conspicuous exemplification of such moral callousness and an important sign of things to come.[21]

In teaching sport ethics to his students, Morgan was concerned that they no longer seemed to have much concern for ethical behavior in their analysis of cases in sports competitions. After analyzing the changes that he had observed, he came to the conclusion that

what had changed was their willingness or capacity (or both) to consider sports from a moral angle. So, instead of considering the effects of their actions on others and on the game itself or, what is the same thing, reversing roles and putting themselves in someone else's shoes, they were playing a cost–benefit language game in which the objective was to further their own preferences and desires. . . . That is, what the students were really saying is that rules should be viewed and treated as egoistic devices, which means that we should follow them when it is in our self-interest to do so and break them when it is not. . . . This brings us back exactly to where we started: the students' unwillingness or incapacity to view sports from a moral vantage point.[22]

This trend, which is also societal, creates a real concern about the survival of our society because it suggests that the society no longer shares a common view of ethical or respectable behavior toward each other. This leads us to an examination of the place of ethics in our field, a look at some reasons why sport has a poor reputation, and some suggestions of what ethical values we should be teaching and learning.

How Does Ethics Relate to Exercise Science, Physical Education, and Sport?

Ethics is a study of ideal conduct and of the knowledge of good and evil. It seeks to determine which actions are right and wrong and which course of action should be taken. The greatest problem in discussing ethical problems is that no single perspective is absolute. Each person may have a different belief about right and wrong, and there are no objective standards by which to judge some issues. For this reason, you need to understand that the ethical standards discussed in this chapter reflect the ethical views of the author.

Ethics is vital to the successful functioning of any society; that is, people must have standards of value by which they live. The development of ethical standards has long been a prominent part of the educational process. The Greeks spoke of the development of character as one of the most vital concerns, if not the most vital concern, of education. Many educational goals were optional, but character was a goal that could never be dropped.

If we agree that we need to develop character, or ethical standards, what does that need have to do with our field? Sport and physical education often are referred to as a laboratory of human experience because there, more than in any other organized area of the educational process, students are likely to show their inner selves. Sport and physical education challenge the student both physically and intellectually, and in the heat of intense competition, a person's true values often show through. One person may be more concerned with fair play, while another may try to win in any possible way. This is the ultimate test of ethical standards, and no other area of educational endeavor is so likely to put the student to the test.

A major difference between physical education and sport is that physical education is concerned with personal outcomes, with learning, with development. Thus, its ethic is different from that of sport, which is concerned with competitive success, rather than the overall improvement of the individual. In physical education, ethical learning has to do with learning what is right, with how to interact and cooperate with others, with how to make decisions. In sport, ethics deals with the concept of fair play.

Sport poses a dilemma in modern life, no less than in ancient times. H. A. Harris discussed the problem in the conclusion to his book *Greek Athletes and Athletics*:

> *Not only are games pleasant to play but many of them afford great enjoyment to spectators; all the problems of modern sport spring from this simple fact. In logical language the essence of sport is the enjoyment of the players; the pleasure of spectators is an accident. . . . So long as sport is true to itself, the only purpose of the organization of it is the enjoyment of the players; as soon as the interests of the spectators are*

*allowed to become predominant, corruption has set in and the essence
of the game has been lost. In other words, sport can be an entertainment
for spectators, but what is primarily entertainment for spectators can
never be sport in the true sense of the term.*[23]

Originally sport was for competitors, but in modern times the influence of
television has vastly increased the problem of the entertainment dilemma. When
sport is still purely for the athlete, however, it is an excellent test of ethical behavior. Because sport and physical education can provide such a fertile ground for
learning and testing ethical behavior, the next question is: Should physical educators teach ethics and values?

Should Ethics and Values Be Taught in Physical Education and Sport?

If physical education and sport really are a "laboratory of human experience" as
is claimed, what better place could be found to try to teach ethics and values to
the future leaders of the world? Delbert Oberteuffer suggests that this issue is a
major area of concern in contemporary physical education.[24] Whenever lists of
objectives for physical education have been prepared, the development of social
and moral qualities is included. The supporters of sports programs argue that the
major contribution of the programs is character development.

It would be more accurate to suggest that sport provides the opportunity to
display character rather than to develop it, but the ties between ethical character
and sport and physical education are strong and of an ancient heritage. As physical educators and coaches, we have an obligation to try to teach ethics and values. Ultimately, it may be the most important lesson we teach.

How Do We Teach Ethics and Values?

We teach ethics and values largely by example. Although they may talk about
living by rules and treating others fairly, students and athletes will be far more
influenced by coaches' and teachers' practices than by what they say. People's
true ethical beliefs are reflected in their daily actions. It does a teacher no good
to tell a class to treat everyone fairly if the teacher does not treat the students
fairly. The old saying that "actions speak louder than words" is very true of ethical behavior. Educators and coaches are unlikely to teach good character if they
exhibit poor character. Teachers and coaches must be constantly aware of the
effect of their actions on their students and athletes because young people will
imitate them because they believe that their actions are examples of accepted and
proper conduct and ethics.

Today the concern over ethical behavior is rising as society becomes more
aware of the need for ethical character in its members. The increasing consciousness of the need for the development of the older concept of ethical character is

reflected by the appearance of texts specifically related to ethics, character development, and sport.[25] Programs need to stress character, ethics, and sportsmanship again. Shields and Bredemeier give suggestions for how to do this in their text.[26]

The "Ethic" of Big-Time Sport, or Why Sport Has a Poor Reputation

Students and athletes learn many lessons from competitive sports. Not all of them are good lessons.

During an interview, Chris Evert, an all-time great in women's tennis, was asked "What are the qualities that make a champion?" Her response was blunt:

> *They're all negative qualities. At least they were for me. When I look at the players who have made it year after year . . . I see intensity. And again, that might come from a negative—from insecurity, from seeking attention. . . . You have to have an arrogance to maintain a high level of confidence. . . . I was totally selfish and thought about myself and nobody else, because if you let up for one minute, someone was going to come along and beat you. . . . I didn't like the characteristics that it took to be a champion.*[27]

Competitive sports do not have a very good reputation today, particularly in the areas of ethics and values. When people think of sports, they often think of Big-Time Sports; that is, top-level competition combined with very large budgets. Whether we look at such competition in terms of professional athletics, or perhaps college or high school sports, whatever the level of competition, many lessons can be learned.

Sport has developed a poor reputation for many reasons. Which philosophies and practices have given sport this questionable reputation? One is the fact that coaches and athletes at lower levels of competition try to imitate the practices they see in the Big-Time Sports programs. However, practices that might seem acceptable in professional athletics (which is essentially entertainment) often are inappropriate in amateur athletics. Unfortunately, we see many of the ideas of professional athletics at the lowest levels of competition. That such ideas reach lower levels of sport and remain there is the responsibility of the teacher–coach. Unless the teacher–coach opposes those practices, they will continue to spread. The following ideas or thumbnail philosophies are examples of practices that should be discouraged if sport is to be educational and part of a consistent system of values.

The Supreme Importance of Victory

Two aspects of the overemphasis on victory might be called the *winning is the only thing* ethic and the *agony of defeat* syndrome. The *winning is the only thing* ethic comes from the popular coaches' saying that "Winning isn't everything, it's the *only* thing." This idea (often attributed, probably incorrectly, to professional football coach Vince Lombardi) has been used by many coaches to justify questionable practices ranging from mistreatment of their athletes to outright violations of the rules of sport. The basic idea expressed here is that the only point of athletics is victory so that the end justifies the means. At best, this is a gross abuse of the idea of sport as a contributor to the educational process. If this philosophy is the philosophy of a school's coach or teacher, the school should have no sports program because this motto does not have the slightest pretense of moral or educational values or ethics.

The *agony of defeat* syndrome covers the total range of sports, which according to television is "the thrill of victory, the agony of defeat." One small question arises in response to this view: *Why* should we think that defeat must result in agony? We compete with the hope of winning, but if we have given our best and still lose, why should we feel agony? One dictionary definition of agony is "intense suffering." Should this realistically be our response every time we lose? Sport is called a "training ground for life" by many coaches, but if agony is a person's response to every defeat in life, would that person be considered well adjusted? Defeat is a disappointment, sometimes an intense one, but the idea that it should be agony is another abuse of the place of sport in education and in life. Indeed, there is value in failure for the lessons that it teaches us.[28]

People who coach or compete in sports want to win. Winning, or trying to win, is a natural desire of the human race. Life is like a competition, but if we make victory with no holds barred the goal of life, we have removed most of the potential quality of that life. If victory is the ultimate lesson in school athletics, there is no lesson worth teaching because the desire to win is inherent. No one *wants* to lose. The value of sport in the school curriculum lies in the *other* values that are taught or promoted during teaching, training, and competing. Victory is neither the only goal nor the highest goal in educational sport and physical education.

The Drug Culture of Sport

As bad as many factors that hurt the reputation of sport may be, the widespread drug culture may be the worst. The use of substances to improve performance is not new to sport; it can be traced in some form back to the ancient Greeks. Often the substances were dietary, with special diets that were strange by any standards (such as beer and stale bread, popular around the 1860s). But sometimes genuine drugs were used. Arsenic was used as a stimulant for some sports in the 1800s—and like some of today's drugs, too much might kill the athlete. Today we see a boom in the sale of energy drinks, designed to mimic the effects of amphetamines. In 2011, the use of energy drinks sent about 20,000 people to hospital emergency rooms.[29]

We have become accustomed to having to rewrite our record books because of failed drug tests.[30] There have been changes in the world and Olympic championship medalist lists in recent years in a number of sports. The rise of designer drugs, mostly reengineered steroids that are difficult to detect, has played havoc with the sense that a championship was won fair and square or that a record is legitimate.

Bicycle racing events, such as the Tour de France, have been riddled with doping scandals. It is not simply an unfair performance by a surprise winner. An unusual number of professional cyclists in their late teens and 20s have died of cardiac arrest in recent years, likely an effect of overuse of EPO and similar substances that increase the oxygen-carrying component of the blood, but as a result may make it too thick for the heart to push through the cardiovascular system. The removal of Lance Armstrong's Tour titles in 2012 was made worse by the reality that in too many cases no one could inherit his titles because so many of the riders had been barred for drug usage at one time or another. In the 2013 voting for the Baseball Hall of Fame, no major eligible star from the "steroid era" was selected for the Hall.

Ignoring the health risks of drugging, including the use of so-called nutritional supplements (which are not tested for safety or effectiveness by the Food and Drug Administration, and which often result in athletes failing drug tests), a greater problem is that this cheating discourages potential champions from continuing in sport. Ben Johnson, who lost the 1988 Olympic gold in the 100 meters because of steroid use, took the drugs on the advice of his coach, who told him that if he did not use drugs, he could not win. Other athletes feel that the hope of their setting an eventual world record is pushed out of sight by athletes who cheat to achieve their marks. And too many people today just assume that an athlete who is unusually successful is a drug cheat.

Poor Sportsmanship

Sportsmanship has been used for many years as an example of the best trait that athletics can develop.[31] Unfortunately, there is no evidence that participating in competitive sports really does develop sportsmanship. We *do* have some evidence that sports competition can bring out sportsmanship or can inhibit or lessen it.[32] Poor sportsmanship may be primarily a result of the examples given by coaches and teachers (and some parents) to their teams and to other students as they pursue victory and fame.

Because of this influence, schools increasingly are looking for ways to teach sportsmanship.[33] In 1999, a youth athletic league in Florida added a requirement that all parents take a 1-hour ethics course before their children can play. The move was in response to conduct problems among parents at games.[34] The North Carolina High School Athletic Association now has a written policy on unsportsmanlike conduct, allowing serious penalties for offending players or coaches. It also gives an annual sportsmanship award.[35]

We also now see poor sportsmanship at the highest level of sport. In the 1932 Olympic Games, American Ralph Hill finished second at 5000 meters. The winner had run wide on the last lap of the race, forcing Hill to run extra distance to pass. The race was a photo finish. When the crowd booed the winner for his racing tactics, Hill objected to their booing. He was willing to accept the silver medal. On the other hand, in the 2010 Winter Olympics the silver medalist in men's figure skating tried to climb to the top of the awards podium, claiming he was a better skater than the winner. He then put a notice on his website that he was winner of the "Platinum Medal" (more valuable than gold). Even at the Olympic Games some athletes act like spoiled children.

The proverb that "nice guys finish last" is a good example of what is wrong with educational sport. Too many coaches and athletes have tried to live up to this motto. The idea is that decency is a sign of weakness, that a person who shows signs of character probably does not have the force of will to become a champion. The result is coaches who abuse their athletes and any ethical standards to pursue victory because they do not think they can win if they play by the rules. If nice guys finish last, sport will finish in that position in the list of educational priorities.

The other aspect of poor sportsmanship is the idea that the coach loves a poor loser. We are increasingly treated to the spectacle of athletes who throw temper tantrums whenever they lose. This action is then cited by the coach or sports announcer as a sign of competitiveness or spirit. Let's be honest: It is nothing more than a sign of childish immaturity. Most people are expected to have outgrown such behavior by the time they enter elementary school. Coaches and athletes do not like to be referred to as cases of retarded emotional development or childish behavior, but poor losers are just that. A person who cannot lose with dignity is not psychologically prepared, is too immature to benefit from a competitive experience. Whether or not we can teach sportsmanship in the schools, we should at least demand that it be shown (as a sign of maturity) by every person who wants to compete or to coach.

Lack of Joy in Sport

Traditionally, sports are thought of as activities that people enjoy or that are fun to do. One aspect of contemporary sport seems to be the idea that sport should not be fun because winning or losing is too serious to permit enjoyment.[36] One example is similar to the last point made under poor sportsmanship. "Show me a good loser, and I'll show you a loser," as some coaches put it, is another example of an immature approach to sport.[37] When we believe that only winning has a value, we are ignoring an important point: Everyone loses at some time. Philosophies of this sort are self-defeating because they turn everyone into losers. If all participants in athletics end up being called losers, who will want to participate? Sport becomes futile or pointless under those conditions.

Another view of the no-joy-in-sport philosophy is expressed by the coach who says, "We're here to win, not to have a good time." If that is the coach's philosophy, the team has already lost because the education such a program will produce is entirely negative. We have all seen examples of the coach who believed that smiling was a sign of a poor competitive attitude. Whose attitude is really the poor one in this case? If there is no fun in sport, what will competitive athletes be like in the future? Will they continue spreading the idea that success equals misery? Is that why we see problems of drug use or of serious disorders such as anorexia and bulimia in athletes? Is that why there are problems of violence and abandonment in personal relationships of athletes?[38]

The Place of Education in Sport (Dead Last)

Actually, it would be more accurate to refer to the place of the *educator* in sport because the concern here is with the coach's dedication to teaching. Most coaches will say that sport is an important part of the educational process. The question is whether their practices uphold their claim of believing the statement. An example could be the not-so-dedicated-teacher syndrome, or the coach whose educational approach is best reflected in his defensive statement, "I get paid to win, not to teach." The most obvious fact in the statement is that this coach is not a teacher and does not consider himself a teacher. Moreover, the statement makes the observer suspect that the coach has never been interested in being a teacher. The statement itself is, in some cases, undoubtedly true, but it is not a very support-able defense for doing a poor job of teaching. Coaches with this philosophy teach athletes far more than they realize—primarily things schools would prefer not to have taught. Is that why we have academic fraud in college credits for athletes?[39]

Sports as Money

Money is the greatest force affecting athletics today because it lies at the heart of so many abuses of the educational goals of sport. The problem is a form of the Midas touch: Athletes hope that everything they touch will pay off in dollars and cents. It is reflected in the coach whose primary concern is his salary and fringe benefits. It is seen increasingly in the high school athlete whose college motivation is "What will you give me?"

Many of today's high school athletes are about as interested in the ethics of scholarships and fringe benefits as a professional athlete: *not at all*. Too often, we can see the picture of a functionally illiterate all-star high school athlete who, after barely escaping high school, suddenly acquires a car, an improved ward-robe, perhaps a well-paid summer job, and the status of amateur college athlete. Too many coaches and athletes today believe that the cardinal rule of athletics is "money talks." What lessons are they teaching to their athletes and to the public?

Perhaps this attitude is reflected in the opposition of some coaches to stronger academic requirements for college athletic scholarships, particularly because those higher standards are low compared to those for the typical college student. Perhaps this attitude of professional athletics in the colleges plays a part in the epidemic of sports gambling on college campuses.[40]

We see that greed reflected in the recent college conference realignments, where schools leave their traditional and regional conferences and create "super conferences" so large that they cannot play all of their conference members in football in a single season. The reason for the expanded conferences is simple: Greatly increased television income distributed to the schools.

At the same time, the money chases the most successful college football and basketball coaches. In most cases, these coaches are paid salaries far larger than the heads of their schools receive. We see the spectacle of coaches jumping to new schools for larger salaries, breaking their contracts and abandoning their athletes, who are restricted in their ability to follow the coaches who recruited them.

We also see a demand for more public money for ever-larger sports stadiums, aimed to increase athletic profits, with no money returned to the public that helped to pay. Finally, college students themselves are forced to help pay for the growing sports programs through increasing fees attached to their school tuition.

Although the major cases of fixing college sports competitions by gambling interests appears to be far in the past, we still stumble upon the fixing of sports competition by gamblers. In 2013, professional soccer was dealing with match-fixing so widespread that cases had been found in 50 nations.[41]

The Nutcracker Reflex

A favorite saying of coaches is that "when the going gets tough, the tough get going." The sentiment is worthy because it teaches the rewards of sticking with a task until it is completed. Unfortunately, it also may be the catchphrase signaling the abuse and dehumanization of a coach's athletes. Teachers and coaches should be sure that the student–athlete goal is worthy of the effort required. Abuse simply for the sake of proving toughness or motivation is never justified in an educational context.

The Culture of Abuse and Violence

Sadly, sports too often allows a culture of abuse and violence to survive among its players and coaches. Although violence against women by professional athletes is a well-known problem, too often local tales of abuse and violence by high school and college athletes are minimized. The sexual abuse of a girl with mental disabilities by high school football players in New Jersey took years to prosecute, even as many supporters of the team fought the idea of any charges being brought. Another case of sexual abuse of a young girl by football players in Steubenville, Ohio, resulted in death threats against both the accusers and the accused.[42]

Not all violence is against women. The conviction of Jerry Sandusky, for many years an assistant football coach at Penn State, for the sexual abuse of a number of young boys over a period of years shocked the nation.[43] The NCAA levied heavy penalties against the institution for its failure to deal with the issue. Several top administrators were charged with crimes, based on evidence suggesting that they covered up the crimes and did not remove the coach. Many fans were more outraged by the penalties on the football program than they appeared to be over the treatment of the boys.

Why the Coach Gets No Respect

Perhaps the greatest failing of physical educators has been the anti-intellectualism of athletics and coaches. People usually do not think of sport in an educational or intellectual sense because of the actions of coaches. In the United States, the coach is seen as dedicated, but not at all intellectual. Coaches are perceived as relatively ignorant people who have little interest in educational matters and even less understanding of education. Unfortunately, because coaches and teachers of physical education often remain apart from the rest of the school staff, many teachers hold this low opinion of their coaching colleagues. Although much of the responsibility for this view lies with poor public relations, actual abuses are also at the heart of the matter.

Coaches who try to have an athlete's grade changed to make the student eligible are showing fellow teachers that they have no concern for education or the primary task of the institution. Teachers who automatically give athletes good grades perform the same negative task. College coaches who enlist their all-star recruits as physical education majors regardless of the students' qualifications or interests show their own lack of respect for physical education's integrity as a field of study.

For many years, educators and citizens outside the field of physical education have been popularizing the notion of the physical education major as a dumb athlete. One reason for the poor reputation of the physical education discipline is the number of major students who are not in college to gain an education, but rather to participate in athletics. Physical education has suffered from the perpetuation of this sort of ignorance.

A psychological study of successful coaches shows that a common characteristic is conservatism, or a resistance to change that is greater than that of the average person.[44] Coaches tend to be inflexible in their practices, so they are likely to come into conflict with other teachers who do not share their opinions. However, such inflexibility does not have to be a negative trait. If physical education teachers and coaches will work with colleagues in other areas, demonstrate interests beyond the gymnasium and playing fields, and maintain academic integrity, they can gradually overcome the often negative image of our teacher–coaches.

We have taken decades to achieve our current position, and changing that position will be neither easy nor quick. Now that we have examined some of the things that have hurt our field's reputation, we need to look at the positive side of the task: our challenge. If we agree that physical educators should try to teach ethics and values, what ethical and value concepts should we be teaching as a part of the task?

What Ethical Values Should We Teach?

Perhaps our first ethical concern is a dual one: What values *do* we teach to our athletes and students, and what values *should* we teach to them? To answer the first part of this question, we must return to our earlier discussion of teaching by example. Regardless of what we say, the people we influence are watching what we do to see whether our practices live up to our theories.

Teachers and coaches were soundly criticized in the past for being hypocrites, pretending to believe in one thing, or teach it, while doing something that contradicts what they teach. If teachers do not live up to their ideals, they will have a negative influence on their students. Educators must *live* what they teach.

To answer the second part of the dual ethical problem posed (what values should we teach our students and athletes), many different values or aspects of ethical character could be suggested. Instead, five basic areas of ethics or values are discussed: (1) justice and equality, (2) self-respect, (3) respect and consideration for others, (4) respect for rules and authority, and (5) a sense of perspective or relative values. This list does not cover everything. It is simply a sampling of some major areas that the teacher–coach should keep in mind.

Justice and Equality

Probably the greatest wish of any student or athlete is a simple one: fair and equal treatment. Students want a genuine opportunity to learn, to be exposed to what the teacher is teaching, as well as a fair opportunity afterward to show what they have learned. Too often, the average or poorly skilled student in physical education is neglected in favor of the gifted student. Educators should assist all students, regardless of their relative ability. Physical educators most often fail to help the students of lesser ability in physical activities by neglecting them. This practice constitutes unjust treatment of the student by the teacher.

Educators can fail to treat students equally for a number of reasons. These can include differences of race, in social or economic background, or of sex. Teachers can also fail to treat some students fairly by giving them less attention because their level of physical ability, whether high or low, is different from that of the rest of the group.

The problem is complicated in athletics because coaches have a tendency to give more attention to the more gifted athletes. This tendency is natural because the ultimate success of the team likely rides more heavily on the shoulders of the most able athletes. Even so, all athletes should be treated equally, regardless of their respective ability. The coach should work with each athlete as much as possible. Athletes will remember how the coach treated them long after they have forgotten what the coach taught.

Self-Respect

A coach who demeans an athlete on a team or a teacher who does the same thing to a student diminishes that individual's chances of success. A student or athlete needs self-respect and a positive self-image to be a success. The teacher/coach who treats all students equally takes a major step in this direction because no student will feel unimportant or undeserving in the eyes of the teacher.

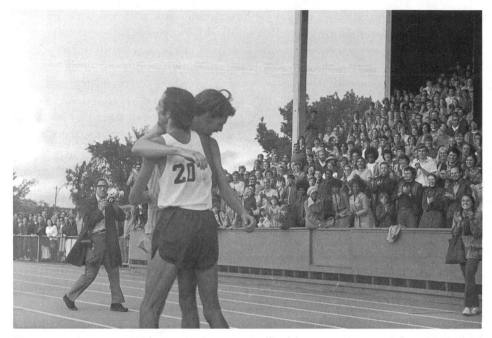

Treating opponents with respect increases all athletes' enjoyment of competition.

The teacher–coach should remember several guidelines that relate to building students' self-respect. First, if the teacher or coach demands that the students give their best, they will very likely give it. However, a class or team that gives its best and still loses should not be abused. If a runner competes and runs faster than ever before, does anyone have a right to complain if the runner still lost the race? Teachers cannot expect more than students have to give, although they can raise the goals of the students to a higher level.

A second concept related to self-respect is a paraphrase of the Golden Rule: Treat others as you wish to be treated. This applies to teachers, coaches, students, and athletes. Self-respect is a sensitive area, and students often feel insecure in the educational or athletic environment. The teacher can reduce the insecurity and help the student develop a sense of self-respect leading to greater self-confidence and self-reliance.

Respect and Consideration for Others

Students and athletes need to respect other people, whether their classmates or competitive counterparts, teachers or coaches. They need to learn the value of treating other people with respect. An athlete who treats an opponent with respect is far more likely to receive the same treatment in return, and the competition will be much more enjoyable for everyone involved. We have grown too accustomed to the idea that opponents are supposed to be abused. Coaches are failing in their ethical duties if they teach that type of conduct. Coaches should, instead, encourage students to extend respect to everyone, including parents and teachers.

We need to remember that many athletes and students learn about respect from their coaches' behavior. A coach who screams at officials when his team receives an adverse call is destroying any real opportunity to teach respect. Athletic competition may seem like war at times, but it is not war. An opponent or official who makes a judgment call against a team will not be a target for abuse in a sports program that teaches ethical character. Coaches must *show* respect in order to *teach* it.

A teacher and coach must always be concerned with the students' and athletes' rights and feelings. A student should not become a target of ridicule because of an error, nor should the athlete accept a coach's abuse. The climate of respect disintegrates when a teacher or coach in a position of authority ridicules or abuses another person.

This is why some state high school athletic groups are getting tougher on bad conduct by athletes and coaches.[45] For example, the North Carolina High School Athletic Association has increased its focus on behavior by listing eight values as "core values and beliefs": sportsmanship, integrity, fair play, honesty, respect, equity, fair competition, and development of student athletes. The organization recognizes and gives awards for outstanding examples of its core values.

Respect for Rules and Authority

Students and athletes need to respect rules and authority because without them a society will not function. The first requirement is that the rules need to be worthy of respect. The teacher–coach who makes ridiculous rules only complicates matters. A teacher–coach should set no requirements except those that genuinely contribute to the task at hand.

Rules are designed as a guideline of conduct in sport. The teacher or coach can abuse the rules without explicitly violating them by pushing them to the allowable limits. We sometimes hear a distinction made between the *letter of the law* and the *spirit of the law*. The letter of the law refers to what the law says shall be done, but underlying the law is the spirit of the law, or the intent. What is the *purpose* of a rule? If a rule is designed to make basketball a noncontact game, why should a coach hunt technicalities that may help the team physically abuse an opponent? If an educator teaches the rules and then hunts ways to break them without detection, what is he or she teaching? The object of all rules and laws is justice—to allow each person *on both teams* a fair opportunity.

We have to realize that living in a democracy requires respect for other people and respect for the rules. If we do not respect other people, we will not be able to get along with them. The result is conflict. If we do not respect the rules of society, the result is anarchy, or disorder. A life of freedom and democracy is based on respect for our fellow citizens and our laws.

A Sense of Perspective or Relative Values

Several questions related to the value of sport need to be considered. This chapter does not seek ultimate or final answers because these questions require much thought and study.

The first question, and perhaps the most important one, is *How important is sport?* Where do we rank sport in the educational spectrum and in our lives? What part does sport play in life? For each of us, the answer will give some indication of the part sport plays in our educational philosophies. Some answers may indicate that sport is more important than it really should be, but as educators, we need to place sport in a proper perspective.

A second question is *What is the proper relationship between sport and physical education?* We must determine the educational relationship between physical education and sport in order to give sport the proper emphasis in an educational program. This is a very difficult question.

A third question is *How necessary is victory?* Should one believe in the idea of victory at any price? The value placed on athletic victory, which can be a choice between means and ends in education, reflects our ethical standards in sport. Educators must decide whether victory is more important than the educational values of competitive sports.

Finally, *What is our academic integrity?* As educators we must decide what we stand for. Are we semi-educators who will bend the academic rules to gain a valuable athlete? Do we want our school to bend the rules to allow us to enroll an unqualified student or one who is unprepared for the academic work? Are we really educators if we encourage the academically inept to attend school as a reward for athletic prowess? We might consider the comments of Jacques Barzun: "The analogy to athletics must be pressed until all recognize that in the exercise of Intellect those who lack the muscles, coordination, and will power can claim no place at the training table, let alone on the playing field."[46]

Toward an Ethical Future

People believe that ethical character and strong values are important aspects of education, but they are not certain how important they are, where they fit in, or exactly what we can do about them. Delbert Oberteuffer commented on our need to learn more in this area:

> *What we needed in physical education was full blown research and clinical experience in the relation of movement to the teaching of ethics and morality, to the improvement of psychological states, and the cultivation of social gain between people and groups. . . . What kind of manpower does our society need for its preservation? This is the compelling question from the standpoint of national need and people in physical education had better have an answer or they will be lost in the oceans of sweat recommended by the muscle-building anti-intellectual.*[47]

The future national leaders in physical education and sport will determine future ethical practices and the subsequent reputation of sport and physical education. Whether physical educators are looked upon as a group of not-too-bright, not-too-ethical jocks (as they sometimes are seen) is up to future teachers and coaches. We need to see a major improvement. Let us hope that the next generation of teachers will be more committed to the ideals of education and therefore more concerned with their own and their students' and athletes' ethical practices.

As Robert Simon writes:

Sports properly conducted provide values of enduring human significance. Through sports, we can learn to overcome adversity and appreciate excellence. We can learn to value activities for their own sake, apart from any intrinsic reward they provide, and learn to appreciate the contribution of others, even when we are on opposing sides. Through sports we can develop and express moral virtues and vices and demonstrate the importance of such values as dedication, integrity, fairness, and courage.[48]

As educators and coaches, we should have positive standards that show our respect for ourselves and others, our interest in fairness and justice, and our commitment to a strong sense of ethics. When we teach and coach, we can do no better than to convince our students and athletes that the often-quoted lines by the sportswriter Grantland Rice are the best judge of our ethical behavior:

For when the One Great Scorer comes
To write against your name,
He marks—not that you won or lost—
But how you played the game.[49]

Summary

Ethics is a study of ideal conduct and of the knowledge of good and evil. Good character includes four virtues: compassion, fairness, sportsmanship, and integrity. Physical education and sport often are caught in ethical dilemmas, unsure as to the best choice of actions. The chapter looks at some current problems, then discusses ethics in physical education and sport, with an emphasis on the sport setting.

Problems in sport and physical education include (1) the abuses of sport, (2) an overemphasis on school sports, (3) an overemphasis on competitive sports in physical education, and (4) the difficult relationship between physical education and sport. Among the questions we face are (1) how does ethics relate to physical education and sport, (2) should ethics and values be taught in physical education and sport, and (3) how do we teach ethics and values? Recent decades have shown a disturbing change in the world of sport and in society: an increasing disregard for fair play and the traditional rules of society. This raises the question of whether the idea of sportsmanship is no longer accepted. This trend creates a real concern about the survival of our society because it suggests that the society no longer shares a common view of ethical or respectable behavior toward each other.

Big-Time Sports does not have a good ethical reputation. Among the reasons are (1) the supreme importance of victory, (2) the drug culture of sport, (3) poor sportsmanship, (4) the lack of joy in sport, (5) treating education as less important than sport, (6) focusing on sport as money, (7) the nutcracker reflex (abusing the athlete), and (8) coaches who are unethical. In response, we should teach at least five areas of ethics or values: (1) justice and equality, (2) self-respect, (3) respect and consideration for others, (4) respect for rules and authority, and (5) a sense of perspective or relative values.

As educators and coaches, we must have positive standards that show our respect for ourselves and others, our interest in fairness and justice, and our commitment to a strong sense of ethics.

Further Readings

Alberts, Carol L. 2003. *Coaching issues and dilemmas: Character building through sport participation*. Reston, VA: NASPE.

Arnold, Peter J. 1997. *Sport, ethics and education*. London: Cassell.

Baker, William J. 2007. *Playing with God: Religion and modern sport*. Cambridge, MA: Harvard Univ. Press.

Beamish, Rob, and Ian Ritchie. 2006. *Fastest, highest, strongest: A critique of high-performance sport*. New York: Routledge.

Branch, Taylor. 2011. The shame of college sports. *The Atlantic,* October.

Clifford, Craig, and Randolph M. Feezell. 2010. *Sport and character: Reclaiming the principles of sportsmanship*. Champaign, IL: Human Kinetics.

Corbett, Doris R. 1998. Civility in physical education and sport: The glue to society's moral and professional conduct. *Quest* 50: 307–318.

Denison, Jim, and Zoe Avner. 2011. Positive coaching: Ethical practices for athlete development. *Quest* 63 (2): 209–227.

Dombrowski, Daniel A. 2009. *Contemporary athletics and ancient Greek ideals*. Chicago: Univ. of Chicago Press.

Ennis, Catherine. 1996. Student's experiences in sport-based physical education: [More than] apologies are necessary. *Quest* 48: 453–458.

Epstein, David. 2010. Sports genes. *Sports Illustrated,* May 17, 53–60, 62, 64–65.

Epstein, David. 2013. *The Sports Gene: Inside the Science of Extraordinary Athletic Performance*. New York: Current.

Farber, Michael. 2010. The devil is in the details. *Sports Illustrated,* May 17, 66.

Feezell, Randolph M. 2006. *Sport, play, and ethical reflection*. Urbana, IL: Univ. of Illinois Press.

Fraleigh, Warren. 1982. Why the good foul is not good enough. *JOPERD (Journal of Physical Education, Recreation and Dance)* (January): 41–42.

French, Peter. 2004. *Ethics and college sports: Ethics, sports, and the university*. Lanham, MD: Rowman and Littlefield.

Gillespie, Michael Allen. 2010. Players and spectators: Sports and ethical training in the American university. In *Debating moral education: Rethinking the role of the modern university*, ed. Elizabeth Kiss and J. Peter Euben, 296–316. Durham, NC: Duke Univ. Press.

Gough, Russell W. 1997. *Character is everything: Promoting excellence in sport*. Fort Worth, TX: Harcourt Brace College.

Hardman, Alun R., and Carwyn Jones, eds. 2011. *The ethics of sports coaching*. London: Routledge.

Hellison, Donald. 1995. *Teaching responsibility through physical activity*. Champaign, IL: Human Kinetics.

Hoffman, Shirl James. 2010. *Good game: Christianity and the culture of sports*. Waco, TX: Baylor Univ. Press.

Holowchak, M. Andrew, and Heather L. Reid. 2011. *Aretism: An ancient sports philosophy for the modern sports world*. Lanham, MD: Lexington Books.

Hunt, Thomas M., and John Hoberman. 2011. *Drug games: The International Olympic Committee and the politics of doping*. Austin, TX: Univ. of Texas Press.

Hyman, Mark. 2009. *Until it hurts: America's obsession with youth sports and how it harms our kids*. Boston: Beacon Press.

Jenkins, Lee. 2012. The virtual program. *Sports Illustrated*, August 27, 46–51.

Levy, Ariel. 2009. Either/or: Sports, sex, and the case of Caster Semenya. *The New Yorker*, November 30, 47–59.

McIntosh, Peter. 1979. *Fair play: Ethics in sport and education*. London: Heinemann.

Miller, Glenn A., Rafer Lutz, and Karen Fredenburg. 2012. Outstanding high school coaches: Philosophies, views and practices. *JOPERD (Journal of Physical Educator, Recreation and Dance)* (February): 24–29.

Morgan, Bill. 2010. Sport, wholehearted engagement and the good life. *Sport, Ethics and Philosophy* 4: 239–253.

Morgan, William J. 2006. *Why sports morally matter*. New York: Routledge.

———, ed. 2007. *Ethics in sport*. 2nd ed. Champaign, IL: Human Kinetics. Powell, Shaun. 2008. *Souled out? How blacks are winning and losing in sports*. Champaign, IL: Human Kinetics.

Reid, Heather. 2002. *The philosophical athlete*. Durham, NC: Carolina Academic Press.

Rosen, Daniel M. 2008. *Dope: A history of performance enhancement in sports from the nineteenth century to today*. New York: Praeger.

Sailors, Pam R. 2010. Mercy killing: Sportsmanship and blowouts. *Journal of the Philosophy of Sport* 37: 60–68.

Schneider, Angela J., and Jim L. Rupert. 2009. Constructing winners: The science and ethics of genetically manipulating athletes. *Journal of the Philosophy of Sport* 36: 182–206.

Schneider, Robert C. 2008. *The ethics of sport and athletics: Theory, issues and applications*. Philadelphia: Lippincott Williams and Wilkins.

Shields, David Light, and Brenda Light Bredemeier. 2011. Why sportsmanship programs fail, and what we can do about it. *JOPERD (Journal of Physical Educator, Recreation and Dance)* (September).

Simon, Robert L. 2010. *Fair play: The ethics of sport*. 3rd ed. Boulder, CO: Westview.

———. 2013. *The ethics of coaching sports: Moral, social and legal issues*. Boulder, CO: Westview.

Tufte, John E. 2012. *Crazy-proofing high school sports*. Lanham, MD: Rowman and Littlefield Education.

United States Anti-Doping Agency. 2012. *Reasoned decision of the United States Anti-Doping Agency on disqualification and ineligibility*.* Colorado Springs, CO: USADA. http://apps.washingtonpost.com/g/documents/sports/decision-of-usada-on-disqualification-and-ineligibility-of-lance-armstrong/72/

Wetzel, Dan, and Don Yaeger. 2000. *Sole influence: Basketball, corporate greed and the corruption of American's youth*. New York: Warner.

Young, Alison. 2013. The supplement danger zone. *USA Today* (July 25): 1A, 6A–7A.

Zeigler, Earle F. 2006. *Applied ethics for sport and physical activity professionals*. Victoria, BC, Canada: Trafford.

Discussion Questions

1. List and explain briefly some of the major problems we have today in physical education and sport. What approaches might we take in solving those problems?

2. Briefly define ethics. Explain the part ethics plays in teaching and coaching, and explain why teachers need to be concerned about ethical problems.

3. David Sarnoff stated that "the problem with competition is that it brings out the best in products and the worst in men." Explain what he meant, then show how his statement relates to ethics and character development in physical education and sport.

4. Compare and contrast the meanings of sport, sports, and athletics.

5. Discuss briefly how physical education and sport can be used to teach ethics and values.

6. Briefly form the arguments both for and against the statement that "Sports builds character," then explain which you consider to be the more accurate answer and why.

7. Discuss the effect on the ethical and values education of the students whose teacher–coach believes the following statement: "I get paid to win, not to teach."

8. Jacques Barzun wrote that "in the exercise of Intellect those who lack the muscles, coordination, and will power can claim no place at the training table, let alone on the playing field." Explain what he meant, then give and defend your reaction to his statement.

---

*202 page document giving evidence against Lance Armstrong, available online at agency website.

References

1. Kretchmar, R. Scott. 1993. Philosophy of ethics. *Quest* 45: 3–12.

2. Shields, David Lyle, and Brenda Jo Bredemeier. 1995. *Character development and physical activity*. Champaign, IL: Human Kinetics, 192–195.

3. Doucet, Hubert. 1991. High performance sport in present-day context: Considerations for ethical analysis. In *Sport . . . the Third Millennium, Proceedings of the International Symposium, May 21–25 1990*, ed. Fernand Landry, Marc Landry, and Magdeleine Yerlès, 445–453. Quebec City, Quebec: Les Presses de l'Université Laval.

4. Gebauer, Gunter. 1991. Citius–altius–fortius and the problem of sport ethics: A philosopher's viewpoint. In *Sport . . . the Third Millennium, Proceedings of the International Symposium, May 21–25 1990*, ed. Fernand Landry, Marc Landry, and Magdeleine Yerlès, 467–473. Quebec City, Quebec: Les Presses de l'Université Laval.

5. Schudel, Matt. 1986. Kevin Anthony, former athlete. *News and Observer* (Raleigh, NC), March 4.

6. Sports Features Syndicate, March 1986.

7. Sargent, Dudley A. 1972. History of the administration of intercollegiate athletics in the United States. In *Chronicle of American physical education: Selected readings, 1885–1930*, ed. Aileene S. Lockhart and Betty Spears, 272. Dubuque, IA: Brown.

8. Savage, Howard J. 1929. *American college athletics, bulletin no. 23*. New York: Carnegie Foundation for the Advancement of Teaching; Hanford, George H. 1974. *A report to the American Council on Education on an inquiry into the need for and feasibility of a national study of intercollegiate athletics*. Washington, DC: American Council on Education; Knight Foundation Commission on Intercollegiate Athletics. 1993. *Report of the Knight Foundation Commission on Intercollegiate Athletics, March 1991–March 1993*. Charlotte, NC: Knight Foundation Commission on Intercollegiate Athletics; and Thelin, John R. 1994. *Games colleges play: Scandal and reform in intercollegiate athletics*. Baltimore: Johns Hopkins Univ. Press.

9. Rostaing, Bjarne, and Robert Sullivan. 1985. Triumphs tainted with blood. *Sports Illustrated*, January 21, 12–17.

10. Lemonick, Michael D. 1998. Le tour des drugs. *Time*, August 10, 76.

11. Brubaker, Bill. 1985. A pipeline full of drugs. *Sports Illustrated*, January 21, 18–21; and Todd, Terry. 1983. The steroid predicament. *Sports Illustrated*, August 1, 62–66, 68–71, 73–75, 77.

12. Schneider, Angela J., and Robert B. Butcher. 1993–1994. Olympic athletes should avoid the use and seek the elimination of performance-enhancing substances and practices from the Olympic Games. *Journal of the Philosophy of Sport* 20–21: 64–81.

13. Miracle, Andrew W., and C. Roger Rees. 1994. *Lessons of the locker room: The myth of school sports*. Amherst, NY: Prometheus Books.

14. Nack, William. 1986. This case was one for the books. *Sports Illustrated*, February 24, 34–36, 41–42.

15. *New York Times* News Service. 1986. Georgia report says university chief knew athletes were favored. April 4.

16. Werthheim, L. Jon, and Don Yaeger. 1999. The passing game. *Sports Illustrated*, June 14, 90–92, 95–96, 98, 101–02; and Yaeger, Don. 1999. Black eye for the Buckeyes. *Sports Illustrated*, June 14, 96.

17. Kane, Dan, and J. Andrew Curliss. 2012. Records: UNC players needed help. *News & Observer* (Raleigh, NC), September 30, A1, 8; Kane, Dan. 2012. UNC tolerated cheating, insider says. *News & Observer* (Raleigh, NC), November 18, A1, 4.

18. Kneer, Marian E. 1986. Physical education and athletics need a divorce. *JOPERD (Journal of Physical Education, Recreation and Dance)* (March): 7.

19. Brown, Lyndon, and Steven Grineski. 1992. Competition in physical education: An educational contradiction? *JOPERD (Journal of Physical Education, Recreation and Dance)* (January): 17–19, 77; and Hager, Peter F. 1995. Redefining success in competitive activities. *JOPERD (Journal of Physical Education, Recreation and Dance)* (May–June): 26–30.

20. Cheffers, John. 1996. Sport versus education: The jury is still out. *International Journal of Physical Education* 33: 106–109.

21. Morgan, William J. 2006. *Why sports morally matter*. New York: Routledge, x.

22. Ibid., xiii.

23. Harris, H. A. 1966. *Greek athletes and athletics*. Bloomington, IN: Indiana Univ. Press, 189.

24. Oberteuffer, Delbert. 1963. On learning values through sport. *Quest* 1: 23–29.

25. Clifford, Craig, and Randolph M. Feezell. 1997. *Coaching for character: Reclaiming the principles of sportsmanship*. Champaign, IL: Human Kinetics; Gough, Russell W. 1997. *Character is everything: Promoting excellence in sport*. Fort Worth, TX: Harcourt Brace College; and Hellison, Donald. 1995. *Teaching responsibility through physical activity*. Champaign, IL: Human Kinetics.

26. Shields and Bredemeier, *Character development*, 197–225.

27. Jenkins, Sally. 1992. "I've led a charmed life." *Sports Illustrated*, May 25, 64.

28. Thomas, Carolyn E. 1991. The value of failure. In *Sport . . . the Third Millennium, Proceedings of the International Symposium, May 21–25 1990*, ed. Fernand Landry, Marc Landry, and Magdeleine Yerlès, 615–620. Quebec City, Quebec: Les Presses de l'Université Laval.

29. Burle, Garance. 2013. Energy drinks put more in ER. Associated Press, reprinted in *News & Observer* (Raleigh, NC), January 13, 5A.

30. ESPN.com. 2012. Steroids loom large over programs. December 20. http://m.espn.go.com/ncf/story?storyId=8765531&wjb=

31. Beller, Jennifer M., and Sharon Kay Stoll. 1993. Sportsmanship: An antiquated concept? *JOPERD (Journal of Physical Education, Recreation and Dance)* (August): 74–79; Rosenberg, D. 1993. Sportsmanship reconsidered. *International Journal of Physical Education* 30 (4): 15–23; and Hon, Jeanne, and Bob O'Connor. 1994. Teaching fair play: The essence of sport. *JOPERD (Journal of Physical Education, Recreation and Dance)* (September): 70, 72.

32. Ogilvie, Bruce C., and Thomas A. Tutko. 1971. Sport: If you want to build character, try something else. *Psychology Today* (October): 61–63.

33. Green, Tomas, and Carl Gabbard. 1999. Do we need sportsmanship education in secondary school athletics? *Physical Educator* 56: 98–104.

34. Associated Press. 1999. Youth league requires training for parents. *News & Observer* (Raleigh, NC), November 19.

35. Stevens, Tim. 1999. Sportsmanship takes center stage. *News and Observer* (Raleigh, NC), August 29.

36. Ferguson, Andrew. 1999. Inside the crazy culture of kids sports. *Time*, July 12, 52–60.

37. Parker, Rosemary. 1993. Learning by intimidation? *Newsweek*, November 8, 14.

38. Chaikin, Tommy, and Rick Telander. 1988. The nightmare of steroids. *Sports Illustrated* October 24, 82–88, 90, 92, 94, 97–98, 100–102; Noden, Merrell. 1994. Dying to win. *Sports Illustrated*, August 8, 52–56, 58–60; Ryan, Joan. 1995. *Little girls in pretty boxes: The making and breaking of elite gymnasts and figure skaters.* New York: Doubleday; Nack, William, and Lester Munson. Sport's dirty secret. *Sports Illustrated*, August 31, 63–70, 73–74; and Wahl, Grant, and L. Jon Wertheim. 1998. Paternity ward. *Sports Illustrated*, May 4, 62–71.

39. Wolff, Alexander, and Don Yaeger. Credit risk. *Sports Illustrated*, August 7, 46–48, 53–55.

40. Layden, Tim. 1995. Special report: Campus gambling. *Sports Illustrated*, April 3, 69–74, 76–78, 80, 82, 84–86, 90; Ibid., April 10, 68–70, 73–76, 79; and Ibid., April 17, 46–48, 51–55.

41. Norman-Culp, Sheila. 2013. Match-fixing pervasive in soccer; organized crime making billions. Associated Press, reprinted in *Oregonian* (Portland), February 14, A1, A6.

42. Hanley, Robert. 1993. 4 are convicted in sexual abuse of retarded New Jersey woman. *New York Times*, March 17; Michelle Dean. 2013. The lessons of Steubenville. *New Yorker*, January 11.

43. Carter, Andrew. 2012. Penn State saga hits home with ACC: "It's a tragic situation." *News & Observer* (Raleigh, NC), July 24, 1C, 3C.

44. Ogilvie, Bruce C., and Thomas A. Tutko. 1966. *Problem athletes and how to handle them.* London: Pelham, 23–24.

45. Stevens, Tim. 2012. Fights and taunts: Players not always good sports. *News & Observer* (Raleigh, NC), October 2, 3C.

46. Barzun, Jacques. 1959. *The house of intellect.* New York: Harper and Row, 95.

47. Oberteuffer, On learning values, 23, 29.

48. Simon, Robert L. 1991. *Fair play: Sports, values, and society.* Boulder, CO: Westview, 200–201.

49. Rice, Grantland. 1941. *Only the brave, and other poems.* New York: A. S. Barnes.

PART 4

Careers for the Future: Where Do You Go from Here?

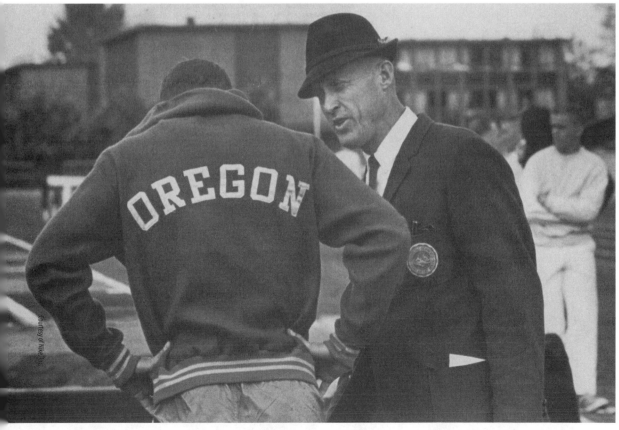

Preparing for a Career

10

Success in any field depends on a high level of knowledge and skills related to that field. Too often outsiders think that success is mostly a matter of time spent on the job, knowing the right people, and good luck. The result is careers that do not reach the levels of success that meet your goals and dreams.

This chapter looks briefly at two major elements of success in any field: developing high-level knowledge and skills, and developing the basic traits that lead to success.

Developing the Knowledge and Skills for Success

Success Follows Preparation and Opportunity

Success in any field requires ability, preparation, and opportunity. You need the opportunity to gain experience and to show what you can do, but before that you need to develop a level of knowledge and skill that will prepare you to take full advantage of that opportunity. An athlete does not win an Olympic medal simply because of the opportunity to be on an Olympic team. Before that opportunity come many years of preparation, learning, and training. Without those years of preparation, the opportunity is meaningless because you will not be capable of succeeding when the opportunity arises. Jobs and careers are the same. To be prepared to succeed at a high level requires years of learning and skill development.

Malcolm Gladwell studied success, trying to determine (1) who succeeds and (2) why they succeed. As he writes,

> *People don't rise from nothing. We do owe something to parentage and patronage. The people who stand before kings may look like they did it all themselves. But in fact they are invariably the beneficiaries of hidden advantages and extraordinary opportunities and cultural legacies that allow them to learn and work hard and make sense of the world in ways others cannot. It makes a difference where and when we grew up. The culture we belong to and the legacies passed down by our forebears*

shape the patterns of our achievement in ways we cannot begin to imagine.[1]

He points out that a large majority of hockey all-stars are born in the first 3 months of the year, not because of an advantage in those months, but because under the definition of age in youth hockey, they will be the oldest athletes in each new group, thus a bit more physically mature than their potential teammates. The result is that from the start they have a physical advantage, which gets them more playing time, resulting in greater skill development than their teammates.

Other sports show similar all-star effects, if they have a highly organized youth competition program based on each year's birth dates starting at a certain point in the calendar. The group born shortly after that date will have an advantage over the other athletes in their year's group.

The importance of that opportunity as an advantage is seen in sports where youth sport is not as big a factor, such as in track and field. The top Olympic athletes often were not the top high school athletes. The weaker high school athletes (less matured) eventually mature and catch up to the athletes who matured early. While some high school all-stars eventually reach the top, many others fall by the wayside as their early maturation disappears as a success factor.

When it comes to careers, you take advantage of your opportunities, whatever they may be. Bill Gates was able to get access to a mainframe (very large) computer at a time when personal computers did not exist. As a result, he had a huge advantage in his early experience with computers. But he still had to put thousands of hours into developing the knowledge needed to gain the full benefit from his opportunity.

The author of this textbook had the opportunity to work with an Olympic track and field coach as a graduate assistant. This was not my goal, but it was an unexpected opportunity. Fortunately, years of reading track and field literature, coaching journals, and rule books gave me the background knowledge to take full advantage of the opportunity. The timing factor was also important because soon after I began working with the coach, that coach (Bill Bowerman of Oregon) was selected to be head Olympic coach, and his school was selected to host both the NCAA National Championships and the U.S. Olympic Trials.

As a result of prior preparation, I was able to perform successfully as Director of the Combined Events competitions (men's decathlon and women's pentathlon and heptathlon) for three U.S. Olympic Trials and half a dozen NCAA Championships. I was also able to serve as coauthor with Bill Bowerman for a textbook on track and field coaching[2] that led to the eventual writing of the *First Edition* of this textbook.[3] Each of those successes depended upon an unexpected opportunity. Each opportunity was meaningful only because years of preparation prepared the author to take advantage of the opportunity.

Success does not happen simply because you have a great opportunity. Success happens because when the opportunity appears, you are prepared to take advantage of it and meet the knowledge and skill requirements needed for success. Without diligent preparation, opportunity is worthless.

Success Results from the Right Habits

Some habits contribute to success, while others interfere with it. You need to develop your good habits and work to overcome your bad habits. A very popular book on developing those habits is Stephen Covey's *The 7 Habits of Highly Effective People*.[4] Covey's idea is that effectiveness should be centered on principles and personal character. The goal is to benefit from interdependence, recognizing that people today must cooperate to achieve things that cannot be achieved independently. In our complex world, success lies in recognizing the reality of our interdependence with others.

Covey begins with three habits that develop independence: (1) be proactive (change starts from within, so learn to assess problems and develop solutions on your own), (2) begin with the end in mind (determine what you want to accomplish, then set long-term goals), and (3) put first things first (prioritize your goals, then create the conditions to achieve them).

The next three habits deal with interdependence: (4) think win–win (try to find solutions that are mutually beneficial, rather than competitive), (5) seek first to understand, then to be understood (try to understand the other person before you try to get that person to understand you), and (6) synergize (work to harness individual differences in a way that the whole together is greater than the sum of the parts).

The final habit, (7) sharpen the saw, is to continue to pursue your personal growth in every element of your being.

The counterpoint to Covey's work on good habits that lead to success is James Waldroop and Timothy Butler's book titled *The 12 Bad Habits That Hold Good People Back*.[5] Their approach is to understand the habits that make it harder to succeed so you can work on overcoming them. Their 12 bad habits are: (1) never feeling good enough (being insecure about your abilities), (2) seeing the world in black and white (not being able to understand that the world is not always perfectly rational and objective), (3) doing too much and pushing too hard (sometimes you need to back off and relax), (4) avoiding conflict at any cost (avoiding conflict can hurt relationships and prevent finding the best solutions), (5) running roughshod over the opposition (you may fail to see the truth in a situation, and you will be unable to achieve genuine cooperation), (6) being a rebel looking for a cause (confrontation and an inability to recognize authority can destroy the feeling of being part of a team), (7) always swinging for the fence (too often not grounded in the real world), (8) putting fear in the driver's seat (too much of a worrier or pessimist), (9) being emotionally tone-deaf (unable or unwilling to recognize the feelings of others), (10) believing no job is good enough (never making a serious effort to achieve or accomplish anything), (11) lacking a sense of boundaries (unable to distinguish between the public and the private, or failing to understand appropriate actions toward other people), and (12) losing the path (losing a sense of the direction you want to be going in your career).

These two books give a sense of the importance of understanding yourself: knowing your strengths and weaknesses, learning how to improve your personal as well as your professional skills, and knowing how best to work with others. This area deals with your personality and behavioral patterns, your personal skills, rather than your knowledge. It is critical to success, but you also need a solid base of knowledge of your field if you hope to succeed at a high level.

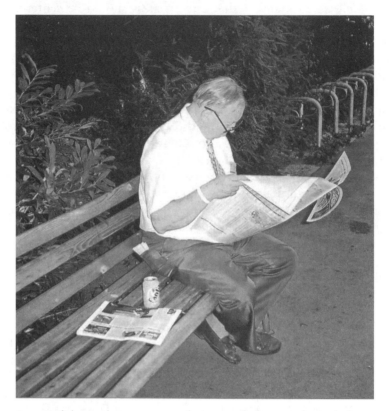

Successful people never stop their search for new knowledge.

Success Results from the Long-Term Building of Your Knowledge

I am making a distinction here between knowledge and expertise. You can have knowledge of your field at many levels, even great knowledge, without necessarily being considered an expert (thus possessing expertise, the knowledge of a genuine expert).

Educators who are concerned about teaching for the future emphasize that in school we are preparing students to be able to learn jobs that do not currently exist, to acquire knowledge that does not yet exist. David Warlick writes of "redefining literacy," of trying to improve the ability of students to learn and benefit from new information technologies as they appear in the future.[6] Knowledge is not static. A textbook is revised with each new edition; research changes or modifies what we discovered through earlier research.

The field of exercise science today is radically different than its parent, physical education, was 50 years ago. At that time, much of the knowledge to be gained was of methodology and performance skills. The scientific and theoretical knowledge that was taught was very limited. Today's knowledge foundations are far more broad and far deeper than in the past. Thus, there is much more to learn before you become knowledgeable in your field.

The process of building knowledge, and at the same time benefiting from already-present knowledge in an organization, is critical. David DeLong writes of the critical threat of the loss of aging workers in businesses.[7] As he points out, experienced workers have much learning based on their years of experience. When they retire, the benefit of that knowledge is lost to the business. There is also a loss of "institutional memory," the understanding of past actions, of why different things were done, of earlier experiments and their outcomes. It is critical to the survival of companies that they find ways to pass that knowledge from retiring workers to the young workers who will determine the future success or failure of the operation.

Along the same line, Dorothy Leonard and Walter Swap developed their concept of "deep smarts," or "enduring business wisdom," through the study of many successful businesses.[8] Their concern, similar to DeLong's, is preserving the personal expertise developed by company leaders over a period of many years. This "experience-based wisdom" is critical to the long-term survival and success of any operation. If it can be passed on to each new generation of employees, it can help them to avoid many years of mistakes and bad choices that might destroy an organization.

The people who possess deep smarts can address practical, real-life problems quickly; can understand the relationships within complex systems (so they can predict the effects of changes in any part of the system); have a large store of knowledge that is not always easy to pass on to others; and because of their years of experience can quickly evaluate a critical situation, sort through the options, and determine an appropriate response to that situation.

Success Results from the Development of Expertise

This reality of experts leads us to the other element of success: the development of expertise. The development of expertise is an interesting research area for psychologists. For exercise science, we think of expertise in the cognitive area (the original focus of research) but also in physical skill development (motor behavior and learning). A chess player requires many years of learning and practice to become a grand master; the learning is primarily cognitive.[9] A world champion athlete also requires many years of training to reach the level of an expert. In this case, we tend to think primarily of physical skills, but there are also tactical and psychological skills that must be developed.

The first studies of expertise were by Herbert Simon and focused on the variations of expert memory, eventually broadening out to multidisciplinary creativity.[10]

Over time the area of research spread from studies of memory or cognitive expertise to include physical or skill expertise. It also discovered several interesting aspects of the development of expertise.

The first element in developing expertise is time and practice. This has become known as the *10 year or 10,000 hour* rule. What this means is that to rise to the level of an expert requires a large quantity of practice, roughly equivalent to 10 years or 10,000 hours of practice time. Note that this does not mean the time from first beginning to compete or train. This is the time needed from the start of serious training; that is, training under expert guidance and with a very well-organized and thorough process laid out over a long period of time. Most world champions first reach that level of competition a decade after beginning focused training. The exceptions are when there are other circumstances that permit earlier success (this is rare).

A second element is called *chunking*. This is the brain's pattern of putting knowledge together in related chunks, so the analytical process does not search through all memories, but through a small number of the most relevant chunks of related knowledge. The result is that "much of the chess master's advantage over the novice derives from the first few seconds of thought."[11] The master can access the critical knowledge far more quickly than the less expert opponent can.

A third element is that development of expertise may result less from talent than from training. Again, this means very focused, wisely planned training, not simply putting in many hours of kicking a ball or running. The critical factor is meaningful training: wise, well-thought-out training appropriate to the current level of skill and the long-term goals of the athlete.

Although this example is of sporting expertise, the essential process and its elements are the same regardless of the type of expertise being developed, whether cognitive, physical, or a combination. This is why the wisest athletes and coaches never stop learning. They continue to experiment, evaluate, and modify their methods, seeking to make them just a little bit better, a little bit more effective. I call it tweaking the system.

Developing the Basic Traits of Success

Career planning is difficult even when you know exactly what you want to do. However, many students change majors and career paths within their first 2 years of college. You may discover that your original interest has lost its appeal or that it is not what you expected. You may find that your academic preparation has been inadequate for the level of work needed to enter your prospective field. You may also discover a new field that is more interesting and appealing to you. I moved into this field while doing doctoral work in another field. Most students realize only gradually how wide the potential career choices of a field can be.

Michael Wade and John Baker suggest that a student should ask four questions when choosing a future career:[12]

1. Am I one of those people who enjoys, prefers, and in many instances seeks personal interactions?
2. Does an undergraduate degree in [this field] commit me to a career path from which I am not able to change in the future? What if it does not work out?
3. What is the breadth of opportunity afforded me with a degree in [this field]?
4. Where eventually do I want to work and live?

These questions concern whether your personality is a match for the type of work, how easily you can change fields if you want to change your career path, how good your options are in your major, and whether you have a preference for where you live. Students often neglect examining one or more of those questions and as a result may encounter difficulties later.

Many books are available to give you guidance in finding a job. Dorothy Zakrajsek and William Pierce argue that many students in our field have difficulties in their careers because their preparation is too narrow to meet the broader needs of the real world of work.[13] Darrell Crase has studied highly productive scholars, trying to determine why they are so successful, and he argues that the highly successful scholars are well prepared, committed to their work, and have effective work habits.[14]

Rather than give a mini-course in job hunting, I want to describe the basic traits that I believe lead to success in our field—indeed, in any field. My list includes seven broad skills:

1. Broad knowledge base (cultural literacy)
2. Communications skills
3. Technical skills
4. Research skills
5. Job-hunting skills
6. Health and fitness
7. Focus

Broad Knowledge Base (Cultural Literacy)

The starting point for any career is to develop a broad knowledge base, sometimes called cultural literacy. This means more than simply having a good preparation in your major field. You should educate yourself in a broadly based program of study in the liberal arts and sciences. You need to be exposed to and understand the breadth of human experience and knowledge. This broad educational background will help you to understand the people with whom you work and the work that they do. It will give you a common basis of communication with other people. It will show you other career options as you study other subjects.

A major value of a broad education is that it will increase the ease with which you can change careers. Most people change careers at some time during their working lifetime. Some will do so more than once. A broad education will increase your awareness of other possible career directions, and it will also give you the background education that you need for studying another field. No one knows what the future holds. A broadly based education will give you the best opportunity for a good future, regardless of your career.

Your educational background is also critical to the next trait, communications skills. You need a good education to improve your ability to communicate with others. You need the knowledge of what to communicate and how to communicate it.

Communications Skills

Every highly successful person is skilled in both verbal and written communication. You must be able to express yourself clearly, to be able to explain your thoughts and ideas to other people. The modern world is a world of reports, both oral and written. Just as you need to be able to read and understand written reports, instructions, and research, you must be able to produce well-written reports yourself. You may have to instruct others on how to perform their jobs. You may write reports to explain how your department or business is performing. You may have to give a formal speech on your work. Because most jobs involve a number of people, you must be able to communicate well with others. Those skills include both speaking skills and writing skills.

Spoken Communication Skills

Most of the information that we share daily is through speech. We talk about what we are doing, how we are feeling, how our day is going. We communicate almost constantly, usually without realizing what we are doing. As we talk to others, we develop our speaking communication skills—or we fail to improve them.

Everyone speaks to other people regularly, yet many people are fearful of giving a formal speech (or even an informal talk) to a group of people. Even so, the basic skills are the same. We organize what we want to say. We learn to follow our audience's reactions. We learn what works and what does not work in getting people's attention.

You can improve your speaking ability through informal and formal methods. You can pay more attention on your own to how you speak to others—how clear your speech is, whether your meaning is easily understood, whether your longer comments show a progression, following an organized or logical approach. You can practice speaking to yourself, then try speaking to a mirror. Some excellent speakers practice very little, but many good speakers practice extensively and have to work to overcome their nervousness, but they still become excellent speakers.

You can also improve your spoken communication through more formal means, such as classes in public speaking or debate. Those classes help you to understand speaking from the inside. You learn how to compose a speech, how to prepare for the presentation, how to deliver the talk, and how to evaluate it and learn from the experience. A class makes the process easier because you have an objective teacher to assist you, and the other speakers are learning just as you are. It creates a nonthreatening environment so you can learn that speaking to groups is not difficult.

Speaking skills are extremely important because often they are your first (sometimes your only) chance to communicate with someone. You may be trying to sell a service or a product, to recruit an athlete, or to convince someone to hire you. The impression that you give, the information that you pass on, the sense of who you are and what you can contribute are extremely important. A good speaker is already a step up on the way to success.

Written Communication Skills

In a physical field we often overlook the importance of writing skills. Yet students must write term papers and research reports. Teachers write reports, researchers write reports, business people write reports. Very often you cannot try new things without producing a strong proposal to convince others of the value of your idea. Writing is a regular part of life in the real world, so you need to develop your writing skills.

Every college student takes courses in English composition. Too often students view such courses only as a barrier, rather than as the opportunity that they represent. You must learn how to put words together in a way that makes your meaning clear. Good writing does not have to be flowery, nor does it require long words. The critical part of good writing is clarity: People must understand what you are writing.

You may benefit from other formal courses, such as courses in technical writing or report writing. You may simply practice on your own, spending more time with the organization and wording of your reports and term papers. You might ask for more feedback from your instructors, a more thorough evaluation of how well you met your objectives in a paper for one of your courses. Just as with your physical skills, you must write if you want to improve the quality of your writing.

Technical Skills

Technical skills are also important to success. The necessary technical skills vary from one occupation to another, but every occupation involves some technical skills. In most cases, these include the ability to use computers in doing your work. This may include using word processing programs to write memos and reports, a spreadsheet to develop and implement budgets, a database to handle inventories or records of people, graphics to supplement presentations or produce newsletters or catalogs, and communications to send or receive information to or from outside sources or customers. Coaches need some skills in athletic training, fitness specialists need skills in measuring body fat, and so on, throughout the range of every field of work.

Developing your technical skills first requires you to evaluate the job that you hope to do, and then to find out which technical skills are needed to do the job.

Once you understand the range of skills that you need to develop, you can approach the task on both the formal and informal levels. You can study and practice the skills on your own, and you can take courses or attend clinics that teach the skills.

The critical thing to remember about technical skills is this: Most schools and businesses will not teach technical skills to you after you are hired. If you want a good job, you should already have the skills when you start job hunting. Otherwise, the jobs will go to the people who already have the skills.

Research Skills

You need research skills in every type of job. Many college teachers are expected to conduct research, so most students are required to take a course in research methods or one that includes research methods. What many students do not realize is that every job includes doing some research.

Not all research is a formal, discovery-of-new-knowledge process. When you are asked to locate potential athlete recruits, your assignment is research. When you are asked to find a better way to conduct an office function, your assignment is research. When you are asked to plan a new program, your assignment is research. When you are asked to create a new product, your assignment is research.

In short, you must know how to find information, how to process it, and how to report it. Although the Internet is a massive source of information, many people do not use it effectively. Why? They do not know how to evaluate and use what they find. They do not have the research skills. You must learn how to conduct basic information gathering and reporting. It is something that you do every day, but you must go beyond the simple level and take your skills to a higher level as you learn more about your chosen field. This is where you apply your skills in critical thinking.[15]

Job-Hunting Skills

Job-hunting skills are often neglected by students. They assume that if they earn a degree, they will be hired. Most students start to pay attention to the process only when they become seniors. You need to be conscious of job-hunting skills earlier because you can be improving those skills throughout your college years.

The first source of information is at your school's placement office. Though many names are used by different schools to describe this function, the essential job of the office is to assist students in finding jobs. Many students are confused by this function, so you need to be clear about it: *Finding a job is your responsibility*. Your school is not responsible, your department is not responsible, your teachers are not responsible. Colleges are not employment agencies. They act only as go-betweens, offering helpful information and in some cases bringing prospective employers to campus. They will not find you a job, and it is not their responsibility to do so.

However, they will provide information on how to hunt for a job. They may provide career testing and counseling. They may offer short classes in interviewing skills.

They may offer help in preparing a resume. They will have information on the tests needed for entry into graduate school. The services vary widely from one college to another, but the office should be an early stop for every serious student.

Find out what services are offered, and use them. Learn how to write a resume, and write one now. You never know when it might be useful. Learn how to conduct yourself in an interview. If the placement office offers practice interviews, do it. Some people will interview for jobs they do not want, simply because they want to practice and improve their interviewing skills.

When you become a senior, create a placement file. It will include records of your studies at your college, a resume or other information on appropriate nonclass activities, and personal letters of recommendation. You should have a recommendation from your advisor or a teacher who can convincingly attest to your abilities and dedication. Ideally, you should include recommendations from people outside your field, such as other teachers or your coaches, as well as people who are not from the academic world. You might include someone for whom you have worked, a professional who has known you on a personal basis for a number of years, or someone in your church. Having a wide range of recommendations is valuable because it gives a prospective employer more of a sense of who you are and what kind of person you are.

Health and Fitness

In our field, we should not forget the importance of health and fitness. In some jobs, your fitness level is critical; if you are not fit, you will not be able to do the job. In some cases, if you are unfit, you will be a poor example to your students or coworkers. It might prevent your employment or limit your chances of promotion. Basic health is always important. Healthy, fit people do a better job because there are fewer limiting factors on their performance. They have fewer sick days, and their performance is not lowered by fatigue.

This does not mean that you must be a great athlete or a hard-core fitness buff. It simply means good health, a good diet, regular exercise, and good sleep habits. A balanced lifestyle is the most likely way to guarantee a long, healthy life. It is also the best way to guarantee your fitness to do a good job, regardless of what that job is.

Focus

This last point is not always easy for people to understand. I call it focus: It is your clarity of vision, combined with the seriousness of your intentions. Are you clear about your goals? Do you take your work seriously? Are you committed to what you are doing? Or are you easily distracted? Some might think in terms of commitment, but I think *focus* is a clearer term.

I have coached many athletes, including performers at the national and international levels. Without exception, the most successful of them had focus. They had a very clear, intensely strong sense of what they wanted to achieve, and they let nothing interfere with that goal. If it required sacrifice, they made the sacrifice. If it took time or energy, or if it was a struggle, they allowed no obstacles to stand in their way.

They were focused on a goal, focused as if on a burning light far away in the dark. They never lost sight of their goal, and they never let anything come between them and that goal. They took no chances with their preparation—they did not want to wake up and wonder if the workout they skipped or the special preparation they skimped on was the reason they failed to reach their goal.

Most people are not that dedicated; they lack focus. They have a goal, but they are not that fixed on it. They do not analyze what it takes to achieve the goal, so their preparation is spotty, and their progress is haphazard. Usually, they end up settling for something less than their goal, and they assume that it is because the goal was unattainable. Often, the problem is not the loftiness of the goal, but the lack of focus in the person.

In an interview after being awarded the Nobel Prize in Medicine, Duke University's Dr. Robert Lefkowitz made this comment about the research process: "Good research . . . requires four things: focus, focus, focus and focus."[16]

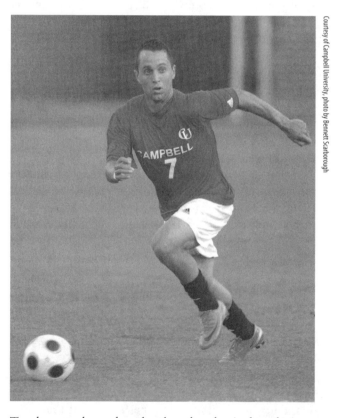

Courtesy of Campbell University, photo by Bennett Scarborough

Teachers and coaches develop the physical, technical, tactical, and psychological skills of athletes and students.

You must have focus. You must be serious about what you want to achieve. You must analyze what your goal requires for success, then carefully plan how to do what it takes. And you must not skip or stint, you must not let obstacles cause you to lose sight of your goals. The average Olympic competitors have trained seriously for 8 years before appearing in the Olympics. They did not get there simply by having talent. They had focus. They worked long and hard. That is what success requires. Success is not an accident. But with focus, you can succeed.

Summary

Success in any field depends on a high level of knowledge and skills related to that field. In developing the knowledge and skills for success, (1) success follows preparation and opportunity, (2) success results from the right habits, (3) success results from the long-term building of your knowledge, and (4) success results from the development of expertise.

Stephen Covey's 7 good habits are: (1) be proactive, (2) begin with the end in mind, (3) put first things first, (4) think win–win, (5) seek first to understand, then to be understood, (6) synergize, and (7) sharpen the saw. Waldroop and Butler's 12 bad habits to overcome are: (1) never feeling good enough, (2) seeing the world in black and white, (3) doing too much and pushing too hard, (4) avoiding conflict at any cost, (5) running roughshod over the opposition, (6) being a rebel looking for a cause, (7) always swinging for the fence, (8) putting fear in the driver's seat, (9) being emotionally tone-deaf, (10) believing no job is good enough, (11) lacking a sense of boundaries, and (12) losing the path.

Career planning is difficult even when you know what you want to do. Many students change majors and career paths within their first 2 years of college. You should ask four questions when choosing a career: (1) Do I enjoy, prefer, and seek personal interactions? (2) Does an undergraduate degree in this field commit me to a career path that I cannot change in the future? (3) How broad an opportunity does a degree in this field offer? and (4) Where do I want to work and live?

Seven broad skills lead to success in any field: (1) a broad knowledge base (cultural literacy), (2) communications skills (speaking and writing), (3) technical skills, (4) research skills, (5) job-hunting skills, (6) health and fitness, and (7) focus.

Further Readings

Bell, Martie. 1997. The development of expertise. *JOPERD (Journal of Physical Education, Recreation and Dance)* (February): 34–38.

Burniske, R. W. 1999. The teacher as a skilled generalist: Preserving humanist traditions in an age of technological utopianism. *Phi Delta Kappan* (October): 121–126.

Covey, Stephen. 1990. *The 7 habits of highly effective people: Powerful lessons in personal change.* New York: Free Press.

Crase, Darrell. 1993. Highly productive scholars: What drives them toward success? *JOPERD (Journal of Physical Education, Recreation and Dance)* (August): 80–82.

DeLong, David W. 2004. *Lost knowledge: Confronting the threat of an aging workforce.* New York: Oxford Univ. Press.

Ellis, Michael J. 1988. *The business of physical education: Future of the profession.* Champaign, IL: Human Kinetics.

Gladwell, Malcolm. 2008. *Outliers: The story of success.* New York: Little, Brown.

Lehrer, Jonah. 2012. *Imagine: How creativity works.* Boston: Houghton Mifflin Harcourt.

Leonard, Dorothy, and Walter Swap. 2005. *Deep smarts: How to cultivate and transfer enduring business wisdom.* Boston: Harvard Business School Press.

Ross, Philip E. 2006. The expert mind. *Scientific American* 295 (2): 64–71.

Tan, Steven K. S. 1997. The elements of expertise. *JOPERD (Journal of Physical Education, Recreation and Dance)* (February): 30–33.

Tishman, Shari, and David N. Perkins. 1995. Critical thinking and physical education. *JOPERD (Journal of Physical Education, Recreation and Dance)* (August): 24–30.

Walberg, Marvin. 2012. Use Facebook timeline effectively in job hunt. Scripps Howard News Service, reprinted in *Raleigh (NC) News and Observer,* March 11, 3E.

Waldroop, James, and Timothy Butler. 2000. *The 12 bad habits that hold good people back.* New York: Currency/Doubleday.

Zeigler, Earle F. 1995. Competency in critical thinking: A requirement of the "allied professional." *Quest* 47: 196–211.

Discussion Questions

1. What is the process and importance of developing the knowledge and skills for success in your career? How would you do it for your career choice?

2. The chapter lists seven broad skills needed for success in our field. What are they, and what part does each play in becoming a success?

3. For the career track that interests you, what are the areas of learning (cognitive and physical) needed for success?

References

1. Gladwell, Malcolm. 2008. *Outliers: The story of success.* New York: Little, Brown, 19.

2. Bowerman, William J., and William H. Freeman. 1974/2009. *Coaching track and field.* Boston: Houghton Mifflin. Repr. *Bill Bowerman's high performance training for track and field.* 3rd ed. Monterey, CA: Coaches Choice.

3. Freeman, William H. 1977. *Physical education in a changing society.* Boston: Houghton Mifflin.

4. Covey, Stephen. 1990. *The 7 habits of highly effective people: Powerful lessons in personal change.* New York: Free Press.

5. Waldroop, James, and Timothy Butler. 2000. *The 12 bad habits that hold good people back*. New York: Currency/Doubleday.

6. Warlick, David F. 2009. *Redefining literacy 2.0*. 2nd ed. Columbus, OH: Linworth.

7. DeLong, David W. 2004. *Lost knowledge: Confronting the threat of an aging workforce*. New York: Oxford Univ. Press.

8. Leonard, Dorothy, and Walter Swap. 2005. *Deep smarts: How to cultivate and transfer enduring business wisdom*. Boston: Harvard Business School Press.

9. Ross, Philip E. 2006. The expert mind. *Scientific American* 295 (2): 64–71.

10. Dasgupta, Subrada. 2003. Multidisciplinary creativity: The case of Herbert A. Simon. *Cognitive Science* 27: 683–707.

11. Ross, Expert mind, 66.

12. Wade, Michael G., and John A. W. Baker. 1995. *Introduction to kinesiology: The science and practice of physical activity*. Madison, WI: Brown and Benchmark, 174–176.

13. Zakrajsek, Dorothy, and William Pierce. 1993. Academic preparation and the academic consumer. *JOPERD (Journal of Physical Education, Recreation, and Dance)* (May–June): 20–23, 31.

14. Crase, Darrell. 1993. Highly productive scholars: What drives them toward success? *JOPERD (Journal of Physical Education, Recreation and Dance)* (August): 80–82.

15. Zeigler, Earle F. 1994. *Critical thinking for the professions of health, sport and physical education, recreation, and dance*. Champaign, IL: Stipes; Tishman, Shari, and David N. Perkins. 1995. Critical thinking and physical education. *JOPERD (Journal of Physical Education, Recreation and Dance)* (August): 24–30; and LeBlanc, Hugues. 1998. Critical thinking in physical education in teacher education. Paper presented at the 8th European Congress of the International Council for Health, Physical Education, Recreation, Sport and Dance, St. Mary's Univ. College, Strawberry Hill, England.

16. Price, Jay. 2012. Robert Lefkowitz. *Raleigh (NC) News and Observer,* December 30, 1A, 9A.

Traditional Careers in Physical Education

Physical education is both a discipline and a profession. With the current shift toward a redefined kinesiology as the scholarly focus of a broader, more unified field of study, the acceptance of a research-focused subdiscipline of sport pedagogy has grown. However, I prefer the term *movement pedagogy*, which seems a more accurate name for the subdiscipline. It represents the scholarly side of teaching, the discipline arm of the profession. In short, movement pedagogy includes the study of any organized teaching or learning related to human movement, regardless of where the activity takes place.

This chapter is concerned with the profession and the career options that you can find in physical education and sport. First, this chapter reviews what a profession involves and what constitutes being a member of a profession, followed by a discussion of the professional development of the physical education student and of the different career options in the field.

The Meaning of *Professional*

I use the term *professional* in its academic sense; that is, a professional is a member or practitioner of a recognized profession. In our case, the profession of physical education refers to teachers of physical education. To understand what this means, a brief review of the discussion of the profession is useful.

Abraham Flexner suggested six criteria or characteristics of a profession. Although they were created in 1915, his criteria are still the most commonly accepted in our field.[1] According to Flexner, these are the characteristics of a profession:

1. Intellectual activity (a "body of knowledge")
2. Practical use
3. Research resulting in new knowledge and ideas
4. Self-organization
5. Communication capacity (internal and external)
6. Altruism (dedication to helping others)

Though we may teach physical skills, an intellectual base of knowledge is required if we are to be fully effective teachers. This is a critical point because the body of knowledge should be broader and deeper than that possessed by a non-professional, such as an experienced athlete without an academic base.

A practical use or application for knowledge must exist in a profession. It cannot be knowledge gained purely for its own sake; it must be knowledge that can be applied to some practical use, such as the development and improvement of people's health, skills, or fitness. Research that results in new knowledge and ideas should be found in a profession. True professionals never stop trying to learn more about their field because this search for knowledge steadily increases their effectiveness and level of performance.

Formal self-organization or professional bodies should exist. These professional bodies provide the capacity for communication—usually through professional publications and meetings.

Finally, an important characteristic of a profession is altruism. *A profession exists to help others.* Its members are concerned about the welfare of other people; they work to help protect or to improve the lives of others.

An important distinction to clarify is what a professional is *not*. A professional athlete does *not* meet the criteria for a member of a profession. Often, students are confused about what a professional is because of their familiarity with the term *professional athlete.* In that sense, *professional* is simply a person who performs for money. By *that* definition (lack of amateur status), every employed person is a professional.

It is important to remember this distinction. A professional in the true sense is a member of a recognized profession, not simply a person willing to perform a task for money. A "roll out the ball" teacher is no more a true professional than is the ordinary person on the street. A professional holds *high standards* in a field that meets the criteria presented earlier. Consequently, a true professional takes pride in a chosen profession.

Becoming an Involved Professional: Development and Responsibilities

Becoming an involved, committed member of a profession is an ongoing process. As a student preparing to teach physical education, you need to meet at least the minimal standards for admission to the profession. When you join the profession after graduation, you will work to improve yourself as a professional. The areas of professional concern at both the student and practicing professional levels follow.[2]

School Selection

Your first hurdle is to choose a college for undergraduate or graduate preparation. In many cases students give too little thought to a school and what it has to offer. An undergraduate institution should have a strong major program in your area of interest, whether it be physical education, health education, recreation, safety education, or dance. You can also receive good undergraduate training in the many combined health and physical education major programs that are found in the smaller schools, although you should ensure that a broad, well-balanced preparation is available. Today some programs are majors in exercise science, exercise and sport science, kinesiology, and other titles, with teacher certification or licensure.

Study the requirements for admission to the school's major program. What type of nonmajor courses are required by the department or the school? Who teaches the courses: professors or teaching assistants? What kind of reputation does the school have in the state and region? Are its graduates respected? Are its graduates successful?

There is an additional concern when you prepare to go to graduate school. You should consider the regional and national reputation of the department and school. What do the faculties of other schools think of the school and its graduates? Where do its graduates find employment? What are the admission and retention standards of the school? Are its professors respected specialists with advanced training in their areas of specialization? Where were the professors trained? Remember that many benefits are gained by earning your degrees at several schools, rather than at one. Many graduate schools will not allow their students to earn all of their degrees, bachelor's through doctorate, at the same school because of the risk of developing a narrow, provincial viewpoint.

Developing and Using a Personal Professional Library

This category might be called *developing the tools of the trade* because at the undergraduate level it means building a strong personal library of professional publications and learning to use the school library and its resources. Library skills are critical to success in professional work. At the same time, your personal library should be broad. As you begin to work in specialized areas, however, a more defined outlook of interests becomes evident in the titles in your personal library.

A common complaint is that too many physical educators are nonreaders, often a reflection of a very narrow professional education. You should read widely, including current newspapers and general periodicals, as well as professional publications. Such reading helps to establish common lines of communication with people outside the field.

Professional Preparation

A good program of professional preparation is also essential. The physical educator needs a strong, broad undergraduate education, but the process of education does not end with a bachelor's degree. Many teachers do additional work through continuing education programs. More advanced work helps you to develop expertise in specialized areas. Your professional preparation can take many years, but it should be a challenging, stimulating experience.

Professional Membership

Membership in professional organizations is one sign of true professional commitment. As an undergraduate, you will find student major clubs and professional fraternities such as Phi Epsilon Kappa on campus. You also will find that most state organizations and the American Alliance for Health, Physical Education, Recreation and Dance (AAHPERD) have lower student membership fees. Those memberships include most professional privileges, including subscriptions to the professional publications.

As a graduate and a professional, you should join AAHPERD at the state and national levels. Membership in many other professional organizations can also benefit an active professional. As a physical educator with a genuine commitment to the profession, you want to be actively involved in other professional groups dedicated to advancing the profession.

Professional Meetings

Professional membership shows an interest in the condition of the profession, but a real commitment involves attending professional meetings. Many such meetings occur regularly around the world. They are the most exciting means of communication among professionals because at those meetings you can meet people from many different backgrounds and discuss common problems and discoveries. In many respects, the greatest impetus to change may result from the stimulus and challenge of these meetings.

At the undergraduate level, you may find statewide student major conventions. They can help you to become more involved and to gain valuable experiences and contacts. You also may want to attend the specialized clinics that are held for areas of interest such as sports coaching, officiating, or the clinics of the President's Council on Physical Fitness and Sports. Those meetings are useful because they broaden your outlook and your experiences as a student.

As a practicing physical educator, you will become more aware of the regular professional conventions. Examples are the annual AAHPERD conventions at the state, district, and national levels. You should try to attend one or more of the conventions annually because the experience is invaluable. Most professional groups have an annual convention, for which the members plan the meetings and the programs.

Mere attendance at the professional meetings is not enough, however. For a profession to grow and improve, its members must be directly involved in its activities. Many professionals become involved in high-level organization work simply because no one else is willing to help. There are numerous opportunities for direct involvement at all levels of professional activities. As a student, you should try to become involved. Most larger conventions have special sections and meetings to encourage student participation. There is room for anyone who is willing to help.

Research and Writing

Too few physical educators are involved in research and writing. A profession and discipline need research to extend the boundaries of knowledge and improve practices.

You need to realize that *every* member of the field is capable of conducting research at some level. Lack of time is often used as an argument for not doing research, but the real reasons are usually the lack of self-confidence or of encouragement. Physical educators should feel obligated to conduct regular research, whether or not it is major or significant.

The same reasons cited for failing to do research are also cited for the failure of physical educators to write about their activities or the state of the profession. We must write to share our ideas, our concerns, and our theories. Our writings can show others how we solved the problems that they are facing.

A profession and a discipline develop out of the professional meetings and the written word. Write about your ideas, and encourage others to write about theirs. Do not be afraid to write because you fear ridicule or lack confidence in your opinions. Physical educators must be willing to accept valid criticism if they are to grow as professionals. They also must encourage writing and research on a grand scale. The more work that is done, the greater the odds that a larger number of better scholars and writers will contribute to improve the field.

The national meetings may be flooded with people willing to write and speak; however, this is not often the case at the district level, and only rarely is it the case at the state level. Get involved, and see where it leads you. The field of physical education will be the better for it, and so will you.

Teaching

The public thinks of physical educators as primarily teachers and coaches. Thus, the physical educator should be dedicated to quality teaching, research, and writing. The future of physical education rests largely on the opinions of the future citizens whom we teach in the schools. Coaching is another form of teaching, when it is done well. Educators should provide quality coaching, but it should never interfere with the quality of teaching. Teaching programs are the cornerstone of public relations in the field.

Commitment

If a single word describes the most desirable characteristic of the professional physical educator (or a member of any other profession), it is *commitment*. True professionals must be committed to their fields. Only by being committed and totally involved can physical educators hope to make a real contribution to the profession. Furthermore, commitment is most valuable if it is a commitment to excellence.

Pride

We sometimes forget the importance of personal pride in our field and in our job as a critical factor in personal success. Physical education is a very worthy field that requires high levels of knowledge and expertise for success. At the same time, it can make an extremely valuable contribution to the life of every student or athlete who works with a quality teacher or coach.

What Are the Components of Professional Preparation?

The college training of the physical educator is traditionally called *professional preparation* in the belief that teaching is indeed a profession. Organized collegiate programs designed to train physical educators for teaching are little more than a century old. In the past, the traditional patterns of preparation were teacher oriented. Most programs now offer several options that do not involve teacher training.

The original pattern of professional preparation developed from the early normal schools, which were simply teachers' colleges. The teacher emphasis of those schools had a major impact on how physical educators were trained. Although physical educators have tried to ally themselves more closely with the sciences, the traditional patterns are not easily changed.

Professional preparation for physical educators covers four areas. The first area includes the academic courses required by the college. Called *general education*, it provides the student with broad academic training in the first 2 years of college. It exposes the student to the breadth of human knowledge.

The second area, the *foundation sciences*, concentrates on the biological sciences, especially anatomy and physiology. Increasingly, however, emphasis is directed toward an understanding of chemistry, which underlies biology (particularly in exercise physiology), as well as physics, which provides an understanding of the mechanics of human movement.

The third area is *professional education*, which is entirely oriented toward teaching. It includes the student teaching experience, generally considered the most valuable portion of the area. Student teaching is required for teacher certification below the college level, and in some cases it is required for junior college teaching.

The fourth area is *physical education*, the teaching major. In many colleges it is a combination of health education and physical education, although it may focus on a single area of the broad field, such as physical education itself, health education, recreation, dance, safety education, or any of the newer areas of specialization.

What Is the Job Situation in Physical Education?

Many students are concerned about future job opportunities in physical education. To understand the job market, we need to understand how it has changed over the last 2 decades. The 1980s saw an economic decline that affected the hiring and retention practices of the schools. This resulted in an unstable employment situation in teaching. At the same time, the number of public school students decreased, while the number of teachers increased beyond the needs of the schools. Most subject and grade areas had a considerable oversupply of teachers, and the number of teachers being produced each year exceeded the number of jobs by a large margin.

The drop in the school population resulted from an increased concern with birth control; women preferred having fewer children, so the size of the typical family began to decrease. Although the zero population growth goal of many birth-control advocates did not happen, the number of students hit a high-water mark and then began a gradual decline.

The effect of the declining birth rate on the school population and teacher needs was compounded by another trend: the consolidation of schools, particularly at the middle or junior high school and high school levels. Smaller schools were combined into larger schools to offer a broader educational program, eliminate unnecessary duplication of teachers within the school district, and end the age-old problem of racially segregated schools.

At the elementary through high school levels, the glut of teachers could have produced positive changes in education. The schools had an unprecedented opportunity to hire the most qualified applicants and remove teachers who were poorly qualified or incompetent. Unfortunately, a strong seniority system, not the quality of the teacher, decided who would be released from employment.

The oversupply of teachers could also have been used to make radical cuts in the size of the classes taught by teachers. A commonly held (though unproven) belief of teachers is that students learn more and better in a small class than in a large one. This, also, did not happen. In fact, the financial crunch in many cases resulted in the release of so many teachers that class sizes increased despite the overall teacher surplus.

Today the job market in physical education is erratic. As a result of several years of difficult economic conditions in the United States, many school districts are forced to operate on smaller budgets, which reduces the number of new teacher hires. The circumstances can vary widely from one place to another, so one district may be hiring at the same time that another nearby district is cutting back. Thus, the demand for physical education teachers is difficult to project in the short term. In the long term, job opportunities for the best graduates should rise.

Teaching as a Career: Pros and Cons

Many physical education students give little thought to the pros and cons of teaching as a career. Before discussing the opportunities in the teaching areas of physical education, you need to understand the positive and negative factors that affect one's enjoyment of teaching.

Positive Aspects of Teaching

A teacher traditionally holds a position of respect in the community and makes a significant contribution to society. Teaching is vital to the survival of the community, and a good teacher is a positive influence on many young people.

Teaching offers good job security. Generally speaking, teachers are well paid for their services. Although salaries might be higher (which can be said of almost any occupation), there have been large increases in recent decades. Teachers also generally receive automatic pay raises each year, which is not true of most jobs. Teachers enjoy the benefit of long vacations; they work an average of 9 to 10 months of the year. The extra time may be devoted to an additional job, or it can be available for travel or study. Long vacations make teaching attractive to people who want free time to pursue other interests.

Perhaps the greatest positive aspect of teaching as a career, however, is the personal satisfaction it provides. A person who really wants to teach will find the work rewarding because teaching carries a degree of personal involvement in the success of others that is found in few other occupations. Many teachers continue to teach for this reason alone.

Negative Aspects of Teaching

Too few prospective teachers stop to look at the negative aspects of their prospective career. On the negative side, teaching is an overcrowded field. The competition for jobs is very high, and it becomes more so each year. Each new crop of college graduates is often better qualified than earlier graduates, in terms of educational training, degrees, and teaching experience.

At the same time, many new teachers leave teaching every year. About 9% of new teachers fail to complete their first year of employment, and about 30% of beginning teachers either move to another school or quit teaching at the end of their first year. "Up to 50 percent of new teachers leave the profession within five years of entering the classroom."[3]

Although teaching has traditionally been a respected occupation in the abstract sense, respect for teachers as a group has decreased. Schools and teachers suffer from a lack of public support and from public dissatisfaction with their work. This problem carries over into the area of teachers' salaries. Teachers' salaries are not low, and they have risen rapidly, but they are low compared to the education and expense required to qualify for them. Schools prefer to hire teachers with master's degrees, yet the salary increase gained by earning this degree represents only a fraction of the cost of the degree. Moreover, if the degree is earned in a full-time study program, the loss of a full year's teaching salary must be added to the cost of the degree. The educational requirements for the jobs are not consistent with the salaries offered when the requirements are met.

Finally, today's teachers have increasingly heavy workloads, which makes doing a good job more difficult. Although a large surplus of teachers is available, for financial reasons schools hire fewer teachers. The result is larger student loads per teacher, combined with less time for recovering from and preparing for teaching. The large quantities of paperwork that are a traditional part of the educational bureaucracy make the workload heavier because few school systems provide enough clerical workers or teaching aides to free teachers from nonteaching duties. At the same time, teaching has become more dangerous because of increasing levels of violence in the schools.

To Teach or Not to Teach

As you can see, teaching has both a good side and a bad side. As a prospective teacher, you must look at both sides carefully and decide which aspects of teaching carry the most weight for you. For many students the overall satisfaction of a career devoted to helping people outweighs the negatives, but for others the workload or pay situation is enough to drive them away from teaching. You must decide which of these positive and negative aspects are most important to you as you consider teaching as a career.

Basic Qualities of the Successful Teacher

What makes a successful teacher? What are the basic qualities needed to become a successful teacher? The qualities specific to teaching that produce success are discussed here.

Teaching Personality and Interests

Successful teaching requires a favorable combination of personal qualities and interests. A good personality is needed. Teachers should enjoy people, work well with them, and have a good sense of humor. Teachers must be interested in the educational process and in the needs of the students. Teachers must *want* to teach and must *enjoy* teaching.

Strong Educational Background

In addition to having intellectual ability, the successful teacher needs a solid educational background, which means more than simply having a good preparation in the major field. Teaching requires a broadly based program of study in the liberal arts and sciences. A teacher needs to be exposed to and understand the breadth of human experience and knowledge. The teacher's educational background and intellect are closely allied to the next quality.

Health and Physical Skills

The successful teacher needs to be healthy simply to be able to do a good job of teaching. This is particularly true in an area such as physical education, which involves physical skills. In physical education the teacher must have a good combination of coordination, flexibility, strength, and speed.

The teacher needs to be skilled in performing the activities that are going to be taught for two reasons: (1) The teacher will have to demonstrate the skills in many cases, and (2) the teacher will have a far better understanding of the components of the skills and the problems that may be encountered by the student in learning the skills.

Intellectual Ability

If there is one single, most important quality of the teacher, perhaps intellectual ability is that quality. A person does not have to be a genius to teach successfully; however, a person of poor or even average intellectual ability is at a distinct disadvantage. Successful teachers must be able to understand material at higher levels than that which is presented to their students. Also, the teacher should be an example to the students, which is difficult if the students consider the teacher an intellectual inferior. Education has an intellectual base, and a prospective teacher needs the intellectual ability and intelligence to work at a reasonable level of accomplishment. The teacher must be intelligent and have a strong interest in learning. A person with little respect for learning will not become a good teacher.

Types of Teaching Jobs

Physical Education

Although people usually think that physical education teachers work only with basic activity classes at the high school level, the field offers many other teaching opportunities. The first level of employment (in terms of student age) is in working with preschool and elementary school children. This age group is sometimes broken into two groups, with the younger group referred to as K–3, or kindergarten through grade 3. Teaching at this level is increasingly done by specialists instead of classroom teachers. They most often use movement education and perceptual motor activities, rather than teach games and sports skills. Children at this age benefit more from activities that develop the most basic movement skills.

The upper elementary grades are sometimes combined with the middle or junior high school to cover a range of grades from 4 through 9. For this age group, the teacher includes more games and sports skills. They are not of a strenuous nature because the bodies of these students are developing rapidly. Teachers of this age group find that the wide range in body sizes, strength, endurance, and skills of their students requires careful adjustments in the physical education program. Many teachers who want to teach at the high school level begin their teaching careers at the middle school level, in grades 6 through 8.

The high school level, sometimes referred to as *senior high school*, includes grades 9 or 10 through 12. Teachers at these grades include more advanced skills, more strenuous activities, and some lifetime sports. In most cases these teachers, as well as those at the middle school level, also coach sports. The prospective teacher may find jobs in private schools, academies, or the public schools.

Beyond the high school level there are two basic types of educational institutions. One is aimed at terminal degree programs of a practical nature. These are most often technical schools or community colleges with 1- or 2-year programs. Whether physical education is offered in these schools depends on the educational philosophy and goals of the community, county, or state sponsoring the school.

The other type of institution is the traditional college, such as the junior college (with 2-year programs that are usually liberal arts oriented) and the senior college or university (with 4-year programs). Most of these institutions have physical education programs, and many of them also have programs for majors.

A teacher is more likely to be a specialist at the college level. Some college teachers primarily teach activity classes, so they may do most of their teaching in the narrow range of four to six specific activities rather than teach a little bit from every type of physical activity. Some college teachers work primarily in teacher preparation, teaching coaching theory, professional skills, the scientific foundations, or other theory areas such as administration or measurement and evaluation. Some college teachers work with intramural programs or in research, and others work as program administrators. As the academic level gets higher, the variety of teaching jobs increases considerably.

There are other teaching possibilities in addition to those in public and private schools and at the college level. A teacher may work for the government and teach in schools on armed forces bases, both in the United States and abroad. These teachers enjoy many of the benefits of governmental service employment. A teacher may also be employed under government-sponsored programs such as the Peace Corps.

Health Education

Health education has become a field that is often separated from physical education. Health educators want to improve the health knowledge and practices of all people, though we commonly think of this work being done in the schools. Many schools below the college level hire specialists in health education, rather than have those classes taught by the physical education teacher (who often has limited training in health). Many of the jobs in the field of health education and school health services are nonteaching jobs.

Recreation

Recreation opportunities are growing rapidly, particularly at the community level. The number of recreation teachers is not large, though it is increasing. Recreation is taught primarily at the college and university level to people majoring in physical education or specializing in recreation and recreational services. As many nations become more affluent and leisure time increases, the recreation specialist will gain increasing importance.

Coaching

Coaching athletic teams has traditionally been an important part of the teaching duties of physical educators in American schools. Many people argue over whether coaching is, in fact, a form of teaching. When it is done well and with a regard to more than the immediate aim of victory, coaching is a very important type of teaching. It affects students for much of their lives.

Coaches are hired as teacher–coaches at the junior high or middle school level, at the high school level, and at the college and university level. Many coaches are now hired part time and are not otherwise employed by the school. The larger the college is, the less likely the coach is to be a teacher as well. Coaching is a very popular aspect of physical education work. It has made the field attractive for future physical educators. The importance of coaching can be exaggerated, but one should not overreact by trying to cast out coaches as unworthy physical educators. They have much to contribute to the field.

Safety Education

Safety education includes all areas of safety practices, including driver education. Many states require young drivers to complete an approved course of driver education before they can receive a driver's license. Insurance companies offer lower rates to young people who complete such courses. Bicycle and recreational vehicle safety has been added to many programs of safety education. The field is concerned with developing safety consciousness and an awareness of the dangers that exist in many activities.

Dance

Many students who major or minor in dance activities become teachers either in the schools or by offering private lessons to students. Although more dance teachers are women, the number of men in dance is increasing. Popular activities are folk dancing as a recreational activity and types of dance as exercise, especially for young women. It also may be used as therapy. Dance offers many benefits in the development of coordination and grace.

The Need for Specialists

Physical education teachers and coaches are in oversupply as a group, yet many areas of teaching and coaching are still not crowded. The field of special education needs teachers who can work with the exceptional child. Teaching special education classes, or using *adapted activities*, refers to teaching any person who is unable to benefit from the usual program of physical activities. It can include working with gifted children, whose needs for more intellectual content or approaches to physical activities are rarely met. It can include working with children who have mental disabilities and with children who have physical disabilities ranging from temporary injury to blindness, deafness, and diseases such as muscular dystrophy and polio. The need for people who are skilled in the special education area is great.

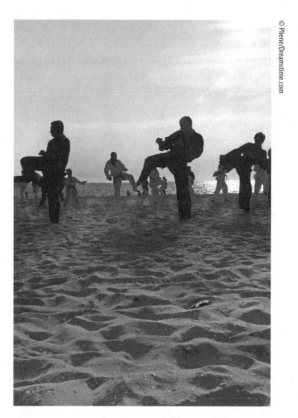

© Pliene/Dreamstime.com

Our concepts of exercise and beauty change
as we encounter different forms of movement.

Specialists are needed in areas such as aquatics and gymnastics because some specialized coaching areas are still far from crowded. The oversupply of coaches is primarily in the so-called major sports, such as football and basketball. Schools offer a wide variety of different sports, but they are handicapped by a lack of trained coaches. Because some formerly regional sports are spreading across the nation, specialists are needed in places where those sports were not common in the past.

Specialists are also needed in the areas of lifetime sports. Many schools have changed the orientation of their programs from fitness activities to lifetime sports, which requires changes in teacher training. At the same time, coeducational activities have become the norm, rather than classes grouped by sex. This change affects teaching content and methods and requires new types of training for different specialties.

Women coaches are a growing group of specialists. The massive increase in the number of women's athletics teams since the passage of Title IX has far outstripped the supply of trained women coaches in most sports. This need, along with the limited number of women physical educators, combines to create a strong job market for women physical educators who are coaching specialists.

Elementary school specialists are also growing in number. They have been in short supply, though some schools have tried to fill that void. More schools are hiring specialists to teach physical education to children or to act as advisors or supervisors to lower-grade-level classroom teachers. The demand at this level is increasing, and teachers of both sexes are needed. The traditional elementary specialist has been female, which has created a greater market for male specialists.

Challenge-oriented specialists are in increasing demand. Examples are instructors in programs such as Outward Bound. These programs, which are designed to challenge the participants, began outside the school, but are now being added to college and high school physical education programs. They provide an extended test of the individual that is difficult to reproduce in the usual school situation. Risk sports are a rapidly growing area of interest.[4]

New areas of scholarship have appeared at the college level, though they are not teacher-oriented activities. Many physical educators specialize in the research areas described in the discussion of disciplines. These areas include motor learning and motor development, sport psychology, sport sociology, sport history, sport philosophy, and new dimensions of biomechanical and physiological sport research. New opportunities are developing in those areas as growing numbers of professionals concentrate in the scholarly studies areas.

This survey is only a sampling of the teaching jobs that are available in physical education and its allied fields. Although the field has an overall surplus of teachers, many areas need more teachers. As a prospective teacher, you can improve your employment potential by developing a specialty in an area of need. The teaching possibilities in physical education are not limited, unless your interests are only in the most common teaching areas.

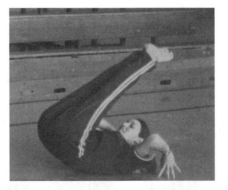

Part of professional development for teachers and coaches is personal skill development, which helps in understanding the learning process and in being able to demonstrate skills to learners.

The Future of Teaching Jobs

As noted, the need for general teachers of physical education is erratic at this time, so the job market in teaching is difficult to project. There is always a greater demand for above-average graduates (the A or B student) than for C students, who exist in considerable oversupply. The teachers with the best chances of finding jobs are those with good grades and at least one area of needed specialization.

Few students realize that many teaching opportunities exist outside the traditional schools. The greatest demands are with recreational activities and services, which in turn create a market for sporting equipment and supplies. By studying the job market carefully and at an early stage in the training process, the student of physical education can find many good potential jobs. However, the student who has only ordinary grades and does not develop a specialty will have a more difficult time finding a job after graduation.

Summary

Movement pedagogy includes the study of any organized teaching or learning related to human movement, regardless of where the activity takes place. It is a profession, and according to Abraham Flexner a profession has six characteristics: (1) intellectual activity, (2) a practical use, (3) research resulting in new knowledge and ideas, (4) self-organization, (5) communication capacity, and (6) altruism, a dedication to helping others.

Becoming an involved, committed member of a profession includes attention to (1) school selection, (2) developing and using a personal professional library, (3) professional preparation, (4) professional membership, (5) attendance at professional meetings, (6) research and writing, (7) teaching, (8) commitment, and (9) pride. Professional preparation for physical educators covers four areas: (1) general education, (2) the foundation sciences, (3) professional education, and (4) physical education.

The basic job situation in physical education is erratic at this time. It is better for women than for men, but there may be exceptions for people with useful specialties.

The positive side of teaching includes respect in the community, making a significant contribution to society, good job security, and the personal satisfaction it provides. The negative side of teaching includes high competition for jobs, a decrease in respect for teachers as a group, low salaries compared to the education and expense required to qualify for them, and increasingly heavy workloads.

The basic qualities needed to become a successful teacher include (1) good teaching personality and interests, (2) a strong educational background, (3) health and physical skills, and (4) intellectual ability.

Types of teaching jobs include physical education, health education, recreation, coaching, safety education, and dance. There is always a need for teaching specialists, who either specialize in teaching at a certain educational level or are proficient in certain subject areas.

Further Readings

Blakemore, Connie L., Nena R. Hawkes, Carol Wilkinson, Maria Zanandrea, and Joyce M. Harrison. 1997. The "Flight" Program: Nontraditional preparation of physical education teachers. *JOPERD (Journal of Physical Education, Recreation and Dance)* (May–June): 56–66.

Burniske, R. W. 1999. The teacher as skilled generalist. *Phi Delta Kappa* 81 (2): 121–122, 124, 126.

Collier, Douglas, and Fred Hebert. 2004. Undergraduate physical education teacher preparation: What the practitioners tell us. *Physical Educator* 61: 102–112.

Cushion, Christopher J., Kathy M. Armour, and Robyn L. Jones. 2003. Coach education and continuing professional development: Experience and learning to coach. *Quest* 55 (2): 215–230.

Drewe, Sheryle Bergmann. 2000. An examination of the relationship between coaching and teaching. *Quest* 52: 79–88.

Floyd, Patricia A., and Beverly Allen. 2008. *Careers in health, physical education, and sports.* 2nd ed. Florence, KY: Brooks Cole.

Giebel, Nancy. 2004. *Great jobs for physical education majors.* New York: McGraw-Hill.

Heitzmann, William Ray. 2003. *Opportunities in sports and fitness careers.* New York: McGraw-Hill.

Lackey, Donald. 1994. High school coaching—still a "pressure cooker" profession. *JOPERD (Journal of Physical Education, Recreation and Dance)* (August): 68–71.

Lounsbery, Monica, and Cheryl Coker. 2008. Developing skill-analysis competency in physical education. *Quest* 60: 255–267.

McBride, Ron E., and Ping Xiang. 2004. Thoughtful decision making in physical education: A modest proposal. *Quest* 56: 337–354.

National Association for Sport and Physical Education. 2006. *Quality coaches, quality sports: National standards for sport coaches.* 2nd ed. Reston, VA: NASPE.

Owens, Lynn M., and Catherine D. Ennis. 2005. The ethic of care in teaching: An overview of supportive literature. *Quest* 57: 392–425.

Rink, Judith E. 1997. Teacher education programs: The role of context in learning how to teach. *JOPERD (Journal of Physical Education, Recreation and Dance)* (January): 17–19, 24.

Sawyer, Thomas H. 2006. Point–counterpoint: The physically illiterate physical educator. *Physical Educator* 63: 2–7.

Sisley, Becky L., and Gwen Steigelman. 1994. From coach to athletic director: A leadership program for women. *JOPERD (Journal of Physical Education, Recreation and Dance)* (October): 62–64.

Stevens, Deborah Ann, and Adelaide Carpenter. 1998. Physical education job security: Saving our jobs and programs. *JOPERD (Journal of Physical Education, Recreation and Dance)* (April): 53–59.

Tinning, Richard. 2010. *Pedagogy and human movement*. New York: Routledge.

Wright, Steven C., and Daniel E. Smith. 2000. A case for formalized mentoring. *Quest* 52: 200–213.

Zeigler, Earle F. 1997. From one image to a sharper one! *Physical Educator* 54: 72–77.

———. 1999. The profession must work "harder and smarter" to inform those officials who make decisions that affect the field. *Physical Educator* 56: 114–119.

———. 2003. Guiding professional students to literacy in physical activity education. *Quest* 55: 285–305.

Discussion Questions

1. What is a professional? Which criteria are used to determine whether a field is a profession?

2. Charles Bucher once wrote of physical education as an "emerging profession." Explain what he meant and why he made such a statement.

3. Among the criteria for a profession are the duties to be selective in admitting members, to require very thorough training for all candidates, and to discipline or expel members who do not meet the standards of the profession. Discuss the field of physical education in terms of those criteria. Does physical education meet those requirements?

4. Briefly discuss what is involved in becoming a committed member of a profession.

5. What functions should professional organizations serve? List three professional organizations in any area of physical education and briefly explain their function or area of interest.

6. Briefly discuss the job market for teachers of physical education. What will the market probably be like in the next decade?

7. Discuss three teaching areas or specializations in which the job possibilities are likely to increase in the future.

8. Discuss the pros and cons of planning to become a full-time coach or professional athlete. What are the odds against finding such jobs, and what qualifications are needed for the jobs?

9. James B. Conant suggested that "the physical education teacher should have an even wider general academic education than any other teacher." Explain briefly what he meant, the reason behind the statement, and its implications for the professional preparation of physical educators.

References

1. Kroll, Walter. 1971. *Perspectives in physical education.* New York: Academic; and in Wade, Michael G., and John A. W. Baker, eds. 1995. *Introduction to kinesiology: The science and practice of physical activity.* Madison, WI: Brown and Benchmark, 123.

2. Seidel, Beverly L., and Matthew C. Resick. 1978. *Physical education: An overview.* 2nd ed. Reading, MA: Addison-Wesley.

3. Eaton, Elizabeth, and Wendy Sisson. 2008. *Why are new teachers leaving? The case for beginning-teacher induction and mentoring.* ICF International. http://www.icfi.com/insights/white-papers/2009/why-are-new-teachers-leaving-the-case-for-beginning-teacher-induction-and-mentoring

4. Greenfeld, Karl Taro. 1999. Life on the edge. *Time,* September 9, 28–36.

Careers in Sport, Exercise Science, and Kinesiology

The majority of jobs in our field today are not in teaching or coaching. Not every student is interested in teaching as a career. Many new careers are appearing, some of which require specialized degrees in other areas, such as recreation or physical therapy. In some areas, a business, communications, or science minor or major may be helpful. A number of books provide an overview of careers in exercise science and sport-related areas.[1] **Table 12.1** shows some of those career areas.

This chapter provides an overview of types of careers within the categories of (1) sport (not including coaching), (2) sport business, (3) sport entrepreneurship, (4) recreational areas, (5) exercise science, and (6) kinesiology (health sciences). These descriptions are necessarily brief because enough potential careers exist to fill several books with detailed descriptions of the jobs, the needed qualifications, and the potential career tracks through a person's career.

Careers in Sport

College Athletic Administration

Work in intercollegiate athletics is a popular goal for athletes, but it is much more complex than it appears to be on the surface. Specialized training in areas of business or promotions is often required for success. Examples of jobs in this area include being an athletic director, director of fundraising, promotions director, director of athletic facilities, director of academic affairs, compliance officer, business manager, sports information director, and coach.

Many college coaches devote their full time to coaching duties, but some coaches also run coaching clinics, schools, and camps, especially during the summer months. This activity has become very popular in the United States, and as the professional sports teams increase in number, more professional coaching positions are becoming available. In fact, this is another area in which training in sport administration is very useful.

Table 12.1 Careers in Exercise Science and Sport

Careers in Sport
College athletics administration
Equipment managers
Facility management
Sport finance
Sport marketing
Scouts
Sports camp director
Sports information
Sports journalism and broadcast media
Sports officiating
Sports statistician
Professional athlete

Careers in Sport Business
Sport management
Sport marketing and sales
Sport financial operations
Sport facility management
Arenas and stadiums
Racetracks
Speedways and dirt tracks
Motor sports management
Concessions operations

Careers in Sport and Leisure Services Entrepreneurship and Consulting
Sports consultant
Athletic scholarship placement services
After school sport businesses
Sports agent
Sports event management
Sport facility design and construction

Table 12.1 (*continued*)

    Sport manufacturing and production

    Sport marketing services

    Sport product and service research and development

    Sport product design

    Sport photography

    Sport media production

    Sport publishing

    Sporting goods

    Biomechanical evaluation and equipment design

    Exercise physiological testing and equipment design

    Software design for training and evaluation systems

    Software design for sports gaming systems

Careers in Recreational Areas

    Campus recreation programs

    YMCA and club sports

    Community-based sport and recreation

    Church recreation programs

    Sports club management

    Aquatics management

    Tennis club management

    Professional golf management

    Teaching professional

Careers in Exercise Science (See Entrepreneurship list also)

    ACSM certification occupations

    Research, basic and applied

    Physical fitness industry

    Fitness testing

    Exercise technician

    Sport nutritionist

(continues)

Table 12.1 *(continued)*

Careers in Kinesiology

Medical doctors

Rehabilitation and injury prevention

   Athletic training and sports medicine

   Physical therapy

   Chiropractic

   Physician assistant

   Other therapeutic areas

ACSM certification occupations

Health education and services

Note: ACSM = American College of Sports Medicine.

Equipment Managers

Equipment managers organize, maintain, and distribute the large quantities of equipment used in a college (or professional) sports program. This includes uniforms, training gear, and equipment used in any sport. This position may also occur in a large intramural or college physical education activity program.

Facility Management

Facility managers oversee the operations of large sport-related complexes. Examples of the jobs in this area include facility director, scheduling director, operations manager, box office manager, personnel manager, stage manager, and concessions manager. Besides training in sport management, you need an understanding of buildings and grounds designs, and the operation of large multipurpose facilities. The facilities may be public or private, ranging from university facilities to municipal facilities to private operations. Public relations skills are critical, as is the ability to work under pressure.

Sometimes event management is a part of facility management. A major facility, such as Madison Square Garden, has a wide variety of events during the year, but it provides its own management for those events. In this case, an understanding of the facility, its staff, and its operations is the critical element. The facility manager works with the sponsors to see that any special needs are met.

Sport Finance

College athletic departments are businesses. In larger schools, their budgets may be run separately from their school's budget, in which case most of the operational funds come from ticket sales, sponsorships, and donations. Effective financial oversight of large athletic programs requires experience and some business training.

Sport Marketing

Sport marketing in colleges primarily involves marketing and advertisement for the school teams. All teams, college and professional, require skillful marketing programs to maximize their income and success.

Scouts

While assistant coaches do most of the scouting for college teams, professional teams hire people to be the scouts who help them locate new talent. This occupation usually requires experience in a sport along with years of experience in learning which traits are needed for success in a sport.

Sports Camp Director

Most colleges now have summer sports camps. Originally, they were small operations designed in part to provide additional income to underpaid coaches during the summer. Today they are sometimes very large operations that provide a significant source of additional funding for athletic departments and colleges.

Sports Information

Sports information is an area of work much larger than people realize. It includes sports information directors and their assistants at the college and professional sports levels, print media sports journalists, broadcast sports journalists, and people working in publishing.

The jobs require a thorough knowledge of sport, a great curiosity about sporting activities, the ability to organize your thoughts well, and good presentation skills in writing and speech. Courses in journalism and communications provide important additions to work in the sports field.

Sports Journalism and Broadcast Media

Sports journalism and broadcast media are the public side of college sports. These are jobs with local newspapers, radio and television companies, and Internet operations. They provide independent coverage of high school, college, and professional sports events to the public.

Sports Officiating

Some people are employed as full-time sports officials, most often by professional sports. Most of the sports officials that we see are officiating as a part-time job because of their love of the sport. Their officiating comes on top of their regular jobs. There are officiating schools to help train potential high-level officials.

Sports Statistician

Most teams use someone to maintain statistics for their teams and athletes. In amateur (school and youth) sports, they are usually volunteers or people with other duties as their primary job requirements. However, at the higher levels of sport large amounts of time may be required to develop, maintain, and publish a team's or league's sports statistics.

Professional Athlete

Like intercollegiate athletics, a career in a professional sport organization is another popular goal for athletes. Examples of jobs in professional sport include general manager, director of promotions, director of public relations, director of facilities, ticket director, travel secretary, sports information director, and coach.

Many high school and college athletes hope to make a career of professional athletics. The one thing to keep in mind is that the competition is extremely keen; the odds against a high school athlete playing well in college and continuing on into professional sports successfully are in the thousands-to-one range. The most unfortunate aspect of the interest in playing professional sports and in coaching at a high level is that too many athletes neglect to prepare themselves to do anything else. As a basic precaution, a student interested in professional sports should be educated for a second career.

Careers in Sport Business

The increased number of people who are interested in activities requiring more formal settings has created a market for administrators of such facilities and programs. Qualifications include an understanding of the facilities and equipment needed for the activities, plus the business skills necessary to handle budgeting, staffing, and other administrative tasks. Many schools now offer programs with a concentration in sport management, which usually involves a combination of exercise science and business administration courses.

Sport Management

Sport management requires the same managerial skills as in the primary sport settings, except that in this case the setting is in a business environment. At one time, managerial theory taught that the basic skills of management were the same regardless of the nature of the operation. Today we recognize that you cannot effectively manage an operation you do not understand, regardless of your general talents as an administrator. A background understanding of sport is essential to success in sport management.

Sport Marketing and Sales

Sport marketing includes jobs such as market researcher, marketing manager, promoter, special event marketer, and work in corporate sponsorship, fundraising, sales, and public relations. As participation in sports and recreational activities increases, so do sales and business opportunities in sporting goods. Private companies hire people with an understanding of physical activities—both competitive and recreational sports. People are needed who are familiar with the equipment needs and changing demands. Many companies are specializing in the design and construction of athletic facilities, and they employ people with knowledge of the requirements of sporting events, participants, and spectators.

Sport Financial Operations

Just as in college sports, there must be people who handle the financial side of the operation. In the business environment, this is more complex because tax issues arise, the effectiveness of production and factors that affect profits are greater concerns, and there may be major financial outlays involved (such as the buying of property or other businesses). At this level, some financial and accounting training is absolutely essential.

Sport Facility Management

At the business level, there are many types of facilities that require expert management. This can include arenas and stadiums, racetracks, speedways and dirt tracks, and even camps. The traits for success are developed through initial course work and years of experience working with experts on the job.

Motor Sports Management

This is becoming a large operation in sports economics. The growth of NASCAR is the most prominent example, but there are racing operations and facilities around the world with various types of automobiles and motorcycles in different race settings, from race tracks to rally cars. There are similar programs with boats and airplanes.

Concessions Operations

Every sports venue offers concessions (food services and souvenirs). Someone must plan and operate them. In some cases, the primary source of profit at a stadium or arena is concessions and parking fees. Concessions stands are the primary source of profit at movie theaters.

Careers in Sport and Leisure Services Entrepreneurship and Consulting

A neglected area of the emerging study of sport business is sport entrepreneurship: starting your own business in the sport and leisure services field. Although this is a multi-billion-dollar market, few universities educate or encourage their students in this direction. The current focus in sport management is on becoming an employee in an NCAA Division I athletic department, with a professional team or in someone else's company. Schools of business have taught courses and offered concentrations in entrepreneurship and small business enterprise for many years. Our field will soon be following in those footsteps (I taught a sport entrepreneurship course for

20 years).[2] Most students have ideas that could become real businesses, but they do not know how to develop those ideas. Although this approach may not be your preferred choice immediately after college, you should not reject it without careful thought. You might start a small business that will become the next Nike, which grew from an initial investment of $1000 to a company with $21 billion in sales and 38,000 employees in 2011.[3]

Sport entrepreneurship has vast potential in our field. The largest number of new jobs in the United States is created by small businesses. One of the reasons for large-scale immigration to this country is the freedom to create new businesses with only limited restrictions. Many companies grew from a small idea of a participant in one sport or another. Nike is the result of a coach who wanted higher quality, lighter, and cheaper running shoes. Moving Comfort grew from a woman runner who was tired of badly fitting running apparel (at that time, women's running apparel was simply smaller men's sizes), so she started making her own. Power Bar was developed by a marathoner as an aid to his own training. Gatorade was the result of a urologist trying to help his school's football coaches with a dehydration problem. A community recreation softball player who liked to hit home runs joined with an engineer to design a better softball bat.

Most small businesses begin as part-time operations. *Runner's World* was originally the hobby of a student at the University of Kansas—he mimeographed two issues a year. Human Kinetics Publishers began when a sport psychology group wanted to publish the proceedings of a conference and asked a local faculty member to oversee the process. Apple Computer (though not sports related) began as a garage hobby. The entrepreneurial genesis can come from anywhere.

All you need is an idea and a willingness to work.

To understand the range of possible businesses, consider P. Chelladurai's classification of sports products into three categories: (1) participant services, (2) spectator services, and (3) sponsorship services.[4] The last two are easy to picture, but the first is more complex. He puts the participant services into three subcategories: (1) the consumer-pleasure and health services, (2) human skills and excellence (which involves teaching and coaching), and (3) human sustenance and curative. Although this is a scholarly description, if you think in terms of potential products and services that can fall into one or another of those categories, you will have an endless supply of business ideas.

Sports Consultant

Sports consultants are often used to provide higher-level expertise in areas such as improving business operations, increasing marketing success, and planning new sports facilities. Most sports consultants have a single specialty (such as building gymnasiums or smaller arenas).

Athletic Scholarship Placement Services

Some former athletes offer athletic scholarship placement services. They meet with a high school student (and parents) who is interested in getting an athletic scholarship but who is not a high-level potential recruit. They analyze the student's level of skills and recommend an appropriate level of school, often with suggestions for particular schools that might be most interested in the student. They may help in preparing recruiting videos and distributing them to appropriate schools. They act as a go-between to match up athletes with colleges.

After School Sport Businesses

This category covers a large range of sport businesses. Essentially these are programs that offer youth and preprofessional sports developmental work. In some cases, they may be full-time sports schools (such as tennis and golf academies) that limit themselves to youths with clear professional potential. They may be regional or local skill development programs offering group and individual instruction. They may focus on physical development or skill development. They may offer evaluative testing, sometimes of the body's level of development, sometimes of biomechanical analysis of skills.

Some of the private sports concerns that run their own schools in a sport require trained teachers, and some organizations have set up resorts dedicated to a single sporting activity that requires highly skilled teachers. Some more general organizations, such as country clubs, also hire coaches to train private sports teams composed of the children of the club members.

Sports Agents

The work of sports agents is now highly visible. Sports agents can work individually or as part of a group. As an individual, an agent usually represents a professional athlete. If the athlete is involved in team sports, the agent begins by negotiating the athlete's contract with a franchise. Beyond that, an agent deals with other potential income areas, such as endorsements and appearances, by negotiating fees and specifying what the athlete will do in return for those fees. The agent may also act as a money manager, handling investments and even paying bills on the athlete's behalf. Today legal training is essential to success as a sports agent.

Some agents work as part of a corporate group. Such organizations can more easily act as full-service operations, with specialists each handling different areas of the athlete's business. One person may be a legal expert handling contracts; another may solicit endorsements and appearances. Yet another may be a financial specialist who can develop an investment portfolio. A benefit of the corporate group is that it represents many athletes, so it can sometimes organize its own sports events—thus creating unexpected opportunities for the athlete to make money. The downside is that a lesser athlete may find his or her needs taking a back seat to those of better-known athletes.

Sports Event Management

Event management involves planning and putting on events ranging from basketball games to road races to Grand Prix races to the Olympic Games. Some individuals or small businesses specialize in a single type of event, such as putting on road races. They provide finish line management, timing and recording of all runners, printed final results, and any other services desired by the sponsors. It is easier for a team of specialists (rather than an individual) to run a competition because a team is usually more experienced with the variables of that activity.

As the use of sponsorships and endorsements has expanded, more special events are appearing. New activities (such as types of risk sports) that televise well or attract a large crowd are being created. Corporations have found that endorsing the right activity can bring much positive attention to their organization, so their sponsorship of sports events continues to rise.

Sport Facility Design and Construction

Facility specialists work with architects to design facilities that take advantage of their knowledge of the needs of a sporting venue. For example, a state-of-the-art running track has the fastest available artificial surface, but for competitive benefits it has shorter straightaways and longer turns so athletes lose less speed fighting the turns. It is located at the most advantageous angle relative to prevailing winds (as are the jumping and throwing areas). A competition surface is harder (more force returned) than a softer training track (to lessen injuries).

Sport Manufacturing and Production

Sport manufacturing is the production of the many sports products that are made for sale by sporting goods stores. This work is either a subdivision of a sport business or work under contract to different sport businesses. As an example, the first Nike running shoes were built by contract by Japanese manufacturers during the early 1970s.

Sport Marketing Services

Some marketing companies specialize in sport marketing, while other companies have their own internal marketing services. This is a much broader form of marketing than found with a college athletic department.

Sport Product and Service Research and Development

This is working to develop new products and services, sometimes for companies under contract, other times provided by the company doing the research and development.

Sport Product Design

This work may be done by a company, but it may also be done by an individual and sold to a company. Tinker Hatfield, a former national class pole vaulter and architecture student at the University of Oregon, designed most of the Michael Jordan line of specialty shoes for Nike.

Sport Photography

Just as college athletic departments have designated photographers, others are hired by newspapers, magazines, and wire services. Other sports photographers are independent contractors, taking pictures at events and selling them to media outlets.

Sport Media Productions

These are primarily operations that produce videos and design and maintain sport-related websites. As the Internet profile exploded since 2000, many sport products and businesses increasingly rely on the Internet for advertising and promotional campaigns.

Sport Publishing

Publishers of books on sports and of textbooks in the area of exercise science and its allied fields need people who are knowledgeable about our field. They need editors who are familiar with the wants and demands for books and magazines in exercise science and sport. This type of job requires knowledge of the field and of writing and editorial skills.

Other people are needed in the sales areas, including direct sales, which often involves traveling across the country to sell books. These jobs require knowledge of exercise science and sport and of the comparative values of the available books, combined with sales ability and an understanding of the available markets for publications in the field.

Companies such as Human Kinetics first produced scholarly books, then moved into textbooks, then the market for trade books (books for the general public). It also expanded into video. Coaches Choice is a publisher that is heavily video oriented (though it publishes books also), producing many instructional DVDs in the areas of sport, physical education, and health education.

Another area of publishing that offers job opportunities for knowledgeable people is that of sporting magazines. Specialty sporting magazines are aimed at people who want in-depth coverage of a single sporting activity. In the 1970s, magazines such as *Runner's World* proved that a sizable market was available to the publisher who knew an area well and was able to predict a great public interest. That growth continues, as magazines and books devoted to newer activities, such as risk sports,[5] have appeared. Though many sporting magazines die almost as rapidly as they are born, a market still exists for knowledgeable people to work as writers, editors, and administrators. A more recent area of publications is sport-themed calendars.

Sporting Goods

Sporting goods is another growth industry. Knowledgeable people can design improved equipment, develop new markets, and test and sell sporting equipment. A specialist in a wide range of activities may be able to determine unmet needs that could result in large business growth. To be very successful in this area, you need considerable knowledge of sporting activities, combined with business acumen and training. An understanding of the working of the human body also is helpful when designing sports equipment because the body determines the manner in which sports equipment must be used.

Biomechanical Evaluation and Equipment Design

Some companies specialize in providing biomechanical analysis of athletes. Others will use their biomechanical expertise to design better sports equipment. Some, such as Dartfish, develop software systems that can be sold to others, who use the software to conduct their own biomechanical analyses.

Exercise Physiological Testing and Equipment Design

Just as some companies provide biomechanical analyses, others provide physiological testing services, such as VO_{2max} or efficiency tests. They may also work to develop better physiological testing equipment and analytical software systems.

Software Design for Training and Evaluation Systems

Software training and evaluation systems are increasingly used by athletes and teams as part of the process of monitoring, evaluating, and improving their training and performance. The most advanced systems use artificial intelligence or expert systems, so they can learn and adapt as they acquire more data.

Software Design for Sports Gaming Systems

Software sports games have become hugely popular. While the code writers do not need to understand a given sport that well, the designers of the games must have an advanced knowledge of the sport. Some sports teams have started to use gaming software to teach athletes tactics.

Careers in Recreational Areas

The recreation area continues to grow. Many small communities are developing programs of community recreation and recreational facilities, just as the large cities did years ago. People are needed to develop and administer recreational programs on a number of levels. Although we most commonly think of community recreation, the government hires specialists for the national parks system and military bases, and many business and industrial concerns hire people to run company programs of intramurals and competitive sports. College campuses often run very large recreation and intramural programs, and many religious groups hire specialists to run church recreation programs.

The growth of the recreational services area in the public and private sectors has created a large market for recreational specialists. More college degree programs are being offered under titles that convey the broad scope of the field, such as recreation and leisure, park management, and leisure services. People are needed to plan, build, and operate parks—large and small, public and private. Leisure services, whether organized community recreational programs, privately financed business or religious programs, or unorganized activities that require maintained facilities (and even businesses that design those facilities and parks), are going to be a strong area of need in the future. This is because the trend is toward shorter working hours and having more leisure time. The broad field of recreation is one of the largest current growth markets for people interested in physical education.

Sports Club Management

With the growth of private sports clubs and health clubs, opportunities in this area are growing rapidly. Jobs include sports club manager, personal trainer, fitness instructor, strength and conditioning coach, exercise physiologist, facility director–manager, program director, and consultant. You may work for a public or private operation or start your own business.

Many health clubs offer to develop and maintain the health of anyone who will pay the bill regularly, and many existing sports clubs are devoted to particular sports, such as golfing, swimming, tennis, skiing, ice-skating, and bowling. Most of the sports clubs hire specialists as club pros who teach or coach the members in the sport. Although the primary prerequisite is a highly developed level of skill in the chosen sport, an exercise science background can be very helpful in this field of teaching. Health clubs can use people with that training, though the dominant hiring interests of some clubs often is simply an attractive appearance and the ability to sell memberships, rather than any evident ability to improve the health of a paying customer.

Training in sport management also can be a useful asset in sports and health businesses. In many cases, the people beginning sports or health clubs are more knowledgeable in sport than in business practices, and as a result, someone with managerial training could help to stabilize the daily operations. Recreation or leisure services training also might enable someone working in sports and health businesses to discover unmet needs. By meeting those needs, the chances of success for the operation are increased greatly. Just as some people want a sports facility where they can exercise, others want organized activities, such as club intramurals, tournaments, or other competitive as well as social activities. Many areas of training and expertise can be useful in such a situation.

Aquatics Management

Aquatics management includes jobs such as aquatics specialist, aquatics program coordinator or manager, and aquatics director or water safety director. These jobs may be with colleges or schools or with public or private recreation or fitness operations (such as local park and recreation districts or YMCAs), or they may be self-employed entrepreneurial activities. Special certifications or licenses are standard requirements for most positions. This is a growing area with a shortage of trained people.

Tennis Club Management and Professional Golf Management

A larger version of sports club management is the management of large single-sport operations. Two of the most common operations are tennis clubs and golf courses. Private tennis clubs include facility management, a sales program, an instructional program, and scheduling operations. The same is true for golf and country clubs. The most common training to work on a golf course is a Professional Golfers' Association (PGA)-approved program in Professional Golf Management.

Teaching Professional

Some sports such as tennis and golf have a higher demand for those in the teaching professions than do other sports. These are usually sports that appeal to a more

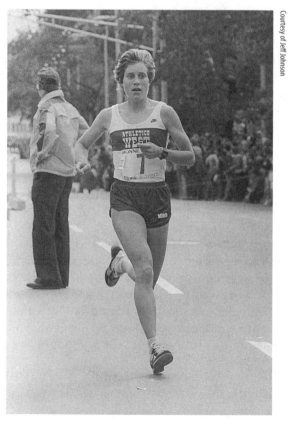

Courtesy of Jeff Johnson

An ongoing issue in school sport is the question of appropriate levels of training and competitive intensity.

well-to-do segment of the population who can afford to pay for individual instruction. Some teaching pros work for a club, such as a country club or a private golf, tennis, or swim club. Others may be self-employed, though this is usually possible only if the pro is well-known.

Some teaching pros or sport coaches also conduct private sports camps. These are very popular during the summer months and range from multisport camps at colleges to single-sport camps run at independent facilities. Some camps are boarding schools with instruction in sports for which there is the possibility of long-term financial gain (or Olympic fame), such as tennis or gymnastics. A growing business is the adult sport camp. These are often held at a resort facility so the customer can have a sport-focused vacation with expert instruction and recreational time, as well as full-service resort options during the rest of the day and night.

Careers in Exercise Science

The need for trained fitness instructors began to boom during the 1980s and continues today, although there are few widely accepted procedures for certifying people. The American College of Sports Medicine (ACSM) is one of the more reliable certifiers of fitness instructors, although it is not the only one. **Table 12.2** is an ACSM list of careers in sports medicine and exercise science. Exercise scientists are concerned about the lack of training of many people who work or advertise themselves as fitness specialists in health and fitness clubs.

Table 12.2 ACSM-Listed Careers in Sports Medicine and Exercise Science

Athletic trainer

Biomechanist

Dietitian/sports nutritionist

Employee fitness director

Exercise physiologist

Group exercise instructor

Medical doctor

Occupational physiologist

Personal trainer

Physical/occupational therapist

Researcher

Strength (sport) and conditioning coach

Teacher

Source: American College of Sports Medicine. *Careers in sports medicine and exercise science.* http://kine.csusb.edu/documents/Exercise_Science_Careers.pdf. Accessed July 23, 2013.

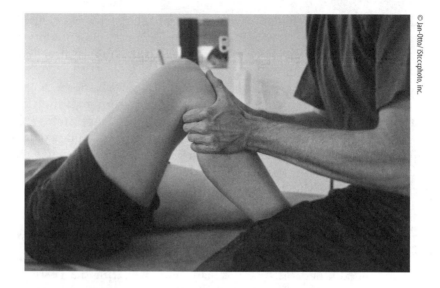

ACSM-Certified Occupations

ACSM certifications are widely recognized and are a good way to quickly be accepted into the job market. **Table 12.3** provides a list of the ACSM certification programs as of 2010. Further information, with details on the occupations, training, and testing requirements, is on the ACSM website. See also the careers in kinesiology.

Table 12.3 ACSM Certifications

Health Fitness Certifications
    ACSM Certified Trainer (CPT)
    ACSM Certified Health Fitness Specialist (HFS)
Clinical Certifications
    ACSM Certified Clinical Exercise Specialist (CES)
    ACSM Registered Clinical Exercise Physiologist (RCEP)
Specialty Certifications
    ACSM/ACS Certified Cancer Exercise Trainer (CET)
    ACSM/NCPAD Certified Inclusive Fitness Trainer (CIFT)
    ACSM/NSPAPPH Physical Activity in Public Health Specialist (PAPHS)

Source: American College of Sports Medicine. Certification. http://www.acsm.org/get-certified. Accessed July 23, 2013.

Research: Basic and Applied

Some people work in areas of specific research, some in basic research (whose primary aim is to advance theoretical knowledge), and others in applied research (whose aim is to solve specific problems or answer particular questions). Although they most commonly work in research university labs, others work for sport-related companies, and some have their own private businesses to conduct contract research for others.

Physical Fitness Industry

The physical fitness industry has grown significantly over the last several decades. Most of the jobs are in the private sector, ranging from health clubs and fitness centers to corporate health and fitness programs to personal trainers to hospital cardiac rehabilitation programs. Many certifications of varying value and authority are available, the best through the ACSM and through the National Strength and Conditioning Association (NSCA). The NSCA certifications are the Certified Strength and Conditioning Specialist (CSCS) and the NSCA-Certified Personal Trainer (NSCS-CPT).

Careers in Kinesiology

Because this text is not designed to address school programs that focus exclusively on academic kinesiology, it does not discuss the potential careers in great detail. As the study of kinesiology has grown in the research universities, it has gradually drawn away from the physical education and sport focus that is traditional to the field. Instead, students of kinesiology are generally interested in careers in the medical and health services field. Examples of some of their career tracks include cardiac and physical rehabilitation programs, physical therapy, sports medicine in medical settings, and testing and research programs in hospitals, medical centers, and research universities. In the private arena, some graduates may operate businesses that provide similar evaluative or rehabilitation services. One of the earliest uses of computerized biomechanical research was by businesses that analyze the performance of elite athletes, who use the analyses to determine how the performance can be perfected.

A good source of information on potential careers for kinesiologists is the ACSM, which is involved in most areas that appeal to the budding kinesiologist.

Medical Doctors and Physician Assistants

We sometimes forget that kinesiology and exercise science majors provide an excellent preparation for medical school. Not only do they provide a strong science background, but there are courses specific to medical and rehabilitative interests that are common in our field but are not taught in the biological sciences.

Rehabilitation and Injury Prevention

Many of the areas of work deal with rehabilitation and injury prevention. Some of those areas are described in the following subsections.

Athletic Training and Sports Medicine

There is a great demand for more specialists in sports medicine (doctors) and for specialists in athletic training (paraprofessionals in sport medicine). The title *athletic trainer* can be confusing because in amateur athletics the athletic trainer does not really train the athletes or plan their program of training. The athletic trainer specializes in the care and prevention of athletic injuries. Prevention may include activities such as providing liquids for athletes to drink during workouts in hot weather or taping ankles for safety or support before practice sessions or contests. First aid and emergency treatment of injuries, as well as planning a program of rehabilitation for an athlete, are all part of an athletic trainer's duties.

The athletic trainer provides an intermediate step between the coach and the physician who specializes in sports medicine. Athletic trainers who are well educated and ethical are needed to prevent the abuse of athletic training and drug-handling practices that can occur in the treatment of athletic injuries. Ethically, the athletic trainer cannot dispense drugs or give injections unless supervised by a physician, but in practice this may not be the case. This is an area of major concern in modern athletics.

Although specialized training is necessary, the need for people in the area of athletic injuries and their treatment is growing rapidly. Many states want to put athletic trainers in the high schools, which would create a huge demand for certified athletic trainers (ATCs), both male and female. Not all high schools have athletic trainers at this time, but a move toward requiring athletic trainers as a safety factor in athletics could make this an area with excellent job opportunities in the future. The National Athletic Trainers' Association (NATA) has information on educational programs and colleges with accredited programs. The number of doctors who handle sports injuries also is limited in most communities, although the addition of certified athletic trainers in the community could improve this situation. The interested student should check with NATA to learn the licensing requirements and to see which schools offer accredited programs.

Physical Therapy and Other Therapies

Although we usually think of therapy as physical therapy, which involves working with people who have temporary or permanent physical disabilities, the areas of therapy are much broader in nature. They can include a wide range of duties in cardiac rehabilitation programs, a growing business sideline for many medical centers. There are four basic types of therapy: physical therapy, corrective therapy, occupational therapy, and dance therapy.

Physical therapy is primarily physical activity planned by a physician to help people to make a physical recovery from severe disease or disability. It might be considered a more narrow area of corrective therapy. Although a physical education degree is helpful, a person needs specialized training before qualifying as a physical therapist.

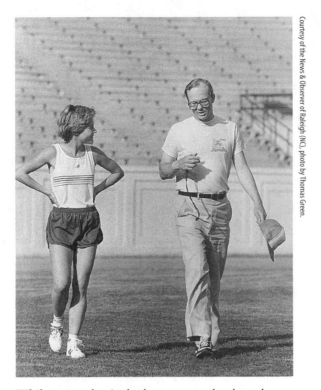

Courtesy of the News & Observer of Raleigh (NC), photo by Thomas Green.

While some physical educators teach a broad range of general skills, others are specialists in a particular skill area and give individual as well as group training.

Broader in scope than physical therapy, *corrective therapy* is concerned with the mental aspects of rehabilitation as well as the physical aspects. It is a team approach to rehabilitating people with physical and mental illnesses. Rather than treat only the physical symptoms, it aims at the mental and social problems that are a result of the disability. This area of specialization has developed largely since World War II. Educational programs in this field are approved by the American Corrective Therapy Association (ACTA).

Occupational therapy involves working with people who are emotionally disturbed or suffer from perceptual motor problems. Physical education activities are often used as part of patient treatment. As with other types of therapy, the occupational therapist needs special training beyond a bachelor's degree.

Dance therapy is a relatively new area. The dance therapist works with people of all ages in programs that use the expressive movement aspect of dance as a means of guidance and improved communication. The dance therapist needs training in dance, movement activities, and psychology to develop the broad background needed to work in this area.

Chiropractic Services

A number of kinesiology students undergo professional training to become chiropractors. Chiropractic services are becoming widely used in the sports world. They are usually found as part of the team health services provided for athletes by medical doctors, athletics trainers, and sports masseurs.

Health Education and Services

Although we think of the health education area as a teaching area, it is closely allied to many activities that do not involve teaching. This area of work includes school nurses and doctors, health specialists in the schools who either provide services or supervise health programs, occupational health workers on the job site, and workers in the many areas of public health services. Health educators may work for local, state, or national governments to provide services, give information, and develop health or health education programs in schools or communities. Many trained administrators are needed for areas of health education work and services.

The field of health education and services has grown rapidly in the last 2 decades. The expansion of local health services has created a need for more specialists trained to work in this area. More schools are offering specialized programs in the health education and services area. Administrators are needed to handle these expanding programs.

There has been a large increase in the number of company groups that combine health care and instruction with recreational and fitness activities. This is a growth area for exercise physiology specialists, recreation majors, fitness instructors, and healthcare and health education specialists. Companies have determined that when such broadly based programs are provided, their overall healthcare costs actually decrease. The combined effect is preventive maintenance for their employees. The growth of health maintenance organizations (HMOs—prepaid healthcare and maintenance programs) has been rapid over the last several decades. The need for unified programs to prevent illness, injury, and poor health has opened another area of potential jobs.

Theory Meets Practice: Student Internships

One of the most useful characteristics of the newer professional programs in our field is the expansion of student internship programs.[6] Many schools provide supervised on-the-job internships in the newer career areas, such as sport management, exercise and fitness management, and cardiac rehabilitation programs. These experiences give students a chance to gain experience in a real setting, develop contacts for job hunting, and gain valuable feedback on their performance at the starting point of their careers. Originally based on the student teaching model, internships are now a critical part of the curriculum in many programs. A well-planned internship experience may be the solution to the difficult job market today.[7]

The Future of Sport Careers

Most of the future growth in the field will be outside the traditional teaching field. Sport business and management careers are expanding rapidly. Many students are not aware of the range of sport-related jobs that are available after graduation. Because of the growth in this market, many schools have added major programs in sport, fitness, and exercise management. Students are encouraged to minor in business, which gives them a much wider range of potential jobs. This is the real growth area in our field today. This is why sport entrepreneurship has a great future.

Summary

The majority of jobs in our field today are not in teaching or coaching. The primary career areas are in sport, sport business, sport and leisure services entrepreneurship and consulting, recreational areas, exercise science, and kinesiology. Most of the future growth in the field will be outside the traditional teaching field.

Further Readings

American College of Sports Medicine. 2012. *ACSM 2012 profiles in sports medicine and exercise science*. http://www.acsm.org/docs/membership-documents/2012_acsm_profiles.pdf

Bolles, Richard Nelson. 2012. *What color is your parachute? 2013: A practical manual for job-hunters and career changers*. New York: Random House. (Updated annually.)

Campbell, Kathy, and Susan K. Kovar. 1994. Fitness/exercise science internships: How to ensure success. *JOPERD (Journal of Physical Education, Recreation and Dance)* (February): 69–72.

Ellis, Michael J. 1988. *The business of physical education: Future of the profession*. Champaign, IL: Human Kinetics.

Erb, Rachel A. 2009. Exercise science: Integrating body and mind. *Choice* (October): 235–238, 240–245.

Field, Shelly. 2011. *Career opportunities in the sports industry*. New York: Checkmark.

Floyd, Patricia A., and Beverly Allen. 2008. *Careers in health, physical education, and sports*. 2nd ed. Florence, KY: Brooks Cole.

Freeman, William H. 1996. Sport entrepreneurship: The missing keystone in the sport management curriculum. In *Proceedings, Fourth European Congress on Sport Management, First International Sport Management Alliance Conference*, ed. Charles Pigeassou and Ronald Ferguson, 254–261. Montpellier, France: European Congress on Sport Management.

Giebel, Nancy. 2004. *Great jobs for physical education majors*. New York: McGraw-Hill.

Hums, Mary A., and Virginia R. Goldsbury. 2011. Strategies for career success. In *Principles and practice of sport management*, 4th ed., ed. Lisa P. Masteralexis, Carol A. Barr, and Mary A. Hums, 543–559. Sudbury, MA: Jones and Bartlett.

McCullick, Bryan, Paul Schempp, Ilse Mason, Cornell Foo, Brad Vickers, and Graeme Connolly. 2009. A scrutiny of the coaching education program scholarship since 1995. *Quest* 61: 322–335.

Miller, Lori K. 1998. Promoting career opportunities for girls and women in the sport industry: Suggestions for existing businesses. *JOPERD (Journal of Physical Education, Recreation and Dance)* (May–June): 32–35.

Rupp, Jeffrey C., Kathy Campbell, Walter R. Thompson, and Donna Terbizan. 1999. Professional preparation of personal trainers. *JOPERD (Journal of Physical Education, Recreation and Dance)* (January): 54–56.

Schneider, Robert C., and William F. Stier Jr. 2001. Recommended educational experiences for high school athletic directors. *Physical Educator* 58: 211–221.

Silvester, L. Jay. 1995. From education to certification. *JOPERD (Journal of Physical Education, Recreation and Dance)* (May–June): 4.

Wong, Glenn. 2012. *The comprehensive guide to careers in sports* (2nd ed.). Sudbury, MA: Jones and Bartlett.

Wright, Steven C., and Daniel E. Smith. 2000. A case for formalized mentoring. *Quest* 52: 200–213.

Zakrajsek, Dorothy, and William Pierce. 1993. Academic preparation and the academic consumer. *JOPERD (Journal of Physical Education, Recreation and Dance)* (May–June): 20–23, 31.

Discussion Questions

1. What preparation is needed for a career in your area of interest? This includes academic preparation, practical experience, and internships.

2. For your intended career, interview two people who are active in that field. How did they get started? What preparation helped them the most? What do they recommend for outside (nonschool) experiences?

3. For your intended career, what are the entry qualifications? Is higher training or graduate study required for hiring, continued employment, or advancement in that career?

4. Is it possible to start your own business in your intended career? If so, what additional skills, training, and/or experiences are needed to improve your chances of success?

References

1. Wong, Glenn. 2012. *The comprehensive guide to careers in sports,* 2nd ed. Sudbury, MA: Jones and Bartlett; Floyd, Patricia A., and Beverly Allen. 2008. *Careers in health, physical education, and sports.* VGM Careers Books; Field, Shelly. 2010. *Career opportunities in*

the sports industry. New York: Checkmark; and Giebel, Nancy. 2004. *Great jobs for physical education majors.* New York: McGraw-Hill.

2. Freeman, William H. 1996. Sport entrepreneurship: The missing keystone in the sport management curriculum. In *Proceedings, Fourth European Congress on Sport Management, First International Sport Management Alliance Conference*, ed. Charles Pigeassou and Ronald Ferguson, 254–261. Montpellier, France: EASM/University of Montpellier.

3. Nike cited at www.statisticbrain.com/nike-company-statistics

4. Chelladurai, Packianathan. 1996. Sport management: Its scope and career opportunities. In *The management of sport: Its foundation and application*, 2nd ed., 13–27. St. Louis, MO: Mosby.

5. Greenfeld, Karl Taro. 1999. Life on the edge. *Time*, September 9, 28–36.

6. Carlson, Judith. 1993. Working to learn—the apprenticeship experience. *JOPERD (Journal of Physical Education, Recreation and Dance)* (October): 57–60.

7. Campbell, Kathy, and Susan K. Kovar. 1994. Fitness/exercise science internships: How to ensure success. *JOPERD (Journal of Physical Education, Recreation and Dance)* (February): 69–72.

PART 5

Today and Tomorrow: Where Is Our Field Going?

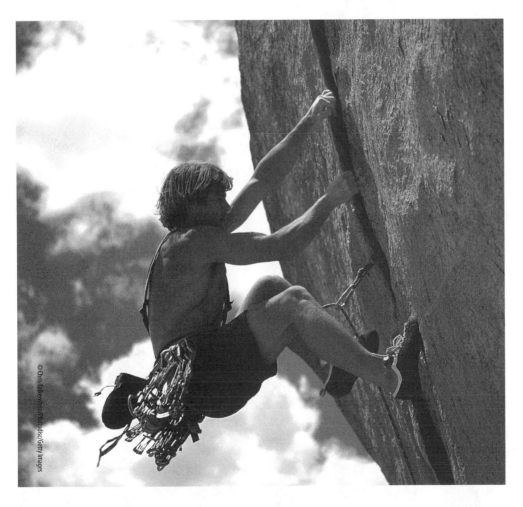

International Exercise Science and Sport Today

The advances in technology during this century have created a shrinking world. We are increasingly caught up in events around the world because communications are almost instantaneous, and travel is not far behind. Nations are forced into contact with each other. The study of comparative physical education, exercise science, and sport is an attempt by exercise scientists around the world to learn about each other and to understand their different national programs.

By studying the exercise science programs and the patterns of physical education teacher preparation in other nations, we can broaden our understanding of the scope of exercise science through many other eyes. International studies can be one more link toward world understanding.

Why Study Comparative Physical Education?

This chapter is concerned with exercise science programs in other nations. Such study is called a *cross-cultural* study of education, or comparative education. Lynn Vendien and John Nixon give five reasons for studying comparative exercise science:[1]

1. We are able to learn about different programs around the world.
2. The studies develop leadership talent by studying other systems in a way that enables us to make comparisons. We can decide whether one system might be better than another one, or whether our own system is best for our society. This process is critical to the improvement of any educational system.
3. We can learn about the goals, ideas, and experiences of other cultures or societies. This knowledge helps us to discover whether our system meets our society's needs. If it does not, the knowledge helps us to decide how our program has moved away from those needs.
4. Comparative studies help us to assess and improve our educational system by allowing us to see how other nations have tried to meet similar educational needs.
5. Studies help to promote international professional collaboration, particularly in research.

Thus, comparative studies of international education are one more facet of international understanding that can lead to better and more peaceful relations between nations.

Assumptions of Comparative Education Studies

Comparative study is based on several assumptions. The first assumption is that an educational system is patterned on the traditional values and practices of its culture. A nation's educational system is expected to be an interpretive reflection of its history, traditions, and cultural practices. The educational system tries to maintain the traditions of a nation and pass them on to the nation's youth.

Second, if the country was once a colony of another nation, we can assume that its educational system was strongly (and perhaps permanently) influenced by the colonial power. Thus, it will be less developed in teaching its own cultural traditions. A colony usually has an educational system similar to the system of the ruling country because the ruling power believes that its own system is the best one. However, because the system is native to the ruling power, it has little regard for the culture or tradition of the colony. It may be useless for mass education of the natives because it ignores their cultural needs and patterns. This pattern is most easily seen in the former colonies of the British Empire, where very English schools were started. Usually, those schools preserved British social class distinctions that did not even exist in the colony schools. The schools were based on the cultural traditions and social patterns of the English, and they had no appropriate cultural function for the natives of the colony.

The third assumption in our comparative study is that if the country is a young nation, it often faces two dangers that put its educational future at risk. The first danger is that the new country will keep its previous educational system unchanged. This perpetuates a system that may be inappropriate to the new nation's culture. The second problem is the other side of the coin: The new nation may drop the old system, but at the same time will simply adopt another nation's educational pattern. The new system also may not meet its own cultural needs. Each country's school system must meet that country's own cultural patterns and traditions to be effective.

Fourth, the young nations may assume that the quality of their new programs is acceptable, thus allowing the new system to stagnate. Any educational system should be in a constant, but gradual, state of change because societies and cultures themselves are in a state of constant change. The system must slowly evolve to meet changing needs and prevent gradual obsolescence. New nations must continually assess and revise their programs to bring them closer to the needs of their own culture, as should the older nations. No educational system can remain static, unless the nation halts progress, because cultural life depends on change and growth. By failing to grow, an educational system begins to die.

Problems of Adopting Western Educational Patterns

Most educational programs now developing in the non-Western nations are influenced by Western ideas and educational patterns. Unfortunately, those patterns are based on Western culture, which may not be appropriate for the cultural patterns and needs of a non-Western nation.[2] When the barbarians invaded the Roman Empire, they wanted to adopt the Roman system, which they considered to be very good. The end result was the destruction of the Roman system because it was not culturally suited to the barbarian nations.

The strength of the Roman system came from the habit of adopting a bit of the native culture of each conquest, while leaving the basic traditional patterns of the conquered people largely unchanged. The Romans were able to strike a happy medium between preserving their own culture and preserving the native culture. This permitted the conquered people to be ruled with greater stability than might otherwise have been the case. Neither the Romans nor those they conquered were expected to adopt a system radically different from the one they had traditionally followed.

Several problems may be created by wholesale adoption of Western educational patterns by non-Western nations. One problem may stem from whether the native country population is either basically competitive or noncompetitive. Many nations are not competitively oriented. If that is the case, adopting Western educational patterns will cause many problems. Western patterns are usually strongly oriented toward competition, both inside and outside the classroom. Another problem involves programs for women. In some cases, the program might simply be a copy of the men's program; in other cases it might be a separately developed program. The difference can be quite important because much depends on the status of women in a particular country. In some nations women do not hold the same rank as or relative equality with men as they do in Western societies.

Schools must reflect the cultural patterns of the native country. If not, the nation may discover that its national system has produced a rapid and very uncomfortable cultural change, as was the case in Iran in the late 1970s. The outcome was a nation in revolt.

A third problem concerns differences in the need for physical activity in different nations. Most Western nations are composed of relatively affluent people who need programs involving more physical activity. Most young nations and many non-Western nations are less affluent, and their people, who are more involved in daily physical labor, need less physical activity in their physical education programs. The educational pattern thus needs to reflect the needs of the local people, rather than the needs of an unseen nation far away.

Dance, which is far more prevalent in non-Western societies than in Western ones, is another potential problem area. Because dance is an important part of the culture of many nations, it should play a much greater part in the physical educational process of those nations. Again, the educational patterns must reflect the nation's own culture and needs.

The Contribution to International Understanding

A comparative study of education around the world can be a major contribution to international understanding. The idea of improving international relations has been a concern for centuries. Baron Pierre de Coubertin of France promoted the Olympic Games to increase understanding between nations. When the games were revived in 1896, a major concern was developing fellowship and understanding among the athletes of different nations. For the ancient Greeks, the Olympic Games were a time of peace and harmony, when people from different states met and mingled in peace.

Coubertin encouraged this aspect of free movement by the athletes—their getting to know their opponents from around the world. As a result of his emphasis on the cultural aspects of the Olympic Games, the modern games include displays of art and other cultural activities. This contribution to international understanding was an important part in the formation of the United Nations in 1945. Previous attempts to gather the world's nations to meet and exchange their views, such as the League of Nations, failed. The United Nations was formed after World War II as an attempt to provide a forum where nations could discuss their common problems and explain their views to each other.

Many of the conflicts in the modern world are the result of misunderstandings or failures of nations to communicate clearly. As the world advances technologically, such misunderstandings become increasingly risky. Aggressive acts can be spotted quickly, and retaliation can be instantaneous. The risk of accidental war in a world filled with guided nuclear missiles is great. The nations of the world need a forum where they can learn about their counterparts from around the world. There must be some channels of communication between nations.

Each of the many international groups in the world today has some particular area of special interest. The primary concern of this chapter is with the international organizations that function in education, exercise science, physical education, and sport. Because there are numerous organizations in those areas, the following sections focus on the larger and more important of the international organizations.

International understanding and goodwill are not the only goals of international relations, especially in the area of sport. Sport is an international language. As such, it can serve many other national interests. International sports competition can be a medium of cultural exchange. Sport also serves as a vehicle of international prestige because individual and team championships at this level can improve a nation's self-image and prominence. Competition also can serve as political propaganda. While winning achieves international prestige, national team tours can be used as a display of prowess, camaraderie between nations, or a desire for good relations. For example, the first improvement in relations between communist China and the United States in the 1970s was the so-called Ping-Pong diplomacy. When the Americans were invited to send their best table tennis players to meet the Chinese in a series of matches, the invitation served notice that China was ready to improve relations with the United States in other areas as well.

International sports competitions can also be a source of national pride. The success of a nation's athletes creates a strong feeling of nationalism, especially for smaller and newly emerging nations. This national pride in successful athletes can be seen at every Olympic Games.

Peter Arnold argues that teaching Olympism, which is an international approach to sport for everyone, is of great educational value.[3] Richard McGehee and Shirley Reekie recommend using international sport in the K–12 curriculum to internationalize school programs.[4] Randall Stewart describes how "Teaching the Olympics in Cyberspace" can use computer, multimedia, and Internet technologies to teach about the ancient Olympic Games, yet the same approach can be used to introduce people to unfamiliar sport and physical education programs around the world.[5]

Orientations of Physical Education Programs

Physical education programs can vary greatly from nation to nation because each nation has its own program goals and orientation. One of the traditional orientations for several thousand years has been toward *military fitness*. This major objective of programs in the past is still seen to some degree today. Historically, it becomes important during times of war when the national goal is to produce healthy young people who will be physically ready for military service. Military fitness is perhaps the most limited goal of a physical education program.

A second program direction is toward *competitive sports training*. Although the objective is partially to develop the skills and fitness of all the students by providing basic training in the techniques of competitive sports, they also can be used as talent hunts, that is, to locate students with the potential to become outstanding athletes. In the past, community programs in the United States were used to locate athletic talent for school teams. Today, these programs are more often on a national scale and are used to locate students with the potential to become national or world-class athletes. The athletes are then trained on a higher level in the hope that they will ultimately bring athletic prestige to the nation.

Another orientation, that of *lifetime sports*, is seen primarily in the more affluent nations. The objective is to teach sports skills that can be enjoyed throughout life. The hope is that the students will take part in physical activities and maintain at least minimal fitness throughout their lifetimes. This approach is seen most frequently in nations where the people have more money and leisure time. A citizen in a poverty-stricken nation generally does not have the time, facilities, or inclination for such activities.

A fourth orientation might be called *cultural fitness*. The emphasis is on activities that are rooted in the culture of the nation. For example, a country might encourage only its traditional activities, such as national dances and sports, and put very little emphasis on activities from other nations, regardless of their world popularity. This type of program is typical of smaller nations or in nations striving to develop their own national consciousness or self-image.

Finally, *total fitness for life* (or sometimes *lifetime wellness*) is sometimes tied into the program as part of the entire educational process. This approach is education both of and through the physical. The emphasis is not on any single area of fitness or training; instead, the concern is for a comprehensive educational process, whether physical, social, mental, or moral.

AEHESIS: European Sport Science Seeks Common Program Outcomes

Curriculum development is always a critical component of a nation's educational system. Curriculum revision is an ongoing concern because the needs of any nation change over time. The educational system needs revision to stay in tune with those needs.

A very interesting parallel to what we need to do is a process currently under way in Europe. Because the continent has many different nations, each with its somewhat unique approach to university education, it is dealing with the problem of creating university degree programs that are transportable in a global economy. More than us in the United States, the European nations are concerned with the ability of their graduates to find employment 100 miles away, in another nation with a different primary language and a different educational design.

The curriculum in exercise science programs changes over time. During the last century, there have been three approaches to curriculum planning: (1) common courses, (2) common content, and (3) common outcomes. The first approach to making college curricula standard was to design a commonly accepted list of courses in the major. That approach was used until the 1960s and 1970s, when the influence of the discipline movement led to new major programs beyond the basic teacher education model.

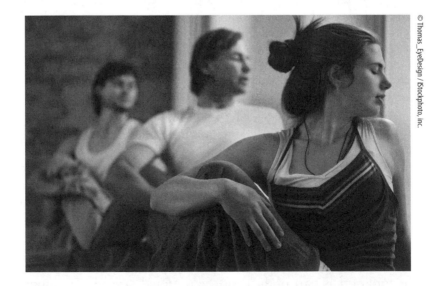

The universities changed to a common content model. Instead of listing the courses that should be required in a major, they developed descriptions of the content that students should learn. From that content list, each school could design its relatively unique list of courses. However, schools tended to interpret each major content component as a course, so major programs were still similar to the older course listings approach.

As the century turned, a newer approach appeared: It is outcome focused, rather than content focused. Instead of examining content options, the focus is on what a graduate should be able to do. This does not mean a small-task focus, but a big-picture look at work in the field. This is what Aligning a European Higher Education Structure in Sport Science (AEHESIS) was trying to do. It is an outgrowth of a larger effort of European universities to prepare graduates for a wide range of fields.

The response of AEHESIS has been to try to find commonalities of goals so it can project what people want to do for a career, understand what types of knowledge and skills they will need, and use those needed outcomes to design their academic programs. As one of the project's documents states:

> *The Bologna Declaration (June 1999) set in motion an agenda of policy reforms with a view to making European Higher Education more compatible and comparable, more competitive and more attractive across Europe. . . . As part of the post-Bologna process . . . an ERASMUS Thematic Network project . . . to "Align a European Higher Education Structure in Sport Science" (the AEHESIS Project), one sector of which is "Physical Education." . . . The sector's prime aim "having in mind the necessity of enhancing the process of recognition and European integration of qualifications" was to formulate a model curriculum for Physical Education Teacher Education (PETE), which would be applicable across Higher Education Institutions in Europe involved with the preparation of teachers.[6]*

As an example of their implementation of the Bologna Process, there is a breakdown of how coach education would be designed (starting with a suggested classification of levels of coaching roles, from apprentice coach to master coach), an outline framework for developing coaching qualifications, a competence framework for coaching (with activities, tasks, and competencies), a general framework for the recognition of coaching competence and qualifications, and a framework for the licensing of coaches.

As an example of the processes that they have set up, figures from their website illustrate the six-step model to collect information (**Figure 13.1**), the overview of the physical education teacher education program of study (**Figure 13.2**), and the competence framework for coaching (**Figure 13.3**).

A major point here is that they are trying to agree on the process. They are not dictating a set curriculum that all schools or nations will follow. Instead, they

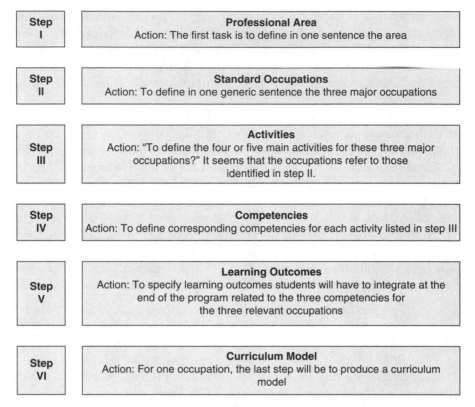

Figure 13.1 AEHESIS Six-Step Model (A6SM)
Klein, G. (2004) AEHESIS Quality Process: Curriculum building, AEHESIS
Management Group, Brussels.

are saying that when graduates leave a university, these are the things they should
know and be able to do, these are the roles they should be ready to fill. How the
students meet those goals is up to the individual university. This project states in
broad terms the outcomes of the major program.

International Organizations

The International Council of Sport Science and Physical Education (ICSSPE) was
founded in Paris in 1958. It serves as an umbrella organization for sport science
(a term more commonly used around the world than *kinesiology*). With offices in
Berlin, it encourages international cooperation across the field of sport science,
while trying to spread the results of research in the field.

The International Association for Physical Education in Higher Education
(AIESEP) is allied with the ICSSPE, but focuses on the field of physical education
and sport at the university level. It holds an annual convention and publishes the
proceedings of the meeting.

Program of Study	
Fields of Study	
Practical Activities (Theory and Practice)	**Outcomes**
Dance Games Gymnastics Outdoor adventure activities Swimming Track and field athletics Other (new and national/local culturally traditional activities)	• Knowledge, understanding and analysis of (motor) skills and performance factors in a range of activities • Teach activities skills/didactic competence combining theory and practice • Teach activities according to principles of horizontal and vertical articulation of the curriculum, respecting principles of inclusion and differentiation of teaching • Have a range of, and apply, practical skills
Educational and Teaching Sciences (Pedagogy/Didactics)	• Knowledge of how to justify the presence of PE in the core curriculum, as well as the importance of physical activity as a health factor knowing how sport contributes to human development • Knowledge of curriculum implementation • Knowledge of education and effective teaching theories • Knowledge of communication and learning processes
Natural and Biological Sciences (General and Applied)	• Knowledge of structure, function, and control of physical systems • Understanding and application of biomechanical principles to movement • Knowledge of human anatomy • Knowledge of the processes of developing pupils' health-related fitness
Social Sciences/Humanities (General and Applied)	• Knowledge of the school as a social institution and contextualization of professional practices • Knowledge of PE/sport in society, including historical and sociological developments • Psychological/sociological knowledge of human movement • Understanding of the concept of culture and application to PE and sport
Scientific Work (PE-related research study: dissertation or project)	• Preparation and conduct of PE project • Ability to generate quantitative/qualitative data • Present written report
School-based Teaching Practice	• Application of teaching skills • Experience content, pedagogical and contextual knowledge • Assessment and evaluation of teaching skills

Figure 13.2 PETE Program of Study and Outcomes
Hardman, K., Klein, G., Carreiro da Costa, F., Rychtecky, A., Patriksson, G. (2005). PE Research Team, AHESIS Project.

The International Council on Health, Physical Education, Recreation, Sport and Dance (ICHPERSD) is the major worldwide physical education group. It represents a wide range of interest in exercise science. Founded in 1958 and headquartered in Reston, Virginia, ICHPERSD works with organizations concerned with the broader international aspects of physical education, including health and recreation, teacher preparation, information exchange between nations, promoting exchange programs in physical education, and conducting special

Activities	Tasks	Competencies
The main activities performed by coaches are as follows:	Within each activity, coaches perform the following tasks:	The competencies needed to successfully perform the tasks related to each activity include:
• **Training:** to prepare sports people for competition by planning, organizing, conducting, and evaluating the appropriate programs and sessions	• **Plan:** ability to put together a step-by-step program to achieve a goal in a session, series of sessions, season, series of seasons	• **Knowledge:** the use of theory and concepts, as will as informal tacit knowledge gained experientially
• **Competition:** to plan, organize, conduct, and evaluate the appropriate events, tournaments, programs, and matches	• **Organize:** ability to coordinate and make all the necessary arrangements to ensure that the goal will be achieved in an efficient and effective way	• **Skills:** the functions (know-how) a person should be able to perform when functioning in a given area of work, learning, or social activity
• **Management:** to lead, direct, or control people related to the sport	• **Conduct:** ability to carry out and execute the planned and organized task	• **Personal, Professional, Ethical:** knowing how to conduct oneself in a specific situation and possessing certain personal and professional values
• **Education:** to teach, instruct, or mentor people related to the sport	• **Evaluate:** ability to study, analyze, and decide on the utility, value, significance, or quality of the above process	• **Generic/Underpinning/Key:** Communication in mother tongue, communication in another language, basic competencies in maths, science and technology, digital competence, learning to learn, interpersonal and civic comptencies, entrepreneurship, and cultural expression
	• Research and self-reflection	

Figure 13.3 Competence Framework for Coaching
Courtesy of Patrick Duffy

international studies and international conferences. It publishes the *Journal of Research* and holds a world conference every year.

The International Federation of Physical Education (FIEP) began in 1923 and has its headquarters in Lisbon, Portugal. Its objective is to promote physical education for all people, regardless of sex or age. It encourages research and the communication of ideas between nations by sponsoring exchanges of teachers and scholars. Its 2011 international meeting was in Brazil. The International Society for Comparative Physical Education and Sport (ISCPES) was established in 1960. Its primary goals are to improve cooperation between all groups interested in physical education and sport and to interpret the cultural values of physical education and sport. It publishes the journal *International Sports Studies* and holds international meetings every 2 years.

The International Olympic Academy was established in 1961 to promote and maintain the ideals of the original Olympic Games. Its headquarters are in Athens, Greece, and it is associated with both the Hellenic Olympic Committee and the International Olympic Committee. The International Olympic Academy conducts annual summer sessions at the site of ancient Olympia. There is an associated U.S. Olympic Academy located in Colorado Springs, Colorado.

The International Association of Physical Education and Sport for Girls and Women (IAPESGW) began in 1953 to bring together women around the world who were working in physical education and sport. It also cooperates with other sports organizations. The IAPESGW tries to improve school programs through international exchanges of people and ideas. It has a world meeting every 4 years.

The European College of Sport Science is an example of an international regional scholarly group. Based at the German Sport University in Cologne, it publishes the *European Journal of Sport Science* and holds a large annual convention whose proceedings are also published.

Some organizations are concerned purely with sports. The major sport organization is the International Olympic Committee (IOC), established in 1894 to revive the ancient Olympic Games. It has conducted the Olympic Games every fourth year since the first modern games in 1896. It encourages sports competitions that are in keeping with the ideals of the ancient Olympic Games. It deals strictly with the Olympic committees of the member nations, such as the U.S. Olympic Committee (USOC), rather than with the national governments. It seeks to keep all political considerations out of the Olympic Games. Some of its intended patriotic moves have gradually led the modern Olympics closer to an international political contest. For example, the use of national anthems and flags at awards sessions recognizes the athletes' home nations as much as their individual skills.

The International Association of Athletic Federations (IAAF), formerly the International Amateur Athletic Federation until amateurism disappeared, began in 1912 to encourage friendly non-discriminatory sports competition among nations. Its emphasis on fair competition has made it the body that creates and revises rules and regulations governing international and Olympic track and field athletics (simply called athletics in most nations outside the United States). It also is the agency that approves world records. Rules are revised at its international meetings, held every 2 years. Like the IOC, membership depends on a nation's chosen representatives being accepted into what amounts to a gentleman's club composed primarily of rich, elderly men. An elitist attitude was seen in many of the organization's regulations relating to amateurism, making it difficult for anyone but the relatively wealthy to be pure amateurs. Consequently, most nations interpreted the rules in this area with considerable latitude, and the IAAF and IOC studiously looked the other way. The amateur standard no longer exists in international sport.

The International University Sports Federation (FISU), with headquarters in Louvain, Belgium, was founded in 1949. It promotes international physical education among students by sponsoring international sports conferences and contests for university students (the Summer and Winter Universiades, and the World University Games, each held every 2 years). More than 9000 athletes competed in the Summer Universiade in 2007, with 174 nations in one of the meetings. The winter meetings have had up to 2500 athletes from 50 nations.

The International Military Sports Council (CISM), organized in 1948, promotes equality within the various armies of the world, while encouraging friendly relations and sports ties among the world's armies. With headquarters in Brussels, Belgium, it supports at least 20 international championships in a number of sports and also holds an annual meeting.

The People-to-People Sports Committee was privately organized in 1956 to advance international understanding and sports competition. It does so by sponsoring touring teams in many sports and by working in other related ways to foster international sports.

The United Nations Educational, Scientific and Cultural Organization (UNESCO) was established in 1945 and has its headquarters in Paris, France. Its goals are to contribute to peace and security in the world through international cooperation in improving education, science, and culture, while stressing a basic respect for justice and individual human rights. It holds an international meeting every 2 years.

The World Alliance of Young Men's Christian Associations, with headquarters in Geneva, Switzerland, first began in 1844. Its goal is to help YMCAs around the world. Its more broadly based work includes the goals of international understanding, basic human rights, and improved social and economic conditions for all people. A large world meeting assembles every 4 years. A similar organization is the World Young Women's Christian Association, which began in 1848.

The World Health Organization (WHO), headquartered in Geneva, Switzerland, was organized in 1948 as an agency of the United Nations. Its ultimate goal is to help all people to attain a high level of health, which it has defined as "a state of complete physical, mental, and social well-being and not merely the absence of disease or infirmity." It meets annually and provides assistance to any world government that requests it.

In addition to these specialized international bodies, which represent only a small number of the many international organizations, there are many international sports organizations. Almost every sport has at least one international organization that keeps its rules updated, verifies world records (if the sport has such records), and sponsors international competition and world championships. These organizations are too numerous to list in a short chapter, but some examples are the International Amateur Basketball Federation, headquartered in Munich, Germany; the International Gymnastics Federation (FIG), located in Geneva, Switzerland; and the International Amateur Swimming Federation, located in Jenkintown, Pennsylvania. Any international physical education or sport organization should have an accessible website.

International Competitions

There are many international sports competitions, but the most important is the Olympic Games. Although the ancient Greek games were dissolved in AD 394, they often attracted scholars' attention over the next 15 centuries.

The International Olympic Committee was formed in the year of the 1500th anniversary of the abolition of the Greek Olympic Games to revive the games. Two years later, in 1896 in Athens, the first modern Olympic competition was held. The games are now held every fourth year, or Olympiad, as were the ancient games. Only world wars caused their cancellation in 1916, 1940, and 1944. Winter sporting events were added in 1908, but the now-separate winter Olympic Games were not held until 1924. In 1994, the dates of the winter games were changed to the even years between the summer Olympics. More nations now take part in the Olympic Games than in any other internationally organized program except the United Nations.

The Olympic competition is open to both men and women in a large number of sports. The number of sports has become so large that suggestions have been made to separate the summer games into several parts and hold them at different sites. The reasons for doing this are that (1) the games represent a tremendous expense for any one city to assume; (2) the large number of competitors and visitors puts an almost impossible strain on the facilities, housing, traffic, and police work of all but the world's largest cities; and (3) the extreme visibility of such a concentrated sports event makes it seem an ideal place for political demonstrations (such as those in Mexico City in 1968) and possible terrorism (such as the murder of Israeli athletes by terrorists in Munich in 1972). The Olympic Games are now facing perhaps their most difficult period. The danger is that their very popularity may destroy them.

A second major world championship event is the Universiade, or the World Student Games, of the FISU. The first competition was held in 1947, and the event is now held in odd-numbered years. Many university students from around the world take part in these games, which include a number of sports.

Another competition, although one of more limited entry standards, is the World Maccabiah Games, patterned after the Olympic Games but limited to Jewish athletes. First held in 1931, this multisport competition takes place every fourth year in Israel.

Many regular regional championships involve only a portion of the world's nations. These contests are frequently patterned after the Olympic Games, although they may not include as many different sports. The oldest example is the Asian Games, first held in 1913. It is now essentially a sports competition for nations in continental Asia, ranging from Turkey to China, but not including Russia. These games now meet every 4 years.

The Commonwealth Games, earlier called the British Empire and Commonwealth Games, began in 1930 and are held every fourth year. Competition is

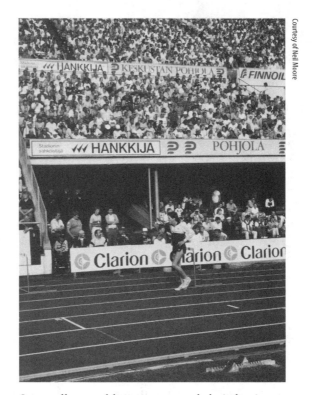

Courtesy of Neil Moore

Sport allows athletes to expand their horizon
across the nation and into other countries.

limited to the present and past members of the British Empire and the countries
in the British Commonwealth.

The Pan-American Games represent a multisport championship for nations
of the Western Hemisphere (North, Central, and South America). First begun in
1951, the Pan-American Games are held every 4 years, during the year before the
summer Olympic Games.

Various European championships, usually involving single sports, also are
held at varying intervals. In track and field athletics, a World Championships is
held in odd-numbered years; they were started in 1983.

Other competitions represent many smaller regions, and some represent individual sports. An example of team sports is the World Cup championships in
soccer. The national teams qualify for the World Cup Final through a series of
playoffs spread over the 2 years prior to the final. The final playoffs involving a
small number of national teams are held every 4 years.

World championships are held at regular intervals for most separate sports,
though not all world championships are designated as such. The rules of the IAAF

state that the Olympic Games also will serve as the world championship event for track and field athletics, although it is rarely referred to in that way. There are, however, dozens of world championships held during every Olympiad, some of which are associated with the Olympic Games and some of which are not.

Summary

Comparative physical education is the study of exercise science and physical education programs in other nations. Reasons for these studies include the following: (1) we can learn about different programs around the world; (2) we develop leadership talent by the comparative study of other systems; (3) we learn about the goals, ideas, and experiences of other cultures; (4) they help us assess and improve our educational system; and (5) they help to promote international professional collaboration and understanding.

Comparative study is based on the assumptions that (1) an educational system is patterned on the traditional values and practices of its culture; (2) the educational system of former colonies was strongly influenced by the colonial power; (3) if the country is a young nation, it faces the dangers of keeping its old system unchanged or simply adopting another nation's system; and (4) young nations may assume that the quality of their new programs is acceptable, thus allowing it to stagnate. The problem of adopting foreign educational patterns is that they may not be appropriate for the cultural patterns and needs of another nation.

Physical education programs may have one of five orientations: (1) military fitness, (2) competitive sports training, (3) lifetime sports, (4) cultural fitness, or (5) total fitness for life (sometimes called lifetime wellness).

The chapter gives an overview of Aligning a European Higher Education Structure in Sport Science (AEHESIS), an attempt to determine the common outcomes desired for different career tracks so graduates of university programs in the different nations will be employable throughout Europe, rather than limited primarily to their own nation.

The chapter introduces a number of international organizations in exercise science, physical education, and sport, as well as a number of high-level international sports competitions.

Further Readings

Bardy, Benoît G. 2008. A European perspective on kinesiology in the 21st century. *Quest* 60: 139–153.

Brownell, Susan. 1995. *Training the body for China: Sports in the moral order of the People's Republic.* Chicago: Univ. of Chicago Press.

Cashman, Richard, and Anthony Hughes, eds. 1999. *Staging the Olympics: The event and its impact.* Sydney, Australia: Univ. of New South Wales Press.

Duffy, Pat, and Liam Dugdale, eds. 1994. *HPER—moving toward the 21st century.* Champaign, IL: Human Kinetics.

Dunning, Eric G., Joseph A. Maguire, and Robert E. Pearton, eds. 1993. *The sports process: A comparative and developmental approach.* Champaign, IL: Human Kinetics.

European Sport Education Information Platform. 2013. Home page. http://www.eseip.eu/

Hardman, Ken, Gilles Klein, Göran Patriksson, Antonin Rychtecky, and Francisco Carreiro da Costa. 2008. Implementation of the Bologna process and model curriculum development in physical education teacher education curriculum. In *Higher education in sport in Europe: From labour market demand to training supply*, ed. Karen Petry, Karsten Froberg, Alberto Madella, and Walter Tokarski; transl. Linda Fragan-Hos. Maidenhead, England: Meyer and Meyer Sport.

Hill, Christopher R. 1996. *Olympic politics: Athens to Atlanta, 1896–1996.* 2nd ed. Manchester, England: Manchester Univ. Press.

Ives, Jeffrey C., and Duane Knudson. 2007. Professional practice in exercise science: The need for greater disciplinary balance. *Sports Medicine* 37: 103–115.

Jennings, Andrew. 1996. *The new Lords of the Rings: Olympic corruption and how to buy gold medals.* London: Pocket.

Klein, Gilles. *Curriculum development strategies in sport education: From the old "six steps model" to the new "five processes framework."* In Petry, et al. 2008 [see ref. below]: 44–55.

Lucas, John A. 1992. *Future of the Olympic Games.* Champaign, IL: Human Kinetics.

McGehee, Richard V., and Shirley H. M. Reekie. 1999. Using sport studies and physical activities to internationalize the K–12 curriculum. *JOPERD (Journal of Physical Education, Recreation and Dance)* (August): 38–45.

Petry, Karen, Karsten Froberg, Alberto Madella, and Walter Tarsky, eds. 2008. *Higher education in sport in Europe: From labour market demand to training supply.* Trans. Linda Fragan-Hos. Maidenhead, England: Meyer and Meyer Sport.

Powell, John T. 1994. *Origins and aspects of Olympism.* Champaign, IL: Stipes.

Pühse, Uwe, and Markus Gerber, eds. 2005. *International comparison of physical education: Concepts, problems, prospects.* Oxford: Meyer and Meyer Sport.

Sanders, Ross H., and John M. Dunn. 2010. The Bologna Accord: A model of cooperation and coordination. *Quest* 62: 92–105.

Schaffer, Kay, and Sidonie Smith, eds. 2000. *The Olympics at the millennium: Power, politics, and the games.* Piscataway, NJ: Rutgers Univ. Press.

Senn, Aldred E. 1999. *Power, politics, and the Olympic Games.* Champaign, IL: Human Kinetics.

Simson, Vyv, and Andrew Jennings. 1992. *Dishonored games: Corruption, money and greed at the Olympics.* New York: SPI.

Svoboda, B., and R. Rychtecky, eds. 1995. *Physical activity for life: Comparative physical education and sport.* Aachen, Germany: Meyer and Meyer.

Wagner, E. A., ed. 1989. *Sport in Asia and Africa: A comparative handbook.* Westport, CT: Greenwood Press.

Discussion Questions

1. Discuss the values and uses of the study of comparative education and physical education.

2. Discuss the problems created when a new non-Western nation simply copies the educational pattern of a Western nation.

3. Name and discuss briefly the different possible major orientations or goals of a national physical education program.

4. What was the purpose of AEHESIS for European sport science? What is the difference between agreeing on a common set of outcomes compared to agreeing on a common curriculum? Why did AEHESIS prefer to agree on outcomes rather than develop a common curriculum?

5. Name and discuss briefly the purposes of three international bodies interested in exercise science and/or sport.

References

1. Vendien, C. Lynn, and John E. Nixon. 1968. *The world today in health, physical education, and recreation.* Englewood Cliffs, NJ: Prentice Hall, 5–6.

2. Ibid., 8–9.

3. Arnold, Peter J. 1996. Olympism, sport, and education. *Quest* 48: 93–101.

4. McGehee, Richard V., and Shirley H. M. Reekie. 1999. Using sport studies and physical activities to internationalize the K–12 curriculum. *JOPERD (Journal of Physical Education, Recreation and Dance)* (August): 38–45.

5. Stewart, Randall. 1995. Teaching the Olympics in cyberspace. *North American Society for Sport History Proceedings* 68.

6. Hardman, Ken, Gilles Klein, Göran Patriksson, Antonin Rychtecky, and Francisco Carreiro da Costa. 2008. Implementation of the Bologna process and model curriculum development in physical education teacher education curriculum. In *Higher education in sport in Europe: From labour market demand to training supply*, ed. Karen Petry, Karsten Froberg, Alberto Madella, and Walter Tokarski; transl. Linda Fragan-Hos. Maidenhead, England: Meyer and Meyer Sport: 56–79.

Current Issues in Exercise Science and Sport

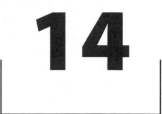

This chapter looks at three broad areas of issues in American exercise science and sport as we enter a new millennium: (1) education as a whole, (2) exercise science and physical education, and (3) sport. It explains what is happening in American exercise science and sport today. Many of these issues are ongoing, although the emphasis changes all the time.

The Focal Issue in Education

One decision lies at the heart of any system of learning: *What education is most worth having?* Certain skills are basic to achievement. The school years are a time of learning and testing to prepare students for advanced levels of training needed in jobs for the future. Even so, as technology leaps ahead, one can see a growing class of hard-core unemployables who have not developed the skills needed for any jobs other than simple, physical ones.

This problem can be prevented with an educational system that sets clear standards and lives up to them, instead of a system of social promotions with the "up or out" rule of education. A society must decide on educational objectives and then enforce those objectives strongly. Unfortunately, in the United States there is no consensus on the goals and objectives of education at any level. Thus, there are no national standards for education.

Two Linked Ongoing Concerns

Americans argue about many education issues, but two have figured prominently for several decades: the back-to-the-basics movement and the problem of the cost of education.

Concerns About the Quality of Education (the Back-to-the-Basics Movement)

The back-to-the-basics movement was a grassroots revolt against the school curriculum. Some parents believed that the schools spent too much time on the nonacademic frills of education and students were not taught the basics, such as reading, writing, and math. The movement's supporters cited the decline in scores on college-entrance examinations as evidence of poor student learning. There are some legitimate excuses for the decline in scores, but it appears that the decline in the level of learning of typical American students is genuine. It is not simply the result of testing flaws, bias, or statistical weaknesses.

Parents suggest several causes for this apparent decline. Television viewing, computer games, time on personal websites, blogging, and cell phone time detract from the amount of time that students spend on homework. Some parents believe that teachers assign too little homework, and others suggest that there is a lack of discipline, including physical discipline and lower grading standards. Criticism of the schools reflects a belief that schools have lost the work ethic, that they no longer teach the value of hard work to achieve success.

In the late 1960s and early 1970s, ungraded classes and more loosely structured requirements became popular in colleges. Young teachers carried this idea into the schools. School districts revised programs by assuming that education would be more successful if the students decided what they should learn and if courses were made more relevant to the students' daily lives. The concept of failure was removed from some programs. The move to an ungraded system was supposed to make students more inner-directed in a noncompetitive atmosphere. They would learn more because they would see the value of what they were trying to learn. At the same time, they would attempt more difficult subjects because there would be no fear of failure.

Problems with this type of educational system were accurately predicted by more experienced teachers. *Relevant* became *easy*; the ungraded approach meant that few people cared whether a student worked or achieved. The system was a failure for the majority of students because it did not require the achievement levels necessary for successful life after school.[1] The disastrous effects of this system became obvious when state legislatures, reacting to parental complaints, set test score standards to be met before a high school diploma could be awarded. Although the requirements were modest, failure rates were startlingly high. Indeed, some teachers failed the student tests. This led to the birth of the high school competency tests.

George Higgins makes these observations about an educational system that claims every student is capable of doing everything equally well:

> If you lie to a kid and tell him that he can do something when he knows very well that he cannot do it, he will try it. And of course he will fail. When you tell him that he has succeeded [schools without failure], he knows you are lying. He will never trust you again. He will be right. [After this happens in several grades] he will get the impression that people lie to him in order to get rid of him. This may be good training for the adult world, but it is poor training for performance in that world.[2]

Higgins points out that students begin to expect people to make allowances for them, which usually will not happen outside the schools. The result is unqualified college students who demand simpler college courses. Without the weaker students, teachers would lose jobs. Higgins paints a discouraging picture of American education today, but it is largely accurate.

Although there are always disagreements over what today's schools should accomplish, people realize that the schools are doing a poor job of basic education. Students cannot read well or perform simple mathematical operations well. This does not refer simply to the weaker students. Today, remedial reading and writing courses must be taken by large numbers of students in many American universities.

This weakness in educational standards in American schools was the reason behind the Goals 2000 legislation proposed by the nation's governors in the mid-1980s and passed into law by Congress in 1994. As David Broder writes,

> The governors' original notion was a simple one: In a competitive world, the quality of the education America's youngsters receive is the prime determinant of the nation's future well-being. So they set out goals for themselves. Among others, they said, by 2000 all children would start school ready to learn and at least 90 percent of them would finish high school. Every graduate would have demonstrated competence in nine basic subjects.[3]

Broder noted that the public has lost faith in educational reforms because they usually fail to ensure that students will acquire knowledge and skills. Yet, even though the nation's governors proposed the program and the president endorsed the effort, by mid-1995:

> only 13 states have standards that are 'clear and specific enough' to guide curricular development. While 33 states have or are developing student assessments geared to those standards, only seven [states] require high school seniors to meet the standards set for 10th, 11th or 12th graders in order to graduate.[4]

Those failures led to the No Child Left Behind Act.

We live in an increasingly technological society. We cannot plan a completely up-to-date, relevant education because technology changes so rapidly that sometimes what is being taught is outdated by the time a textbook is written and published. The basic skills of reading, writing, speaking, mathematics, logic, and mental and social adaptability are important attributes for success in the modern world. Yet the typical American student is weak in those basic skills. As a result, they face the risk of terrible failures in their ability to function efficiently in the everyday world of the technological future.

Endless School Budget Crises

The demands of the back-to-the-basics movement are admirable and understandable in terms of the problems that its proponents are trying to correct. The unfortunate aspect of those demands is that they came during a time of spiraling educational costs and severe budget cuts in most school systems. This combination led to the loss of many program frills that were not believed to be critical to the curriculum.

This is unfortunate because the need to strengthen educational requirements and learning in basic areas does not lessen the value of supplementary areas of education. Although "reading, writing, and 'rithmetic" comprise the cornerstone of education, exposure to the sciences, the arts, business courses, technical programs, physical education, sports, and nonphysical extracurricular school activities can be equally valuable in developing the well-rounded citizen.

Issues in American Education

Table 14.1 is a list of the major issues and subissues in American education today. A detailed discussion of these issues follows.

Table 14.1 Issues in American Education

Issue 1: Quality of education

a.	Who should be educated, and to what degree?
b.	Teacher competence
c.	Teacher preparation
d.	Limited school funding
e.	Decline in breadth of school programs
f.	National versus local standards
g.	Testing controversy
h.	Alternative educational institutions
i.	Privatization

Issue 2: Negative societal changes

a.	Lack of parental involvement in education
b.	Changes in student environments
c.	Changes in study habits and skills
d.	Changes in students' maturation rate
e.	Extreme body images
f.	School violence

Issue 3: Proper educational practices

a.	Elitism
b.	Sexism
c.	Multiculturalism
d.	Education of persons with disabilities
e.	Nontraditional age groups
f.	Bilingual education

Table 14.1 (*continued*)

Issue 4: Expanded applications of digital technologies

	a.	Online education
	b.	Replacing the school book with digital media

Issue 5: Place of sport in the educational process

	a.	Is the school a legitimate place for sport?
	b.	How intensely should school sport be conducted?
	c.	When should students begin competitive sport?

Issue 6: Moral dilemmas in the schools

Subissue 1: Teaching moral education
Subissue 2: Moral standards
Subissue 3: Conflicting philosophies of moral education
Subissue 4: Sport and education hypocrisy

Quality of Education

Who Should Be Educated, and to What Degree?

This is a critical question, but there is no workable policy to answer it. Americans believe that all students should be educated to the limits of their personal potential. Unfortunately, they have never accepted that not everyone's potential is the same. Thus, people of high and low potential are mixed, the more able are held back, and the less able are pushed too hard.

Because we consider elitism bad (except in sports, where we worship it), we have gradually developed an educational system that stresses conformity and mediocrity. We need a clearer national policy for assessing student potential so we can provide appropriate programs. This is the idea behind Goals 2000 and No Child Left Behind. Only then will we be able to achieve the goal of equal opportunity for all students.

Teacher Competence

Weakened college requirements have resulted in many teachers who graduated with limited subject knowledge. More states now require prospective teachers to pass standardized tests to prove their competence. Those test results show that many college graduates do not have the knowledge necessary to teach. Many people oppose standardized testing as a part of teacher certification. Although it is true that standardized tests cannot accurately show which candidates will be *skillful* teachers, such tests *do* indicate which candidates have the *knowledge* needed to teach successfully.

Teacher Preparation

One of the oldest issues in the education of teachers is the question of time. How long should an effective training program last? The minimum is 4 years, although many educators insist that 5 years is a more reasonable period: 4 years to become well trained in the field of specialization, followed by a year devoted to professional training in education. In many cases, the fifth year blends into work toward the master's degree.

Some experts have argued that well-skilled physical education teachers can be produced in 2 years, as they were in the early years of teacher training. They argue that the length of time required to prepare teachers is largely wasted because it keeps younger professionals out of an overcrowded marketplace, while it provides more jobs for college teachers. Although the issue is more complex than this, at its heart lies a growing conviction that the preparation process has expanded to include busy work that serves no practical purpose and does not pay off in increased teaching skill or success.

Another issue is the amount of work devoted to the subject matter versus professional education training. One side contends that we need strong concentration on the subject matter so the teachers will know *what* to teach. Another argument is that professional education is more important because subject mastery is useless unless you know *how* to teach it. This controversy may be the reason for the push toward a fifth preparatory year because it permits more work in both areas.

Should the subject matter be taught with the emphasis on the subject itself, or should students be taught the methodology of how to teach the subject to others? In other words, should the teaching methods instruction be integrated into the subject matter instruction, or should it remain segregated and taught in methods courses outside the subject courses?

The question of whether to emphasize philosophy or science arose early in the twentieth century as educators sought to develop a science of teaching. They never really succeeded, and the issue has not yet been settled. In a way, this controversy is an extension of the liberal arts versus sciences debate, or the practical versus theoretical arguments still prevalent in education.

Another controversy revolves around laboratory experiences, or the time spent observing teaching activities and student teaching. The opinions range from involving the students in small teaching observation experiences regularly from the first year of college, to the more traditional approach of concentrating the experiences during one or more terms of the last year of college, to the idea of requiring a full year or more of successful teaching before awarding certification.

A final concern involves general education. How much time should be spent in areas outside the major field and the other areas directly related to the teaching field? How broad should the general education be? Professional educators argued against additional work in general education because they believed it limited the amount of time devoted to the subject areas.

At the heart of the issue is the far-from-simple question that confronts us all: What is education? What is its ultimate goal? What type of education is most worth having? The question has not been resolved for centuries, nor is it likely to be settled in the near future, but exercise scientists should not be too dogmatic or closed-minded to the views of the liberal arts supporters. By ignoring their views we may isolate ourselves from the other areas of the educational experience.

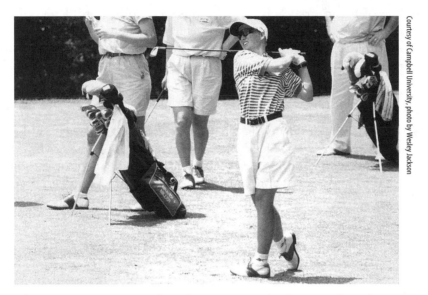

Courtesy of Campbell University, photo by Wesley Jackson

The sport experience and performance are the focuses of much research.

More scholars are calling for changes in teacher education in reaction to changes in the world outside. Other writers criticize the field's tendency to plan training that is too specialized, when most employees need more broadly educated workers.[5] Indeed, college students often receive a shallow, limited education, producing (as two scholars noted) "graduates who are unfinished," or unprepared to do an adequate job in the workplace. Although the field has strengthened the scientific knowledge base, the changes in most programs were made at the expense of other areas of the field of knowledge:

> *These graduates then are seriously lacking in the humanities of the profession such as the historical and philosophical components of sport. Due to this concentration on muscle fibers and distal attachments, the profession is instructing their future professionals to look at each student as a machine and not as a person.*[6]

Limited School Funding

The budget battles show no signs of easing after decades of argument. This creates great problems because balancing the school budget requires cutting back or eliminating valuable programs. As the population ages, there are more voters who do not have school-age children. They are less willing to pay taxes to educate other peoples' children. This dangerous short-sightedness is a growing problem throughout the nation.

Decline in Breadth of School Programs

The decline of broad programs stems from several other problems, such as the budget crunch and the back-to-basics movement. Some voters oppose paying for broad programs, and others believe that nonessential programs dilute the academic focus of the schools. The result is a drawing back from the old ideal of the comprehensive school.

National Versus Local Standards

Another area of controversy is the question of whose standards will be used in setting school requirements. Should the standards be local, set within the state, the school district, or even by the local school? Should there be national standards so that all high school graduates will be comparable, no matter where they live? This question is very controversial. National standards of genuine quality would be very helpful, but the idea runs counter to our national tradition of local control. National standards are a common feature of education in other nations, but they are rarely found in American education.[7] The Core Standards of 2010 is an attempt to deal with this issue.

Testing Controversy

Since the 1990s, we have seen increased student testing, an outgrowth of the earlier use of statewide minimum competency tests leading to high school graduation. This growth has led to what Gerald Bracey calls "testing madness."[8] States are requiring extensive testing of student accomplishment, with a goal of letting it determine student promotion and graduation, but also serving as evaluative data for individual teachers, whole schools, school systems, and the states themselves. The results are then used in budgeting, determining teacher salaries, and deciding teacher retention—they could even determine the survival of an individual school.

Our society has become a numbers-oriented place; we want to believe that raw numbers will answer our questions and solve all of our problems. The real answers are not so easy. We already know that a major factor in test scores is economic status, and that students whose parents are involved in their education will outperform students with disinterested parents. Not all educators are in favor of increased testing.[9] The schools are often blamed for parental shortcomings.

Alternative Educational Institutions

Many different forms of education are available today, some formal, some less formal, and others extremely experimental. Traditional American education is conducted in a formal school setting, with scheduled courses and comprehensive examinations. A record of achievement is kept in terms of course units, hours, or some other unit of quantitative measure. A diploma or degree requires a set quantity of these units.

Alternative private institutions continue to grow in number. Some are religious or political alternatives to public education. These schools were designed to compensate for the failures of the public schools and to avoid problems evident in the public schools. Some of the schools are public or private elite institutions (schools for the intellectually gifted). Other alternative schools emphasize special areas of student talents, such as in the arts or sciences. Other institutions, such as open schools, implement experimental educational programs.

At the college level, since the 1960s the expansion of community colleges has offered credit and noncredit courses for a vast range of interests. Many colleges also permitted students to develop some of their own courses in more specialized or unusual areas. Life experience schools offered college credit and degrees based on a person's personal experiences, rather than formal training. External degree programs expanded, as more colleges and organizations began offering courses, first by mail or television, and now as online courses and programs. Those programs have made college credit and diplomas available to people who are unable to attend college in the traditional manner.

Privatization

Privatization is the ending of public services, which are replaced by private, for-profit businesses. We are seeing a real growth in this area. The benefit is that such programs must meet market demands, which supposedly include better standards of education. On the other hand, these programs may simply give in to paying customers who want their children to receive better grades, regardless of their accomplishments (which is already a problem in the public schools). Privatization ultimately may lead to the weakening or removal of public options. If that is the case, then it would increase the problem of a society divided into the haves and the have-nots: Those with money can pay for a good education; those who are poorer will receive a weak education—or no education at all.

Negative Societal Changes

Today people complain of the changes in society that they consider unfortunate, things that lower the quality of life or that threaten the future. These changes also have an important effect on education.

Lack of Parental Involvement in Education

A common teacher complaint is that many parents no longer play a role in their children's education. Although we see many reasons for this change, the lack of parental involvement is a major contributor to student failure.

Changes in Student Environments

Our society has changed significantly over the last few decades. Broken homes through divorce are common, and many children live with a single parent. In many two-parent homes, both parents work, weakening parental involvement in the life of their children. Drugs have become a highly visible part of life for many students. The problem of student pregnancy is another aspect of high school life. These changes affect the learning patterns and potential of all students, not just the ones who are directly involved.

Changes in Study Habits and Skills

Many students spend more time as observers than as participants in life. They have a very short attention span, poor reading skills, and a limited experience in learning. As a result, it is more difficult to teach students who may have little understanding of *how* to learn and even less interest in making the *effort* to learn.

Interestingly, we have *not* made the same concessions to mediocrity in sport training, where students are still required to make significant personal efforts.

Changes in Students' Maturation Rate

Students grow up faster in our society today. Television, movies, and computer games expose them to violence, drugs, and sex and affect their attitudes and practices. An example of the change is the rising number of unwed parents at the high school level.

Extreme Body Images

Although this trend has been around for many years, its impact on society has sharply risen. Our movie and television programs show men with bodies that are muscular far beyond normal limits, even as it shows women who are dangerously thin and with equally unlikely artificial enhancements. Elements of this were seen a century ago in the physical culture movement,[10] but today's ideal body image often cannot be produced without the use of drugs, surgery, or other abuses of the body. We even see those body images presented in dolls and in children.[11] At the same time, we also see rising physical and mental problems, along with drug-, diet-, and surgery-related problems that accompany the drive of young people to achieve perfect bodies.[12]

School Violence

The school is no longer a safe haven in a dangerous world. It has its own dangers as the world increasingly intrudes behind the walls. School violence is a growing concern of teachers, students, and parents. Incidents of violence against students and especially against teachers lend an air of fear to some schools. Although this issue is thought of as an exclusive inner-city school problem, it is really a more general school concern. Violence has become common in many schools throughout the country, regardless of their location or size.

Proper Educational Practices

Elitism

Another area of controversy is elitism, or education for the superior student as opposed to education for the average or typical student. The dispute over elitism affects subject matter and level, grading standards, educational emphases, and related areas of sexism and education of children with handicaps. For the most part, the American educational program has been designed for the average student. This may work well for the majority, but it sorely neglects the intellectually gifted student, the potential leader of the future. Education primarily for students of average ability carries elements of anti-intellectualism.

Two physical educators expressed their concern over the neglect of intellectual needs at many educational levels. In responding to an article on standards for graduate study in physical education, they wrote that, even though the suggestions were for graduate education, "it is appalling that enhancement of scholarship and research was absent from the list of recommendations."[13]

This problem of intellectual neglect stems partly from the popular idea that *elitism* is a dirty word because it implies that some people are more valuable than others. Our schools should not accept the idea that one person is better than another, but they cannot afford to ignore the reality that one person may be more talented than another. If educators ignore that difference, they deny and suppress that person's talent. The idea of education is to stimulate and expand each person *within the limits of his or her own ability*. Elitist programs should be *required*; the law requires programs for the average and for those who are far below the average, yet the most talented people are often ignored, unless they are athletes.

Elitist views have been condemned for being unconcerned with equality and with treating all students the same. However, people are not intellectually or physically equal, and to deny that is foolish. Equality demands that each person be given the opportunity to reach his or her *full* potential, without that opportunity depending on another person's greater or lesser potential. We already promote elitism in school sport; it is only in matters of the intellect that we argue against it.

Many issues are part of the controversy over elitism. Competition as a part of the educational process is one issue. Some people argue that competition is harmful to education, but others believe it is necessary, beneficial, and normal. There is no denying that people have to compete when they are out of school. Thus, some people consider competition in the classroom to be a necessary preparation for real life.

Sexism

A parallel concern with elitism is sexism. The idea of equality of education and opportunity regardless of sex was guaranteed by law under Title IX. During the 1970s, the greatest impact of Title IX was the expansion of women's school sports. The effects of Title IX were also felt in academic areas because many school courses had been taught primarily to a single sex. Boys took shop courses, and girls took home economics. The reality that as adults both sexes need information in both areas was disregarded.

In a more subtle vein, women were often discouraged from more scientific and technical study because such areas were not considered appropriate for women's talents. Often, women also were discouraged from graduate work because they were expected to get married and leave the job market at an early age. Sexism was only another leaf on the tree of discrimination because minority groups also were discouraged from entering some fields based on assumptions about their talent. The Fourteenth Amendment to the Constitution has been applied in both racial and sex discrimination suits, along with Title IX in sex discrimination suits. However, the survival of Title IX has been threatened in the years since it became law.

Multiculturalism

The nation has concerns about ensuring cultural diversity in its school programs. The population of the United States is increasingly diverse; in a few more decades no ethnic or cultural group will be a majority of the population. Thus, we must have inclusive education to develop an awareness and acceptance of the different cultures that are part of our nation.

At the same time, we face the danger of a fractured society if we have only a collection of independent ethnic entities, but no common American culture. The danger of that direction faces us on the news every day, as we hear of the many internal wars, of nations tearing themselves apart as one group tries to drive out or destroy another group for ethnic or religious differences.

Education of Persons with Disabilities

Under Public Law (P. L.) 94–142, the public schools are required to provide education for people with handicaps because the law guarantees free and appropriate education to all students with disabilities. The law also encourages mainstreaming, that is, putting students with learning disabilities into classes that usually have no students with disabilities. The passing of P.L. 94–142 created many controversial issues in education. These concerns continue with P.L. 99–457.

There is no denying that students with disabilities have been shortchanged in education. Fortunately, new programs for disabled students have been implemented. However, several arguments have been raised against aspects of the new programs. Those arguments are not over the rights of students with disabilities to an education or to increased opportunities. One major concern is cost: Can the schools afford the massive costs of the new programs for students with disabilities at a time when normal school activities are already being dropped from the curriculum? At the same time, many people are concerned that educational mainstreaming, rather than advancing societal mainstreaming, may lower the level of education offered to able students to a level acceptable to students with learning disabilities. Opponents of mainstreaming see this as a denial of the rights of the majority who are not disabled.

Many educators are also concerned that some of the programs for students with disabilities were developed to take advantage of federal grants. Those educators suggest that people who are really interested in helping students with disabilities will help without grants. They believe that many programs will disappear when grant monies disappear. In addition, there is concern over whether students with disabilities are being used or displayed for sympathy and money-raising purposes. This is a dehumanizing process, as Wilfred Sheed pointed out in his essay, "On Being Handicapped."[14]

Non-traditional Age Groups

The concept of adult education as a lifelong process, a never-ceasing continuum from birth throughout adult life and into old age, continues to grow as our population ages. Credit for popularizing this concept must go to the local and community colleges that developed programs to meet the interests of all ages and groups. Courses offered in those programs range from exercise to wine tasting to business to the arts. A brief study of the courses offered at any large community college will give a good idea of the breadth of experience and expansion of education in the modern American community.

Gerontology, the study of aging, is a growing area of interest to educators. As the baby boom generation enters middle age, the average age of the population is rising. Improvements in health treatment and disease control have continued to raise our life expectancy. Consequently, the proportion of elderly citizens is growing. We need to develop educational and physical programs of interest to our older citizens to improve the quality of their lives.

Bilingual Education

Bilingual education affords non-English-speaking students English instruction in their native tongue until they are able to learn equally well in English. The basic concept is sensible, but difficulties have risen with the expansion of the concept. The first difficulty comes from a growing tendency to use the foreign language program not as a temporary measure while English is being mastered, but as a continuing practice that replaces mastering English. This situation has resulted in a great need for bilingual teachers, few of whom are available.

At the same time, bilingual education has created a second difficulty, a growing population that cannot mix with the majority of Americans because its members do not try to learn the language of their adopted country. Bilingual education has caused the weakening of the old concept of the United States as a melting pot of nations, where foreign peoples are all blended together as Americans who speak a common language. People who retain another preferred language without learning the native language leave themselves outside the mainstream of the society in which they live, weakening their chances of success as they weaken the cohesiveness of that society. The controversy over what bilingual education should be in the schools is yet to be solved, but non-English speakers are the fastest growing segment of our society.

Expanded Applications of Digital Technologies

Although computers and digital media have been in use for several decades, we are now seeing a surge in expanded applications of digital media. As download speeds have increased, combined with continued miniaturization of digital components and exponential increases in digital storage capacity, we are now at the point where educational applications have become widespread.

Online Education

Online courses have been used in many colleges, but their use is now becoming widely accepted for broader applications. Early courses had very limited enrollments as colleges experimented with how they could be best used and whether they were worthy of college credit.[15] Now some universities are offering massive open online courses (MOOCs), which may have more than 100,000 students enrolled[16] and are offered free through consortiums such as Coursera.[17]

Replacing the School Book with Digital Media

Elementary and secondary schools are also increasingly using digital media in the classrooms. The rise of hand-held tablets is resulting in a shift from printed books and media to ebooks. Part of the change is the result of a drop in prices, but a major factor is that many children are already familiar with using computers and tablets. Added to the benefit is the replacement of the large number of printed books that students must carry by a single tablet containing all of the books in digital format. Estimates are that 20 million students and teachers are already using tablets.[18]

The Place of Sport in the Educational Process

The place of sport and sporting competition in American education is a continuing issue that raises many concerns. Only a few are addressed here.

Is the School a Legitimate Place for Sport?

Though long-standing tradition and public interest seem to accept sport, there is no genuine agreement about whether the school is a legitimate place for sporting competition. The U.S. tradition of school sport is almost unique among nations. It may be one reason for the weakened focus on education in American society. Schools have become a place where sport is taken more seriously than learning. This tradition affects the public view of education and learning.

How Intensely Should School Sport Be Conducted?

Should the pursuit of success be the major emphasis of a school sport program? Should more attention be paid to the personal development of the students and

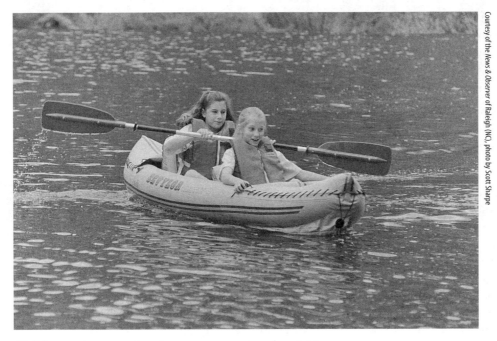

Children enjoy experiencing new recreational activities.

to the lessons learned through competition in sports activities? At this time, the common focus is on elitism and success.

When Should Students Begin Competitive Sport?

At what age should students be exposed to competitive athletics? How great should the competitive emphasis be in the program and how seriously should young athletes train or be made to train? These interlocking issues became more critical with the developments in international competitive sport, particularly after the advances by eastern European athletes in the 1970s and 1980s. Children with athletic potential (some younger than 10 years old) were placed in intensive training schools that were often located in major cities far from their homes. All aspects of the children's education, growth, and development were monitored. In many cases, drugs such as steroids were administered to those children to develop desired physical characteristics. World junior championships in many sports have increased the impetus toward elite sport at a young age.

Currently, most American competitive school sports begin in junior high or middle school (grades 7 through 9), although intramural competitions may occur in the elementary school. Some children begin competitive athletics, through either the schools or community programs, at or before the age of 10 years. Such programs can be beneficial if their administrators and coaches are concerned individuals who realize that young children's bodies are very vulnerable to abuse, overload, and contact injury. The psychological development of the young athlete must be considered by the administrators of these programs. The place of competitive sports and youth sports is still an area of great controversy in American education.

Moral Dilemmas in the Schools

One of the most difficult problems in American education is the question of moral dilemmas, particularly within the school curriculum. American schools have always considered moral education to be important, although religious education traditionally takes place outside the schools. The Constitution requires the separation of church and state. However, that requirement does not affect moral education, such as ethical behavior, or subjects that include moral questions or issues such as sex education.

Teaching Moral Education

The major dilemma is whether such subjects are the proper concern of the schools or whether they should be left to each student's parents. Although moral education is considered extremely important, nobody agrees on what should be taught, how it should be taught, or even whether it should be taught in the school rather than in the home under parental direction.[19]

Moral Standards

If moral standards are included in the curriculum, other dilemmas arise regarding the content and emphasis used in teaching the courses. Should specific moral or ethical standards be suggested or recommended? Should the students simply be directed to develop their own standards as they see fit?

Conflicting Philosophies of Moral Education

Dilemmas in moral education are especially difficult because people have conflicting views. Few people disagree that students need to learn about moral issues and develop standards of conduct. The controversy revolves around what standards to develop, how they should be developed, and who is ultimately responsible for teaching them.

Sport and Education Hypocrisy

There is a large dose of daily hypocrisy in honoring the ignorant athlete while promoting academics. The U.S. educational system worships elitism and accomplishment in sport (which is not its major function), yet does not always encourage the same striving for success in the education of our nation's youth.

The list of issues in American education just reviewed is far from definitive, and there are major areas of controversy. Education is not a placid stream. It is a constantly changing area of modern life. An educator must be aware of the questions that concern fellow educators, parents, and students. At the same time, an educator must be flexible enough to adapt to the changing educational scene.

Issues in Exercise Science and Physical Education

Table 14.2 lists important issues in exercise science and physical education today. A discussion of these relevant issues follows.

Table 14.2 Issues in Exercise Science and American Physical Education

Issue 1: The disciplines versus the profession

a.	Has the discipline movement strengthened our education?
b.	Has the discipline movement strengthened our teaching?
c.	Has the discipline movement promoted our professional unity?
d.	Has the discipline movement improved our public image?
e.	Future directions of exercise science and sport

Issue 2: Is the curriculum too science focused?

Issue 3: Value and quality of the school program

a.	Teacher competence
b.	Loss of the requirement
c.	Decreased teaching time
d.	Difficult learning environments
e.	Teacher–coach role conflict

Issue 4: Emphasis of the school program

a.	Individual versus societal needs
b.	Divisions for group instruction

Issue 5: Proper educational practices

Issue 6: Maintaining quality programs despite budget cuts

a.	Accountability: Demonstrating accomplishment
b.	Developing public relations

The Disciplines Versus the Profession

This subject has been controversial since the 1970s. It has created a conflict over both present practices and future directions.

Has the Discipline Movement Strengthened Our Education?

Is undergraduate education in the major stronger because of the research and changing emphases that result from the discipline movement? It has, in fact, added the equivalent of a second major to what is studied today. Few schools offered courses in most subdisciplines in the 1970s (except for kinesiology and exercise physiology). Is the current program better than the old one?

Has the Discipline Movement Strengthened Our Teaching?

Do educators teach more effectively or do a better job because of the discipline movement? Has the movement contributed significantly to their teaching skills or knowledge? What has been its impact on the job that physical educators do?

Has the Discipline Movement Promoted Our Professional Unity?

Are professionals unified as a group? This question probably creates the most heated discussion because many teachers believe that the discipline movement has split the field into teachers versus scholars and that neither group wants to be associated with the other group. Irwin and Pettigrew argue that "most indicators tend to show it has not been beneficial."[20]

Has the Discipline Movement Improved Our Public Image?

A major goal of the discipline movement was to increase academic respectability in education and before the public. Interestingly enough, after 40 years of the movement, there is little evidence that anything was accomplished toward that goal. Indeed, the field may have lost ground.

Future Directions of Exercise Science and Sport

The focal question is what should be the future direction in exercise science and sport. Professionals in the field need to determine the most useful and effective programs for the future. This is a critical area of concern.

Is the Curriculum Too Science Focused?

Since the discipline movement took over the field, the traditional curriculum has been replaced by a heavily science-focused one. As more science courses were added to the curriculum, older courses in the sociocultural and humanities areas were often removed from the program.

To some exercise scientists, the new program has become unbalanced, too focused on the science courses, while neglecting any learning in the broader concerns of the field.[21] This narrow curriculum can weaken a graduate's ability to perform in the field. It is also destructive to the field that Franklin Henry called for, an "interdisciplinary field," rather than a field of small, autonomous subdisciplines that do little cooperative work beyond their own narrow interests.

Value and Quality of the School Program

Perhaps the most critical issue in American physical education today is a question of value. As budgets tighten and come under close scrutiny, which programs are the most worthwhile? Physical educators must defend the place of their branch of learning in the school program.

Sports are popular in the schools and communities, and many physical educators assume that their role in the curriculum is safe. That is a risky assumption to make. Today a program must demonstrate its value, rather than simply defend its budget request. A quality physical education program must show that it has clear, useful, attainable goals; that it has a well-rounded program to achieve those goals; that it regularly tests to determine that progress is being made; and that it succeeds in meeting its goals.

Physical educators agree that their subject is a vital part of a well-rounded educational program. It contributes significantly to the needs of growing students, and it affects intellectual growth just as it affects the development of physical health and coordination. However, we do too little to sell the value of a good physical education program to the public, and often we ignore what the public wants. Instead, the public often views physical education as the tail end of the athletic program. This weak public relations effort must be corrected.

Teacher Competence

Teacher competence is a concern in all subject areas, so we cannot ignore it.[22] Too often, physical educators are perceived as poorly trained, poorly educated people who are primarily interested in coaching. Coaching is only a small part of the role of physical educators.

Any competent teacher needs a strong academic education because the acquisition of concrete and theoretical knowledge is essential. Some professionals want more emphasis on the discipline of physical education (the acquisition and spreading of a scholarly knowledge), and others want more emphasis on the pedagogical (teaching) side of the field. This conflict has been called teachers versus scholars. However, teachers should be scholars just as the members of the discipline are.

Do people who are trained only in the discipline have the knowledge of teaching theory and the physical skills necessary to teach and coach? Do those who concentrate on teacher education have the content (the scientific knowledge) needed for appropriate, useful teaching and coaching? It is important to solve this nagging problem and to create cohesive programs of professional preparation that will produce legitimate teacher/scholars.

At the same time, we must choose the most beneficial programs. Research is needed to determine and to recommend the most useful national program of physical education for students of various age groups, and evidence should be collected to support the value of the chosen emphasis, activities, and goals. Then the program could be promoted across the country, and local modifications could adapt the national program to meet local needs.

Loss of the Requirement

Another concern is the loss of the physical education requirement in the schools. Since the 1960s, the requirement has been gradually disappearing, until today only one state still requires daily physical education at all levels. In most states, high school students are not required to take any further physical education classes. This trend has been one of the great failures of the profession.

We especially see the effects of these losses in the impact on young children. Many elementary schools no longer have physical education specialists. The shift to classroom teachers having oversight, combined with increasing demands on teaching time, has resulted in the lessening or removal even of recess or playtime for young children. Education and health advocates are calling for increased recess or playtime, noting that it affects not only health but also cognitive function and learning in the classroom.[23]

Decreased Teaching Time

At the same time that the physical education requirement was being cut back (usually with budget problems as an excuse), those costs also produced a tighter schedule, with less actual teaching time. If a daily program is cut to 3 days per week, 40% of the teaching time is lost. With less instructional time to teach skills and knowledge, the students make less progress, and goals become more difficult to reach.

Difficult Learning Environments

Still in the same vein, the learning environments for physical education have become more difficult. When classes are larger, there is less time to help each individual. When classes are made more diverse (or less homogeneous), with a greater range of abilities and aptitudes, the teacher encounters more difficulty in helping each student to reach his or her potential. Factors creating a more difficult learning situation can include larger class sizes, multiple classes in the same setting (such as several classes in the same gym), the addition of students with behavior problems, and mainstreaming. These situations can result in cutbacks in the opportunities for students in each group rather than attempts to improve their opportunities.

Teacher–Coach Role Conflict

Being a teacher and a coach creates many difficulties because the roles are at times in conflict. The coach must be careful to act as she or he would as a teacher, rather than reject the role of educator while coaching. At the same time, there are difficulties in developing an effective and proper relationship with the athletes.[24]

Emphasis of the School Program

The phrase *physical education program* does not refer to a single model used across the country. Each school system (and sometimes each individual school) has its own favored curriculum. The major emphases fall roughly into these four divisions: (1) competitive sports, (2) lifetime sports, (3) fitness and health, and (4) wellness and health.

Some programs focus on *competitive sports*. Classes develop playing and tactical skills in the locally popular sports, such as football, basketball, and baseball. Although efforts may be made to relate the work in these sports to overall physical development, the emphasis too easily turns toward producing strong teams and locating and training young athletes for those sports. Thus, the physical education program becomes a farm system for the athletic department, run by and for the coaches. There is more interest in how physical education can meet the needs of the athletic program than how it can meet the needs of the students.

A second emphasis is *lifetime sports*. A program of lifetime sports includes activities that are appropriate for people of any age. Students are taught skills that they can enjoy through middle age and into later years. For example, few 50-year-olds can play football, but volleyball and badminton are excellent sporting and fitness activities at any age.

A program of lifetime sports does not ignore fitness. The fitness effect of any activity depends on its intensity. For example, a younger person will find that badminton can be an extremely taxing activity from the fitness standpoint. However, an older person can play an enjoyable and competitive game at a lower level of intensity that is more suited to his or her fitness level. This accounts for the popularity of games such as volleyball and slow-pitch softball. They can be enjoyed regardless of the skill or fitness level of the players involved.

A second advantage of lifetime sports is that they are more easily part of coed and mixed-ages classes. Competitive sports and fitness activities require greater homogeneity of skill or fitness levels. Many classes are now mixed, so this point is very important. Games such as volleyball and slow-pitch softball work as well in coed classes as in single-sex classes because neither the less skilled or less fit individuals nor the shorter or lighter individuals are at a great disadvantage.

A third focus is that of *fitness and health*. Its primary goal is to develop a high level of physical fitness in the students. This orientation is especially strong during times of war. Fitness-centered programs tend to ignore basic motor skill development and the more social and intellectual aspects of physical education.

Fitness is a very worthy goal for today's programs. A well-planned program can develop a high level of fitness without emphasizing calisthenics and conditioning in class instruction. However, fitness can become a barrier for a program aimed at the growing student; consequently, a broader goal is called for. Many programs now use a health or wellness orientation to fitness.

A fourth emphasis is *wellness and health*. It has less emphasis on physical training for high-fitness measures. Instead, it focuses more on basic levels of fitness combined with broader concerns of good health and nutrition. It may also use elements of lifetime sports in achieving its goals.

The substance of a program tends to change gradually over a long time. This is not a bad characteristic because it shows that the program is responsive to the needs and interests of the society it seeks to serve. The early emphasis of many programs was on health, leading to fitness. That was gradually replaced by a sports orientation, except during times of war. During the 1970s and 1980s, lifetime sports became most prominent. Now we are seeing a wellness focus. The programs will continue to respond to new leisure patterns of the future, as they have in the past.

Individual Versus Societal Needs

Should a program focus on group or societal needs or on the needs of the individual student? It is much easier to plan a program that takes little account of each individual. In schools with large classes, that is a great temptation. We need to prepare people to fit into society. However, it is important to see that their differing individual needs are also met. The concept of people's needs and potential is changing sharply when we consider what people of differing abilities set as personal goals.[25]

Divisions for Group Instruction

Forming groups for instruction has led to problems as a result of federal intervention in local programs. Far more classes are taught on a coeducational basis than in the past. There is more mixing of age, sex, and ability levels. The introduction of individuals with disabilities through mainstreaming further complicates the picture, as does the introduction of multilingual requirements in areas with non-English-speaking language groups. Physical educators must decide how best to meet those complications of the instruction program so that the effectiveness of the program is not diminished.

Proper Educational Practices

Many concerns fall into this category, but perhaps the primary ones are elitism, sexism, and racism. Elitism returns to the objective of what we want to achieve in our programs. Do we focus only on the most or least talented students or on the norm? Do we encourage people to strive for excellence or settle for average? How do we treat the non-elite students compared to the elite?

Sexism and racism refer again to equality of treatment and of opportunity. Just as in the case of elitism, we want fair and equal treatment, encouragement, and opportunity for all students. With elitism, we are dealing with talent. With sexism, we are dealing with unequal treatment of men and women. With racism, we are dealing with unequal treatment of people from different racial, ethnic, or national groups.

Maintaining Quality Programs Despite Budget Cuts

When the budget crunch hits, does physical education have a place in the school program? People in the field must do more to justify the position of physical education within general education. At the same time, they must find ways to maintain quality instructional programs in times of budgetary crisis. In some cases, the answer is a choice between physical education and competitive sports, with one sacrificed to save the other. However, physical education seeks to help every student, while competitive sports leans toward the most skilled. The most skilled do deserve the chance to develop their talents to the fullest, but that right does not overcome the right of the majority of the students to have their needs met. One complaint against physical education in the past has been that as coaches, physical educators have preferred the elitist approach, neglecting the average students in favor of developing the skills of the talented few who can be successful in competitive sports. This is never a proper direction for a teacher to take.

Accountability: Demonstrating Accomplishment

Educators must demonstrate that their programs are working by highlighting their students' accomplishments. Unless they can clearly show that the programs have useful goals, and that they meet those goals, their programs will be in danger of disappearing.

Developing Public Relations

Physical educators must be more conscious of public relations. This is their weakness in a budget crunch because without favorable public support they risk having programs damaged, if not lost, when the supply of money dwindles. The physical education program must make a strong effort to prove its value and see that the public knows about it, if it hopes to be protected when there are money shortages.

Relationship to Athletics

Athletics is a persistent problem for our field. The issue often becomes teacher versus coach, a question of who controls the overall physical program of the school. Does the physical education program benefit the athletic program, or is athletics simply another facet of the program? If a physical educator emphasizes the sports program, a budget cut may damage the physical education program severely. That would affect the needs of far more students than those affected by the sports program. The intent of this comment is not to suggest that school sports are not a valuable adjunct to the school program; it simply is to point out that sports is a dessert or side dish in relation to the main course, physical education.

Issues in American Sport

Although there are many issues in sport today, this section looks primarily at the problems that are reflected in school sports (**Table 14.3**). The major issue is the growth of Big-Time Sports and of other matters that fall under that umbrella.

Big-Time Sports in the public schools can be compared to baseball played by the cartoon character Charlie Brown and his friends and a highly organized Little League program. It also has been described by many writers as the "professionalization of amateur sports."

Table 14.3 Issues in American Sport

Issue 1: The place of sport in education		
	a.	Maintaining the focus on education
	b.	Using sport for noneducational purposes
Issue 2: Ethical dilemmas		
Issue 3: Growing professionalism of sport at all levels		
Issue 4: Elitism versus sport for all		
Issue 5: Drugs in the sport setting		
	a.	The athlete as junkie
	b.	Alcohol and tobacco sponsorship
	c.	Better winning through chemistry, or the coach as pharmacologist
	d.	Extremism in the sporting body
Issue 6: Violence in sports: Society's mirror?		
	a.	The ethic of approved violence
	b.	Good guys finish last
	c.	Sport as society's steam vent
Issue 7: It's money, money, money that I want		

Sports programs have turned their emphasis from the participants and the benefits they gain to the spectators. Booster clubs donate large amounts of money, facilities become very elaborate (especially for the spectators), the number of coaches and the coaching rewards increase considerably, and often the actual number of sports and participants decreases (to avoid "diluting school efforts" and perhaps fielding weaker teams in the "minor" sports). The ultimate prestige is on the success of a few teams, combined with the revenue they produce. Teams become a public relations and financial venture for the school, rather than a growth experience for the athletes.

The Place of Sport in Education

The issue of the place of sport in education is really a question of what part should it play? What is its proper place in the education of young people? Is it so important that the intellectual education of the students has less value than their striving for athletic excellence?

The state of Texas was the first state to take a hard look at the future of its students and realize that the first task of the school is to educate. A state law now requires a student/athlete to pass every course being taken or be dropped from the athletic program until grades improve.

Among the unique arguments against the law was that a major function of high school was to qualify youth for athletic scholarships to college, regardless of poor grades or academic incompetence. A more understandable fear was that students would avoid the challenging academic courses to protect their chance to play sports. However, this fear (a legitimate one) was weakened by the high proportion of students who failed at least one course, regardless of how easy their academic schedule was. This failure rate said much about their lack of seriousness.

In fact, the United States has developed the reputation of having the least academically strenuous educational program in the world. After a major study of American education, Arthur Powell and his coauthors referred to the "shopping mall high school." They explained that schools try to have something for every level of ability and as a result have no standard education for all students. As one student said, "It's a big job to make up a curriculum that everybody can do."[26]

Maintaining the Focus on Education

Has sport in the schools caused us to lose sight of the major purpose of education? School sport is symptomatic of the problem because too often students (and many coaches) believe that schools should provide a support system for athletic teams rather than the teams' being just a part (and not the most important part) of the educational process.

The ethic of Big-Time Sport (and elitist attitudes) has filtered down to the high schools and even lower. Sports should offer the athletically gifted a chance to achieve, but if sport really is an educational experience, there should be a place for the less athletically talented students. The less intelligent students take classes structured to their level of ability. They are not barred from school.

Using Sport for Non-educational Purposes

The university model of sport is one of entertainment, public relations, and potential profit. The current times are notable for their marketing of sports, even at the public school level. Not only are we selling children's games to the public to raise money, we actually claim that we cannot provide sports otherwise. If we truly believe our own arguments about the educational value of sports, we should be willing to fund them through our taxes, just as we do the other necessary components of a good school system. When we use sport to raise money (usually for noneducational causes), we have left the schools far behind.

Ethical Dilemmas

There are many ethical dilemmas. Do students learn to respect others and to play fairly and by the rules when they take part in school sports? Do they learn good sportsmanship, or do they gradually form a nation of immature sports whiners?

What lessons about life and adulthood do they first learn and then teach through their participation in sports?

Growing Professionalism of Sport at All Levels

This issue reflects another aspect of the Big-Time Sport syndrome, the professionalism of sport at all levels. As noted when discussing the rise of modern sport, professionalism is a characteristic of modern sport. Should an Olympic-level athlete be paid to train or perform? Should a college athlete receive payments? Should high school or lower-level athletes be paid to perform? If so, how can one say that sport belongs in the schools? No one has ever expected payment for learning; it is an obligation and a necessity for survival.

Elitism Versus Sport for All

The Sport for All movement is growing in many nations. It is based on broad participation in sport, moving the focus away from elite competition and the preparation of elite performers. This attitude stands in contrast to providing no sport options other than varsity athletics or to making participation in school sports a "pay or don't play" dilemma.[27]

Drugs in the Sport Setting

Drug use is a huge problem in sport today. Is the use of any type of drug to enhance performance or training *ever* acceptable from an ethical or sporting point of view? Whether it is the use of anabolic steroids, human growth hormone, EPO, or designer drugs by a high-level athlete or the use of stimulants, depressants, or narcotics by any athlete or coach, the problem is critical.[28]

The Athlete as Junkie

There have been far too many cases of athletes failing a drug test, then protesting that the test was wrong or unfair. This was the case with Ben Johnson's loss of his gold medal and world record at the 1988 Olympics in Seoul. As the world soon learned, the test was not wrong. The image of athletes as not-very-bright physical specimens is rapidly being replaced by an image of athletes as drug users and drug abusers.[29]

Alcohol and Tobacco Sponsorship

Alcohol and tobacco businesses deal in drugs that create significant health hazards for our population. Because sports are popular, they spend millions of dollars each year to sponsor sports events as a method of advertising and reaching potential buyers. Is it proper for sports events, which supposedly represent good health and oppose drug use, to accept such sponsorship? Should it be legal because these events are widely watched by children who cannot legally purchase the products? Does this advertising encourage children toward the acceptance of drug use as normal?

Better Winning Through Chemistry, or the Coach as Pharmacologist

Do coaches encourage drug use in athletes, either directly by recommending it (such as steroids) or indirectly by not discouraging its use? What does this say of our personal attitude toward drug use? What does it say about our personal ethical standards?

Extremism in the Sporting Body

As mentioned in the section on societal changes, we are seeing increasingly extreme bodies, particularly in the world of sport. Drugs have played a large part in this trend.[30] The desired bodies are "perfect" bodies for a sport, or a position, or an event within a sport. We see supposedly adult female athletes who weigh less than 90 pounds, and male athletes of average height who weigh more than 300 pounds. We see unusual body shapes, and many of them have long- or short-term health or longevity risks.

Violence in Sports: Society's Mirror?

What is the effect of violence in sports? Is it a reflection of a more violent world? The world has never been peaceful in the past. Has violence become more acceptable in sport? If it has, does it carry over into real life, making violent acts more acceptable off the playing field? The soccer riots of 1985 that killed dozens of people and barred the British professional teams from playing in Europe are not a new problem. However, violence at sporting events seems to be more common. Is sport the cause, or is it just an innocent victim exploited by violent people as an excuse for their acts?

The Ethic of Approved Violence

Do people encourage sport violence by accepting the bad boy as a role model? Do they encourage unnecessarily aggressive acts in athletes? Do they publicize as dedicated those athletes who deliberately attack or belittle their opponents? If they do, their actions signal their approval of violence and improper conduct, regardless of their claims to the contrary. We now see these images regularly on television, with staged wrestling contests and other so-called sports that feature cartoon-like violence and bloodshed.

Good Guys Finish Last

This is a popular saying for people who are poor sports. If coaches instill this adage, we will see the death of good sportsmanship. We will be forced to accept the birth of the new ethic—to be a winner, you must be a loser. Is this the message we want to promote in sports?

Sport as Society's Steam Vent

This is a sociological theory, suggesting that sport gives us a chance to vent our aggression, to attack other people in an acceptable way. If so, it can explain sports riots in which people are sometimes killed. However, is this really a function of sport? Should it be a function? What will be the result if we accept it?

It's Money, Money, Money That I Want

At many (perhaps most) levels of sport today the focus is not on the experience, or the competition, or even the performance. It is about the money. How much money can an athlete, or a team, or a school make? How can we maximize our income?

Universities are in a contest to see which school can build larger, more extreme sports venues, with the idea of attracting more spectators and money to their events. College sport today is a marketing arm of the school, with separate budgets that make its real mission clear: publicity and income. The athlete has become, essentially, a cog in the business machine.

Some universities are able to sell their athletic merchandise around the world, adding millions in potential income. The National Collegiate Athletic Association (NCAA) sells its championships, in some cases, such as basketball, for more than a billion dollars. It now produces video games that use actual student athletes (some of whom are now suing for the illegal use of their images without pay).

Money has become, perhaps, a greater threat to school sports than drugs are. Drugs are dangerous, but they are generally a problem of the individual. The money chase has infected the entire system, from extreme facilities to extreme salaries for coaches.

It is clear that sport is a controversial topic in education and society. Sports professionals need to look at the issues and consider them carefully, not just from the side of the athlete or coach, but also from the side of the fan, the spectator, and the opponent. They all have valid reasons to support and oppose sport. These issues are major concerns, but they are only the tip of the iceberg—and they will not go away. They must be faced now and in the future.

Summary

This chapter examines three broad areas of issues: education as a whole, exercise science and physical education, and sport. The focal issue in education is: What education is most worth having? Linked to this are two ongoing concerns: the back-to-the-basics movement and the problem of the high cost of education.

The major issues in American education today are (1) the quality of education, (2) negative societal changes, (3) proper educational practices, (4) the place of sport in the educational process, and (5) moral dilemmas in the schools.

The major issues in American exercise science and physical education today are (1) the disciplines versus the profession, (2) if the curriculum is too science focused, (3) the value and quality of the school program, (4) the emphasis of the school program, (5) proper educational practices, (6) maintaining quality programs despite budget cuts, and (7) the relationship of exercise science and particularly physical education to athletics.

The major issues in American sport today are (1) the place of sport in education, (2) ethical dilemmas, (3) the growing professionalism of sport at all levels, (4) elitism versus sport for all, (5) drugs in the sport setting, (6) the problem of violence in sports, and (7) the athletic systems' focus on money.

Further Readings

Arum, Richard, and Josipa Roksa. 2010. *Academically adrift: Limited learning on college campuses*. Chicago: Univ. of Chicago Press.

Benedict, Jeff. 1997. *Public heroes, private felons: Athletes and crimes against women*. Boston: Northeastern Univ. Press.

Bennett, Gregg, and Frederick P. Green. 2002. Student learning in the online environment: No significant difference? *Quest* 53: 1–13.

Brackenridge, Celia H. 2001. *Spoilsports: Understanding and preventing sexual exploitation in sport*. New York: Routledge.

Brooks, David. 2012. Measuring what colleges do. *New York Times*, reprinted in *Raleigh (NC) News and Observer*, April 24, 11A.

Buscher, Craig. 2006. Online physical education: Wires and lights in a box. *JOPERD (Journal of Physical Education, Recreation and Dance)* 77 (2): 3–8.

Byers, Walter, and Charles Hammer. 1997. *Unsportsmanlike conduct: Exploiting college athletes*. Ann Arbor: Univ. of Michigan Press.

Festle, Mary Jo. 1996. *Playing nice: Politics and apologies in women's sports*. New York: Columbia Univ. Press.

Gilbert, Bil. 1988. Competition: Is it what life's all about? *Sports Illustrated*, May 16, 86–90, 92, 94–95, 97–98, 100.

Gregory, Sean. 2010. The problem with football. *Time*, February 8, 36–43.

———. 2010. Struck out by béisbol. *Time*, July 26, 45–49.

Holowchak, M. Andrew, and Heather L. Reid. 2011. *Aretism: An ancient sports philosophy for the modern sports world*. Lanham, MD: Lexington Books.

Hudson, Susan O. 2007. Are professional organizations viable in the 21st century? *JOPERD (Journal of Physical Education, Recreation and Dance)* 78 (2): 3.

Hunt, Thomas M. 2011. *Drug games: The International Olympic Committee and the politics of doping, 1960–2008*. Austin TX: Univ. of Texas Press.

Hyman, Mark. 2009. *Until it hurts: America's obsession with youth sports and how it harms our kids*. Boston: Beacon Press.

Mazanov, Jason, and Vanessa McDermott. 2009. The case for a social science of drugs in sport. *Sport in Society* 12 (3): 276–295.

McCallum, Jack. 2000. Gym class struggle. *Sports Illustrated*, April 23, 82–85, 87, 89–90, 92, 95–96.

Miah, Andy. 2001. Genetic technologies and sport: The new ethical issues. *Journal of the Philosophy of Sport* 28: 32–52.

Morgan, Bill. 2010. Sport, wholehearted engagement and the good life. *Sport, Ethics and Philosophy* 4: 239–253.

Norton, Kevin, and Tim Olds. 2001. Morphological evolution of athletes over the 20th century: Causes and consequences. *Sports Medicine* 31 (11): 763–783.

Pauline, Gina. 2012. Celebrating 40 years of Title IX: How far have we really come? *JOPERD (Journal of Physical Education, Recreation and Dance)* (October): 4–5, 56.

Rosen, Joel Nathan. 2005. *The erosion of the American sporting ethos: Shifting attitudes toward competition.* Jefferson, NC: McFarland and Company.

Rosentraub, Mark S. 1997. *Major league losers: The real cost of sports and who's paying for it.* New York: Basic Books.

Ross, Stewart. 2008. *Higher, farther, faster . . . Is technology improving sport?* London: Wiley.

Sabo, Don. 1998. Women's athletics and the elimination of men's sports programs. *Journal of Sport and Social Issues* 22: 27–31.

Sack, Allen L., and Ellen J. Staurowsky. 1998. *College athletes for hire: The evolution and legacy of the NCAA's amateur myth.* Westport, CT: Praeger.

Saunders, Ross H., and John M. Dunn. 2010. The Bologna Accord: A model of cooperation and coordination. *Quest* 62: 92–105.

Sawyer, Thomas H. 2006. Point–counterpoint: The physically illiterate physical educator. *Physical Educator* 63: 2–7.

Spirduso, Waneen W. 2009. Staying afloat in an information-age sea change. *Quest* 61: 5–18.

Thomas, Evan, and Pat Wingert. 2010. Why we can't get rid of failing teachers. *Time,* March 15, 24–27.

Torres, Cesar R., and Peter F. Hager. 2007. De-emphasizing competition in organized youth sport: Misdirected reforms and misled children. *Journal of the Philosophy of Sport* 34 (2): 194–210.

Trudeau, François, and Roy J. Shephard. 2008. Is there a long-term health legacy of required physical education? *Sports Medicine* 38 (4): 265–270.

Tufte, John E. 2012. *Crazy-proofing high school sports.* Lanham, MD: Rowman and Littlefield.

Discussion Questions

1. Briefly discuss three issues in American education, explaining how each affects our planning for the future.

2. Briefly discuss three issues in American exercise science and physical education, explaining how each affects our planning for the future.

3. Briefly discuss three issues in American sport, explaining how each affects our planning for the future.

4. Discuss the reasons behind the back-to-the-basics movement and the problems that it can cause in the educational system. Can you propose and defend a reasonable solution to the question, keeping in mind the severe financial problems facing many school systems?

5. Cite and describe briefly some of the problems in educational accomplishments that may have resulted from earlier educational experiments.

What lessons do these problems suggest for us in planning educational programs for the future?

6. Explain the meaning of equality in education, discussing how it should be provided and what problems it can create.

References

1. Ebel, Robert L. 1980. The failure of schools without failure. *Phi Delta Kappan* 61: 386–388.

2. Higgins, George V. 1980. Clumsy oafs, unlettered louts. *Harpers* (May): 60–63.

3. Broder, David S. 1995. Goals 2000 won't be met if cuts made. *Portland Oregonian*, August 2.

4. Ibid.

5. Feingold, Ronald S. 1994. Making connections: An agenda for the future. *Quest* 46: 364; and Zakrajsek, Dorothy, and William Pierce. 1993. Academic preparation and the academic consumer. *JOPERD (Journal of Physical Education, Recreation and Dance)* (May–June): 20–23, 31.

6. Irwin, Carol, and Frank Pettigrew. 1993. A look back to the future. *Physical Educator* 50:173.

7. Issues: Do you think it is time for the U.S. to implement a national curriculum? 1994. *JOPERD (Journal of Physical Education, Recreation and Dance)* (February): 8–12.

8. Bracey, Gerald W. 1999. The ninth Bracey report on the condition of public education. *Phi Delta Kappan* 81 (October): 147; and Ramirez, Al. 1999. Assessment-driven reform: The emperor still has no clothes. *Phi Delta Kappan* 81 (November): 204–208.

9. Mathews, Jay. 1999. Put more students to the test. *Raleigh (NC) News and Observer*, September 1; Tests are an easy way out. 1999. *Newsweek*, September 6, 50–51; and Walberg, Herbert J., and Rebecca C. Greenberg. 1999. Educators should require evidence. *Phi Delta Kappan* 81 (October): 132–135.

10. Budd, Michael Anton. 1997. *The sculpture machine: Physical culture and body politics in the age of empire*. New York: New York Univ. Press.

11. Takahama, Valerie. 1999. Ab-normal image. *Raleigh (NC) News and Observer*, August 26.

12. Kalb, Claudia. 1999. Our quest to be perfect. *Time*, August 9, 52–59.

13. Blair, Steven N., and Russell R. Pate. 1980. Letter to the editor. *JOPER (Journal of Physical Education and Recreation)* (September): 12.

14. Sheed, Wilfred. 1980. On being handicapped. *Newsweek*, August 25, 13.

15. Lewin, Tamar. 2012. Online courses to be reviewed for college credit. *New York Times*, reprinted in *Raleigh (NC) News and Observer* (November 13): 1A, 10A.

16. Stancill, Jane. 2012. Colleges join in online ed. *New York Times*, reprinted in *Raleigh (NC) News and Observer* (November 16): 1B, 7B.

17. Friedman, Thomas. 2012. A revolution in education. *New York Times*, reprinted in *Portland Oregonian*, May 17, C7; Dan Lyans. 2012. Cheaper than Harvard. *Time*, May 14, 13; and Mary Beth Marklein. 2012. College may never be the same. *USA Today*, September 12, 1–2A.

18. Elliott, Philip. 2013. Schools shift from textbooks to tablets. Associated Press, reprinted in *Raleigh (NC) News and Observer*, March 11, 1–2D.

19. Issues: Sportsmanship—an antiquated concept? *JOPERD (Journal of Physical Education, Recreation and Dance)* (October 1993): 6–7; and Shields, David Lyle, and Brenda Jo Bredemeier. 1995. *Character development and physical activity*. Champaign, IL: Human Kinetics, 197–225.

20. Irwin and Pettigrew, Look back, 173.

21. Ives, Jeffrey C., and Duane Knudson. 2007. Professional practice in exercise science: The need for greater disciplinary balance. *Sports Medicine* 37: 103–115.

22. Sawyer, Thomas H. 1992. The physically illiterate physical educator: What can be done? *JOPERD (Journal of Physical Education, Recreation and Dance)* (January): 7–8; Issues: Should all physical educators be expected to have a common set of performance skills and competencies for teaching? 1992. *JOPERD (Journal of Physical Education, Recreation and Dance)* (April): 9–11; and Issues: Should physical education, dance, and recreation educators be expected to maintain a certain level of physical fitness? 1992. *JOPERD (Journal of Physical Education, Recreation and Dance)* (November–December): 8–10, 73–75.

23. Schoof, Renee. 2013. Bring playtime back to schools, experts say. McClatchy Newspapers, reprinted in *Raleigh (NC) News and Observer,* February 14, 8A; and Schoof, Renee. 2013. Experts want to revive recess. McClatchy Newspapers, reprinted in *Raleigh (NC) News and Observer,* February 17, 14A.

24. Hornak, N. Joan, and James E. Hornak. 1993. Coach and player—ethics and dangers of dual relationships. *JOPERD (Journal of Physical Education, Recreation and Dance)* (May–June): 84–86; and Wolohan, John T. 1995. Title IX and sexual harassment of student athletes. *JOPERD (Journal of Physical Education, Recreation and Dance)* (March): 52–55.

25. Hoffer, Richard. 1995. Ready, willing and able. *Sports Illustrated*, August 14, 64–70, 72, 74–75.

26. Powell, Arthur G., Eleanor Farrar, and David K. Cohen. 1985. *The shopping mall high school*. Boston: Houghton Mifflin.

27. Swift, E. M. 1991. Why Johnny can't play. *Sports Illustrated*, September 23, 62–64, 66–68, 70, 72.

28. Schneider, Angela J., and Robert B. Butcher. 1993–1994. Why Olympic athletes should avoid the use and seek the elimination of performance enhancing substances and practices from the Olympic Games. *Journal of the Philosophy of Sport* 20–21: 64–81.

29. Lemonick, Michael D. 1998. Le tour des drugs. *Time*, August 10, 76; and Williams, Melvin H. 1996. Ergogenic aids: A means to citius, altius, fortius, and Olympic gold? *Research Quarterly for Exercise and Sport* 67 (3 Suppl.): 58–64.

30. Nack, William. 1998. The muscle murders. *Sports Illustrated*, May 18, 96–100, 103–104, 106; and Gorman, Christine. 1998. Girls on steroids. *Time*, August 10, 76.

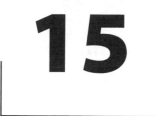

Into the Future in Exercise Science and Sport

After studying the roots of our field, what it is, and how we prepare to work in it, we still face a major concern: What does the future hold for our field? What are the developing trends in our lives, and what effect will they have in 10, 20, or 30 years?

Toward the Future

People have always been fascinated by the future. In literature, many writers express their views of the future, sometimes as a warning and other times as a suggestion of the ideal society. In earlier times, the suggested ideal is found in Plato's *Republic* and Thomas More's *Utopia*. Other futuristic views are found in Aldous Huxley's *Brave New World* and George Orwell's *1984* and in Alvin Toffler's series of books, *Future Shock*, *The Third Wave*, and *Powershift*.

We want to know what the future holds, but our concern about the changes that it may bring sometimes leaves us apprehensive. Changes are a certainty, but we do not know whether the results will be better or worse for the human race. An area of study called futurism or futuristics is a scientific study of the future.

Previous studies of the future were attempts to plan a perfect society (such as the ideas of the Utopians, who took their name from Thomas More's work), but modern study is inclined more toward predicting the future than designing it. Madge Phillips cites Henry Winthrop's contention that sociologists prefer futurism because they believe in a value-free discipline.[1] However, even predictions of the future are based on perceived or inherent value systems. World trends, particularly those relating to population growth problems, climate change, and energy and food shortages, have created widespread interest in predicting the future.

The Problem with Predictions

Educational theorists are usually full of ideas about how to improve education and society, but their record of success has not been good. For decades educators have been putting their theories into action, but the results have not been impressive.

Theorists are becoming more cautious in their predictions of successful, meaningful change because too many of their earlier predictions did not come true.

At one time, the American population was expected to increase indefinitely, as was the school population (and the need for teachers). Many school systems expanded based on that prediction, and a large number of teachers were hired. However, the prediction was incorrect. A change in family habits (the trend toward smaller families) resulted in a drop in the school-age population. That trend has now reversed.

The college population was also expected to increase indefinitely, partly from a population increase, but also from a wider pool of student ages. The population of the United States was once expected to taper off somewhere below 300 million people, but it has grown past that point. At some point it *may* stabilize, though that stabilization is difficult to predict. However, because many other countries have not decreased their growth rate, the world population will continue to rise at a phenomenal rate.

This chapter discusses trends in the United States in three areas: society, education, and exercise science and sport. Societal trends provide a broad picture of what the future may hold, and educational trends give us a bit more specific idea of the factors that may affect our field. A study of the trends in exercise science and sport offers the clearest idea of the implications of the future for the field. These are not the only trends, but they are a group of major currents that could have a critical impact on the future. However, before trying to predict trends, the following section examines the ideas of several scholars in the field.

Scholars Predict Trends in Exercise Science and Sport

We can get a sense of the directions of our field from people who are trying to analyze the major changes of the recent past. Daryl Siedentop suggests 10 themes that he believes define the future of our field:[2]

1. Specialization or integration of the field
2. The split between the discipline and the profession
3. The growing activity and leisure industries
4. Distributing the field's efforts more equitably
5. Wellness as the center of lifestyle education
6. A more broadly based (inclusive) sport culture
7. Re-emphasizing people skills in the human services professions
8. Gender equity in the field
9. The success or failure of school physical education
10. Focusing on new populations

He focuses on the idea of life span involvement; that is, participation in physical activity at all ages in our life. Christopher Edginton lists what he calls "drivers of change," to which we must respond:[3]

1. Life ethic
2. Demographic shifts
3. Independence of action
4. Greater diversity
5. Knowledge and information supermarket
6. Family structure
7. Women's roles
8. Emerging global connectedness

Donald Hellison suggests the following trends in physical education (exercise science), noting that in doing so, he is "basking in unbridled optimism":[4]

1. Physical education in higher education will return to an applied mission.
2. Physical educators in higher education will collaborate with practitioners at work sites.
3. Research in physical education will emphasize application to on-the-job problem solving.
4. There will be a reversal of the trend toward separating physical education from health education and recreation education.
5. Public school physical education programs will have smaller classes. The teacher–coach role conflict will end, and there will be more leadership by physical educators.
6. Physical education practitioners will involve clients more in dealing with their needs.

Sadly, most of his trends have not happened.

John Burt sees a narrow vision in the field. He uses dreams and questions to explain his three broad concerns:[5]

1. Have we compromised our academic birthright and lost sight of our common purpose?
2. Have we failed to make our field an integral part of people's lives?
3. Have we counteracted the inherent good in our goal to improve health by making health seem unpleasant or contrary to pleasure?

Shirl Hoffman refers to our profession as having

organizational Alzheimer's, leaving it confused, disoriented, and unable to put together an effective strategy for accomplishing reasonable goals. . . . It wasn't until 3 years after its passing that word finally reached the AAHPERD, who immediately assigned a committee to study the matter.[6]

This is a recognition of the profession's failure to provide leadership and direction.

Earle Zeigler stresses the need for reunifying the splintered field of allied professions.[7] He argues that each separate area has lost something important by losing contact with the other areas. Part of his effort to show the unity of the field was to develop a list of what he called "Physical Education's 13 Principal

Principles" (**Table 15.1**).[8] These are, in his view, the most important theories or generalizations in the field.

Like Zeigler, Charles Corbin stresses the need for once again unifying the field. The people in the disciplines are largely university based, while the professional people work in the schools and in a wide range of other public and private sector settings. Corbin expected the field of kinesiology to emerge during the 1990s, defining a field as "a discipline that has professionals who use the discipline as the basis for delivering important and needed social services to clients, learners, and patients."[9] Twenty years later, that expectation has not been met.

Sharing a similar point of view, Ronald Feingold argues the importance of the field from a holistic perspective; that is, as it contributes to the health and education of the nation. He broadens our future focus to include "the development of positive, healthful lifestyles . . . wellness programs, development of self-esteem, and values orientation," stressing that as a field we "must reevaluate [our] mission and status. . . . Physical education professionals must recognize that health and physical education is [sic] truly at the center of education."[10]

Feingold's call for the holistic approach to the field echoes Roberta Park as she points out our field's similarities to that of medicine as it made the transition to a science- and research-based field.[11] It had to recenter itself toward a holistic

Table 15.1 Physical Education's 13 Principal Principles

Principle 1:	The Reversibility Principle
Principle 2:	The Overload Principle
Principle 3:	The Flexibility Principle
Principle 4:	The Bone Density Principle
Principle 5:	The Gravity Principle
Principle 6:	The Relaxation Principle
Principle 7:	The Aesthetic Principle
Principle 8:	The Integration Principle
Principle 9:	The Integrity Principle
Principle 10:	The Priority of the Person Principle
Principle 11:	The Live-Life-to-Its-Fullest Principle
Principle 12:	The Fun and Pleasure Principle
Principle 13:	The Longevity Principle

approach that would use the science while focusing on the patient, student, or client. Professionals also must make that transition to a broadly based, holistic field.

Some of these writers paint a grim picture because they are struggling with a reality that has not always been pleasant. Although there are many growth areas, our field is still fragmented in many respects. Instead of a unified field with shared goals toward which all members work, we find an endless number of small, self-important, specialized groups whose primary interest appears to be their own professional aggrandizement, regardless of the cost to the field. There is an oversupply of mice who see themselves as lions.

With that rather pointed thought in mind, let's try to construct an overview of the trends that we see in the field, both today and on into the middle of the twenty-first century.

Societal Trends in the United States

This section briefly examines 11 trends that affect society in the United States (**Table 15.2**). They are not given in order of importance. Each is important, and they are in many cases related to and affected by other trends.

Table 15.2 Trends in American Society

The United States: A New Multicultural Society
Trend 1: Growing language gap
Trend 2: Growing economic inequality
Trend 3: Growth of the underclass population
Trend 4: The New Tribalism: Growing ethnic conflict
The Decline of Personal Responsibility
Trend 5: Declining social conscience and cooperation
Trend 6: Family instability
Trend 7: Growth of the now generation
The Growth of World Change
Trend 8: Growth of a world culture through the online world
Trend 9: Growth of a world techno–industrial economy
Plus ça Change (the more things change)
Trend 10: Changing leisure patterns
Trend 11: Continuing ethical dilemmas

The United States: A New Multicultural Society

The United States has been a nation of immigrants from its earliest days. Many different nationalities and language groups came from the earliest colonial days to the present. However, in the past the nation prided itself on being a melting pot, where immigrants blended together as Americans, sharing a common language and cultural heritage.

The nation is becoming a truly multicultural nation as its native population gradually becomes a minority. Projections indicated that in 2010, for the first time, more minority-heritage babies than white babies would be born, up from 48% in 2008. Other projections suggested that by 2050 there would no longer be a majority racial or ethnic group in the United States, as is already true in several states.[12]

Growing Language Gap

Many immigrant groups maintain their customs, lifestyles, and languages. This creates tension in some communities, where some people may believe that maintaining another cultural identity is un-American. Particularly in some large cities, the growing number of foreign languages used in students' homes creates problems in the local schools. One Virginia high school listed 60 different languages used at home by its students.

Growing Economic Inequality

The United States is a nation of economic class structures, with increasingly distinct differences between the upper and lower groups.[13] The result is a country of haves versus have-nots, those who can afford to live as they wish, compared to those who have little hope for either the present or the future. The poor quality of public education in the United States today has added to the problem. Many students do not learn enough to perform a job at any level other than the lowest skilled task. Unfortunately for them, that type of job is rapidly disappearing. In an increasingly technological world, almost no jobs are that simple. Workers must be able to read and understand instructions so they can operate and repair machinery, and too many Americans cannot read well enough to follow simple instructions.

Growth of the Underclass Population

A growing number of Americans cannot meet their basic needs and live in poverty. They lack health care to treat and avoid disease, and they lack the education to win jobs at wages that allow an average standard of living. For them, there is little hope of rising out of their impoverished state. The size of this group has grown dramatically in the last few decades, and it is a major concern for the future. Their needs are basic, but they have no resources to meet them.

This trend is part of a larger, worldwide population explosion. The greatest rates of increase are found in the nations that are least able to provide for their people. Such growth creates a great conflict within and among nations, as the wants and needs of those people clash with the reality of their shortage of resources.

The mushrooming population has an impact on all other areas of life, both in terms of the ultimate resources available for the earth's inhabitants and in the potential quality of life for them. Many of the earth's resources (such as food supplies) can be replenished, but others (such as fossil fuels) are not renewable. When the planet's petroleum reserves are gone (which is expected within 50 years), alternative energy sources will be needed.

Greater populations mean greater drains on limited resources, such as energy supplies; greater populations also limit the ability of the planet to provide optimum shelter and nourishment. The result is an increasing dichotomy between the haves and have-nots, with the subsequent social unrest created by such division. Many wars result from the basic need of overcrowded societies to provide more room or to find more sources of food. The ultimate impact of the world population increase is critical. Mass starvation is one result of too many people in areas that cannot support large populations. If major climate changes occur, as they did in the Dust Bowl during the 1930s, entire nations can starve.

The New Tribalism: Growing Ethnic Conflict

One of the traditions of American history is the melting pot, America as a place where people from many nations blended together. Whether or not that belief is a truly accurate description, it is accepted American folklore. Today there are more conflicts over ethnic diversity, with groups that want to be U.S. citizens, yet use their native (non-English) language and maintain their native customs.[14] The difficulty is that many of the groups fail to learn English well enough to blend into American culture and qualify for better jobs. This leads to conflict between people who decry their limited opportunities and others who resent the presence of alien elements.

This issue has become a greater concern because in some parts of the nation ethnic groups are a large part of the population. The United States is a mixture of races and cultures that need to be able to work together for the common good. New groups need to learn the language and culture but do not have to throw away their native culture. If we fail to blend, we run the risk of the tribalism that is destroying some other nations.

The Decline of Personal Responsibility

Declining Social Conscience and Cooperation

There has been a growing lack of societal concern about unmet needs over the last 2 decades. In many communities and states, the voters have shown that they will not help the poor, will not pay for better schools, and will not pay for quality-of-life public services. Yet they complain loudly if those services are not provided at a high level. It is an attitude of "I've got mine, so who cares if you get yours." It is a complex problem that relates to most of the other social and economic trends given here. It is causing increasing conflict in communities across the nation.

At the same time, we see a growing intransigence, a lack of cooperation between groups. People no longer seem willing to compromise or work out common problems. Instead, they want total victory. In an overpopulated world, total victory is impossible. The result is hostility, unrest, and never-ending conflict. Groups with different beliefs are unwilling to accept that groups with differing views hold their views just as strongly and have a right to do so. This is one reason why society seems to break down, with increasing violence and lower quality of life.[15] A society that cannot compromise and accept other people's right to be different cannot survive because it cannot work as a unit for survival.

Family Instability

Family patterns today are characterized by changing family roles and a disintegrating family tradition. This is not a simple (or single) problem, but the result of complex changes that are interrelated, but not necessarily causative.

More women are working outside the home, which moves us away from the traditional family pattern. It is not a matter of lack of parental caring. There are more single-parent families, and many families in which both parents work. In most cases, the jobs are an economic necessity, not a parental preference. To add to the parental absence, today's more intensive jobs can keep parents focused on work even when they are at home. Computers increase the tendency to do job-related work during the off-hours at home.

At the same time, traditional sources of family roots are disappearing. There are fewer intergenerational families (several generations living together). More families move from one part of the country to another, away from their ancestral homes. We are becoming a nation of strangers.

Children are growing up faster because of outside influences: television, mass advertising, movies, drugs, less family stability, less sense of their family roots. This trend is characteristic of larger communities with less adult supervision, coupled with a declining religious influence. The weakened religious influence adds to the growing lack of an overriding ethic to provide stability and guidance not found in the home.

Growth of the Now Generation

We see a growing demand for instant gratification. People are unwilling to take a long-term approach. Businesses fail because their primary goal is immediate profits, rather than long-term growth and survival. The quality of social services is declining because people are unwilling to forgo any immediate wants in return for long-term benefits. The nation's massive debt is the result of a buy-now, pay-later philosophy that guarantees serious large-scale problems in the future, when those debts fall due. Indeed, we see the same problem in sport, by overtraining athletes to get immediate results, even though it will probably shorten their athletic careers and perhaps even lessen the highest level of performance that they can achieve.

The Growth of a World Culture

The Online World and the World Culture

World culture is growing through technology. The world has become a connected place, with instant communications and knowledge of worldwide activities. This creates a world culture, rather than a national culture. Because we are more aware of the greater world, we tend to work and react in terms of that world, rather than simply our own nation or narrower focus of interest. We saw the blurring and disappearance of many regional differences in the post-television decades. We are now seeing the next phase, moving from a national to a world culture.

The World Techno-Industrial Economy

We are developing an interconnected world of technology and industrialism. This trend has led to have-not nations: Their people have limited education, so they cannot be competitive in a high-tech world. The United States faces this same risk as it fails to educate enough of its citizens to the needed level of ability. Some technological businesses have higher incomes than many nations. People need higher levels of education to take advantage of the opportunities that this trend represents, but the failure to educate means that many people are left behind in the world economy.

The industrialized world has become a high-tech world. The knowledge explosion forces people to specialize because no individual can hold the broad store of the world's knowledge. The world is increasingly computerized and miniaturized, so many of the older distinctions between regions and people no longer hold true. Many of the old regional differences among areas of the United States are almost impossible to discover today. The influences of satellite television, instant world news, and increasing wealth at many levels of society have done more in a generation to make the United States homogeneous than all of the other changes of the past 2 centuries.

Plus ça Change (The More Things Change)

Changing Leisure Patterns

Experts predicted far more leisure time in an increasingly technological world. We expected work hours to continue to decline, leaving more hours for leisure activities. Instead, we may be seeing the death of the idea of the leisure generation. The predicted growth in leisure did not happen. Instead, workers are finding that the difference between work and leisure is disappearing as technology moves into the home. It has become a 24/7 world, where we are busy 24 hours a day, 7 days a week.[16] The computer allows working at home, just as the cell phone allows it to continue in the car. People can work anywhere now, and they do.

Indeed, their job success increasingly requires it. The result is less leisure, rather than more. Added to that, companies in the United States allow less vacation time than any other industrialized nation. There is a failure to provide sufficient leisure, which is a significant factor in people's long-term health and longevity.

Greater world wealth increases our ability to provide leisure activities for the general population, particularly in the United States. We need people who can teach and direct recreational programs, and we need more emphasis on teaching recreational skills and exercise in the schools. At the same time, we need to shift our focus toward activities that require less time rather than toward time-intensive, long-term programs that conflict with today's short-term focused lifestyle.[17] Programs of relaxation skills and tension relief are growing rapidly, especially in more technological and complex areas of society.

Continuing Ethical Dilemmas

We will continue to face ethical dilemmas involving questions for which there may be no clearly right or wrong answers. For example, the booming growth in the world population is a serious threat to the ability of the world to support its citizens. There is a natural need for a world policy on birth control, but many newly emerging nations see such a suggestion as a threat to their power. They believe that it will keep their nations small and weak. Such nations face the dilemma of having a small population that they can feed or a large population that will face starvation.

A similar ethical dilemma is in the environmental debate over economy versus ecology. The ecology of a nation may be hurt by industrialization, yet the effect of strict ecology laws may be a weaker economy. The issue in some cases has been simplified to a choice of one or the other. Some people believe that any possible compromise will hurt both sides to some degree. There may not be a right answer, but if this generation cannot solve the problem, the next generation will have much greater problems to solve.

Ethics are vital to the successful functioning of any society; that is, people must have standards of values by which they live. The development of ethical standards has long been a prominent part of the educational process. The Greeks spoke of the development of character as one of the most vital concerns, if not the most vital concern, of education. Many educational goals were optional, but character was a goal that could never be dropped.

Educational Trends in the United States

This section briefly examines 12 trends that affect education in the United States (Table 15.3). As in the social trends, they are not given in order of importance. Each is important, and they are often connected to other trends.

Table 15.3 Trends in American Education

Trend 1:	Disagreement about educational priorities
Trend 2:	Education for a technological world
Trend 3:	The future curriculum: Narrow or broad?
Trend 4:	Changing educational priorities
Trend 5:	Declining student knowledge levels
Trend 6:	More accountability
Trend 7:	More testing
Trend 8:	Changing school populations
Trend 9:	Teacher education: Specialist or generalist?
Trend 10:	Whole-school involvement in teacher education
Trend 11:	Higher teacher education standards
Trend 12:	Privatization of education

Disagreement About Educational Priorities

As a nation we are not in agreement on our educational priorities. The United States has traditionally attempted to educate a larger proportion of its people to a higher level than most other nations. However, that raises critical questions. Should every person be educated? If so, what should be the process, what should be the content, and to what level should they be educated? There are no correct answers to these questions. Each nation must make its own educational decisions for the future, but as the world changes, those decisions affect the rest of the world. Conflict over what the schools should teach has increased community involvement in the schools. More citizens are interested in what is happening in the schools and are working to make the school programs more responsive to community needs.

The knowledge explosion has created educational conflicts: What knowledge is most important? In recent decades, we have seen a massive disagreement over what people expect from their schools. The result of that discord is confusion. Different schools are trying different approaches to education. The results tend to be confusing rather than enlightening. The question is asked and repeated: What knowledge is most worth having? Educators do not agree on the answer. This is an area of conflict that will remain for some time.

Education for a Technological World

Today's high-tech world is a complex one. The person who hopes to survive and perform well needs many skills.[18] Our education must meet those technological needs so our schools can prepare tomorrow's citizens to fulfill their roles in society. The old-fashioned education was designed to prepare a person for a civilization that was also old-fashioned. We must prepare people to live in the future, rather than in the past or even in the present. Our decisions have a critical impact on our nation's economic future.

The Future Curriculum: Narrow or Broad?

During the mid-twentieth century, the school curriculum became broader, and more areas of study were included than in the past. The narrow bounds of traditional educational subjects and interests weakened as interdisciplinary studies crossed the old subject boundaries. More electives were permitted in the schools, although the idea of a totally elective program showed little sign of public acceptance. That era of a broad curriculum is ending, as parents call for more accountability and demand a return to the core subjects of education.

In 1978, the broader curricular pattern led to Richard Gross's suggestion of seven new Cardinal Principles of Education to replace the 1918 list.[19] His revision put the principles into today's world. To show how they contrast to the original list, they are placed side by side (**Table 15.4**).

As we can see, the old and new cardinal principles are equally broad, yet the new principles are a bit more in touch with what are seen as necessary functions of education in a modern world. One question for the future is how those principles will be applied in the school program.

Table 15.4 Seven Cardinal Principles 1918 and 1978

Seven Cardinal Principles (1918)	Gross's Cardinal Principles (1978)
1. Health	1. Personal competence and development
2. Command of fundamental processes	2. Family cohesiveness
3. Worthy home membership	3. Skilled decision making
4. Vocation	4. Moral responsibility and ethical action
5. Civic education	5. Civic interest and participation
6. Worthy use of leisure	6. Respect for the environment
7. Ethical character	7. Global human concern

Changing Educational Priorities

Our nation's education priorities are changing. There is a battle for educational dominance between the cognitive and affective domains, a focus on relevance in education, a growing interest in career preparation before high school graduation, and attempts to humanize the curriculum.

A struggle has developed between the cognitive and affective domains of educational objectives. Under the *taxonomy of educational objectives* (a way to classify the objectives of education into more exact types), the objectives of education fall into three broad categories, or *domains*: cognitive, affective, and psychomotor.[20] The cognitive process is a means of determining factual knowledge. It includes intellectual abilities and skills. The affective domain includes feelings, emotions, and attitudes. Bloom also refers to the psychomotor objective as the "manipulative or motor-skill area,"[21] which involves the development of the motor skills of the student.

Although most education is traditionally in the cognitive domain, the affective domain is increasingly important. However, attitudes and emotions are not only difficult to teach but are more difficult to test quantitatively or objectively. The idea of precisely putting a feeling into words or numbers is a contradiction in terms. The interest in the affective domain rises from the feeling that people need a greater concept of values and that a vital part of the educational process is the development of attitudes and appreciations consistent with those of society in general. This interest in what might be called *moral education* is an attempt to re-create a lost culture of responsibility in the midst of what Christopher Lasch called a "culture of narcissism."[22] It is a desire to produce a society that understands that citizens in a crowded society have certain responsibilities to each other, rather than an unimpeded right to do as they wish, regardless of the effect on others.

Proponents of affective learning sometimes overreact by rejecting the cognitive domain, without realizing that the affective cannot survive without the cognitive base. Facts must come before theories and values if the theories and values are to survive. For an education to be well rounded, however, *both* areas need to be developed. There is no reason for a tug-of-war between the cognitive and affective domains.

People want education to be functional, to be relevant to their needs outside of the school. Those concerns are part of the demand for accountability of schools and of teachers, who are expected to prove that they are indeed accomplishing something, and to show that it is *worth* accomplishing. There is massive public resistance to the old idea of the school as an ivory tower where reality and the outside world never enter. Today the outside world is moving into the school and the educational process.

A greater consciousness of a future of work is being developed in students through career training. Students are shown the place of work in society and are introduced to many career options at an early age. It is intended to counteract the problem of students who graduate from school with absolutely no idea of what they want to do in the future, and in many cases, with no idea that they *need* to do anything.

One complaint about education is that it dehumanizes students or puts them into a lowly position of feeling that they have little human value. Humanizing education and the curriculum is one aspect of the affective concerns. It puts increased emphasis on the idea of caring for the students. The curriculum has become more flexible with an increasing variety of options designed to fit the needs of the individual student rather than bend the student to fit the curriculum.

Declining Student Knowledge Levels

Today's student has poorer language and math skills than the typical student of 20 or even 50 years ago. Among the reasons given for this decline are the rise of permissive education, a lack of discipline in the schools, and the greater emphasis on the affective domain (attitudes and appreciations) rather than knowledge and skills.

The accountability movement continues to grow. Students are asked to prove their knowledge by passing basic competence tests. Meanwhile, teachers must show precisely what changes they expect to produce in students and how they will test those changes. Teachers also must prove that they are sufficiently skilled or knowledgeable to produce the desired changes in their students.[23]

More Accountability

A major concern is that there is too little accountability for student education and achievement. Three efforts to improve school accountability are the Goals 2000: Educate America Act, signed into law in 1994; the No Child Left Behind Act of 2001; and the Core Standards of 2010.

Goals 2000 recommended educational goals to be met by that date. The goals were not met. No Child Left Behind set new standards, but added accountability by requiring regular standardized testing. By 2010, there were questions about whether that bill had led to genuine student progress. Core Standards was an attempt to get the individual states to adopt rigorous standards that were set by a group of governors and education leaders.[24] (See www.corestandards.org.)

More Testing

To determine real accountability leads to testing. Although student testing has been in the schools for many decades, only in recent decades has it become a factor in promotion to higher grades and graduation. Unfortunately, increased focus on those test results has also had negative side effects: teaching to the test rather than focusing on broader education, and cheating by students and in some cases teachers and school administrators. While testing is a necessary part of accountability, the nature of the testing is a controversial issue.

Changing School Populations

The school population today includes a wider range of ages and experiences, from preschoolers to senior citizens. We find different cultures and nationalities and also encounter more instability. Many students are from single-parent homes. Many children do not see a parent when they return home from school. The number of students who come to school hungry or in poor health is increasing. A change in our attitude toward post–high school education and the radical growth of 2-year schools in the United States during the 1960s and 1970s resulted in a much greater variety of programs for postschool adults and retirees.

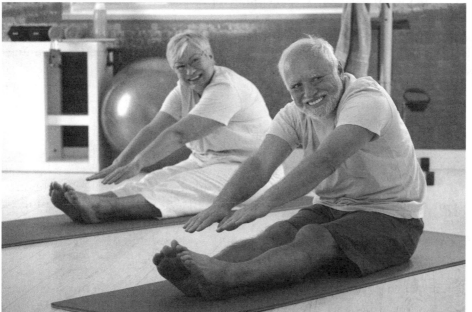

The population concentration of the United States is shifting toward more adults and elderly citizens, which creates new challenges in society, education, and physical education.

The dissatisfaction of many parents with today's public education has led to rising attendance at alternative institutions. The number of these public and private schools has increased. The first alternative schools were started to provide a more humanistic or free-form educational environment, but the term is now used for almost any school that differs from the typical public school in method or emphasis. Some alternative schools are designed to provide students with more discipline and direction, others are planned to re-emphasize basic education, and still others (primarily private schools) wish to provide a more religious or patriotic environment. This movement also may be partially a result of the modern homogenized school, which tried to remove anything that might be considered the least bit controversial from the educational program. The rise of special-interest pressure groups who attack anything in the schools that conflicts with their own personal values has sometimes created an atmosphere similar to the red scares of the 1920s, 1930s, and the early 1950s.

Teacher Education: Specialist or Generalist?

Although in the past we saw an increase in teaching specialists who had narrow areas of focus, we now are seeing some hesitation in that trend.[25] The issue is whether schools are more likely to employ a large number of specialists at great cost or a smaller (thus less expensive) number of generalists, each of whom can teach several areas. This situation is not the case in technology, yet it may happen in education, which is not a profit-driven field. This trend can affect areas such as health education, recreation education, safety education, dance, athletic training, coaching, and adapted and therapeutic work. We may see a movement in teacher education toward returning to the traditional combined health and physical education degree.[26]

Whole-School Involvement in Teacher Education

Who decides and enforces the standards for teacher education? The professional schools of education failed to produce effective teachers despite a free hand in applying their theories. An ongoing trend of involving all branches of the university in planning the teacher training process is a reaction to the isolation of specialists in education and physical education. Departments of education try to do everything, including academic preparation, which limits teachers' exposure to their subject matter. Involving the entire campus in planning the teacher preparation program and its content ensures that the educator's concern for methodology will not replace the fact that teachers must actually know something to teach.

Higher Teacher Education Standards

Grade standards for teacher education are rising, which is critical because teacher education students traditionally are among the weaker students in any school. At the same time, many schools have become open-admissions colleges. Any student may be admitted, regardless of ability. There are many reasons for the increase in open-admissions schools, but the major reasons are to limit questions of discrimination in admissions and maintain student enrollment during a time when fewer students are available.

In an open-admissions school every person has a chance to demonstrate the ability to do college work. This does not make higher standards impossible, or even necessarily more difficult to attain. The school can require that the bulk of the general education and foundational sciences coursework, along with some introductory

409 **Trends in Exercise Science**

areas of physical education theory courses, be completed with set grade restrictions before the student is admitted to the professional preparation program. Although this work should be the equivalent of 2 years of college work, the student is not limited to 2 years to meet the requirements. Time can be permitted to make up for academic deficiencies in addition to taking the required programs.

Privatization of Education

There also is an increased demand for private schools. This is a complex issue. One motivation is to improve educational standards at a time when the public schools often seem inadequate to serious education, but there are other factors involved in the trend. Some people send their children to private schools for a more religious atmosphere. Some are seeking a different mix of educational and social experiences. Still others are simply trying to leave schools that they consider dangerous. The risk of this privatization is that a two-tier educational program is developing in the United States: Those with good incomes will get better schools, while those who are less privileged will have poor-quality, dangerous schools.

Trends in Exercise Science

This section briefly examines nine trends that affect exercise science in the United States (**Table 15.5**). As in the societal and educational trends, they are not given in order of importance. Each is important, and they are often interconnected.

Table 15.5 Trends in Exercise Science

Trend 1: New lifestyle needs for old lifestyle failures

Trend 2: Fatter kids and less PE in the schools: Is anybody listening?

Trend 3: Holistic goals

Trend 4: The discipline morass

Trend 5: The field moves closer toward the real world

Trend 6: Expanding the service focus

Trend 7: The service shift from public to private sector

Trend 8: Inequality of services

Trend 9: The continued decline of school service programs

Trend 10: Our failure to provide leadership

New Lifestyle Needs for Old Lifestyle Failures: The United States and the All-You-Can-Eat Buffet

We have a growing population that is aware of the importance of lifestyle to health and longevity. This is evident as we enter a new millennium. Restaurants are offering more health-conscious meals, and hotels are featuring exercise options. However, some people work at maintaining a healthy lifestyle, but many others do not. John Burt asks if we have discouraged many people by making a healthy lifestyle and regular exercise seem unpleasant.[27]

Unfortunately, this lifestyle awareness trend seems to have developed largely despite our field's efforts. It is market driven, and the major practitioners are not within our formal organizations. Thus, our field's influence has been minimal.

Fatter Kids and Less PE in the Schools: Is Anybody Listening?

The rise in childhood obesity in the United States over the last few decades is remarkable. At the same time, physical education requirements in the schools have lessened, and fewer physical education specialists are provided, especially at the critical elementary school level. We have already noted the disappearance of not just physical education, but even recess, from many schools.[28] So far, state legislators and local school boards have shown little interest in attacking this problem, perhaps because they consider physical activity a "frill."

Holistic Goals

We are seeing a growing societal use of wellness as the focus for health and fitness. Health and exercise science appear to be drawing closer together around a wellness concept. Earle Zeigler has called for reunification into the larger field.[29] It would be a return to the cradle, so to speak: a return to a century ago, when our field was first focused on whole body health. The theory then was that healthier, fitter students learn more effectively. In reality, it applies to all people. That message seems to be reappearing as the focus on instruction in competitive sports and physical exercise structures shifts to a broader-based health consciousness.

The Discipline Morass

The discipline movement continues, but the problems of specialization are becoming more noticeable. The individual disciplines and specialized areas continue to split from the field, fragmenting into small, self-centered, self-important focus groups with little impact or importance outside of their own group. The movement has elements of a misguided attempt to gain prestige, rather than an attempt to improve the value of the field.[30]

Many practitioners have expressed concern that the discipline movement did not truly contribute to the advancement of the field. As Frank Rokosz wrote:

Several decades ago physical education made the mistake of entering the academic arena with the intention of competing with the likes of biology and physics for academic credibility. It did so, I suspect, out of an inferiority complex. Now, the profession and those we serve are paying for that mistake. . . . My eyes and ears tell me that the physical education literature is rife with distortion. . . . As a thoughtful, responsible physical educator [I] am being held to professional standards that have been established by people who are often out of touch with reality.[31]

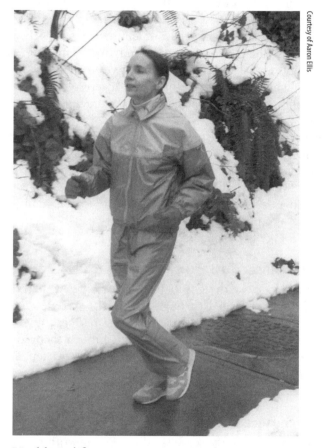

Courtesy of Aaron Ellis

Health and fitness are major contributors to success at all ages.

Expressing a similar concern, Harry King notes that

university scholar–theorists . . . have been generous in giving advice to practitioners (i.e., teachers) . . . who must directly provide instruction in physical activities. Holding a privileged place in their access to and control of the media of communication—scholarly and professional journals, textbooks, and professional meetings—the scholar–theorists' prescriptions have often been unexamined and unchallenged. . . . The public school teachers' rejection of the advice of the scholar–theorist has been a wise one. . . . [Those] recommendations have simply been inappropriate and out of touch with the practitioner's reality.[32]

The damaging aspect of the discipline movement is that it did not contribute to scholarly acceptance by the outside academic world, which was its primary goal. Instead, the apostles of the movement tend to draw closer to groups outside the field, huddling for implied status based on their proximity to more prestigious groups. That tendency weakens our claims of scholarly value, even as it removes presumed scholars from professional involvement in the field. At the same time, we may not be improving our image in the outside world of scholars. For example, why would physiologists be interested in a physical education or sport-trained physiologist? What is there to offer that nonsport physiologists would otherwise not encounter?

We can see two results of the ongoing struggle. First, the holistic people (those who are more interested in developing the field as a whole) will draw together and become stronger. Second, the discipline hard-liners may organize themselves out of existence, eventually disappearing into the larger subject areas to which they have allied themselves. We are already seeing this as many research university kinesiology programs have become entirely health science programs, more closely allied to biology departments.

The Field Moves Closer Toward the Real World

There is still a need to close the gap between our current methods and what we have discovered about our field through research.[33] We need to bridge the gap between the researchers and practitioners so our research gives meaning to our field. We have suffered from the weakness of too much theorizing based on limited real-world experience. At the same time, we have a tendency to train our graduate students for specialties with limited job opportunities so we can maintain our own narrow research interests.

Expanding the Service Focus

The service focus (the people we serve) will expand in both population and range of services provided. We are reaching the younger (preschool) and the older (gerontology) generations, in addition to school-age students.[34] At the same time, we are moving away from providing only school and public recreation services, adding a mix of health, lifestyle, fitness, and sport services that can be utilized separately or as an overall way of life by clients. We are losing the distinction between health, physical education, exercise science, recreation, and sport. This change is to our benefit.

The Service Shift from Public to Private Sector

Demographic and economic trends are limiting what can be done with public funding and shifting services to the business arena, a trend called privatization. There is a governmental trend toward funding public services with users' fees instead of taxes. Our field is moving (largely without our direction or influence) from a public institution base to a private institution base.[35]

The greatest problem with this service shift is that it creates a have and have-not culture in health and wellness because lower-income people are unable to gain access to services that are available only to private subscribers. This leads to increased resentment and class conflict in a supposedly classless society. We are also reacting to the marketplace rather than leading the way. If we do not face the reality of how this marketplace works, we may lose our influence in it.

Inequality of Services

With the service shift to the private sector, we may see conflict within the same community. There is a growing separation between the quality of services available to the well-to-do versus the lower incomes, the aware versus the unaware. This creates even more problems in a nation that is becoming more culturally diverse than in the past. People should not promote an access to health- and longevity-related services based only on the ability to pay for those services. If we provide no public options, we are stepping onto very shaky moral ground.

The Continued Decline of School Service Programs

This trend is the result of a century of failing to sell our programs or provide meaningful results to the public. Though the reasons for the decline are tied to economics (lack of money for complex, broad programs) and academics (declining reading and math scores), our failure to sell the value of our work to the public has cost us dearly. Surprisingly, even athletic programs face the axe for the same reasons. We must show their value, or our programs will be included among the frills that disappear when school budgets are cut. We must be more conscious of budgets and more careful of our spending habits.

A newspaper article that appeared late in 1990 dramatizes the risks we face. The school board of Pittsfield, Massachusetts, decided to drop a required physical education program that was considered a model for teacher training by the University of Massachusetts. The school board declared it to be an unneeded frill, and instead required students to read an article or booklet about fitness every 2 weeks. They considered the actual instruction, activity, and testing unnecessary. As a spokesman said,

> *Kids should be encouraged to participate in sports . . . but the school day is too short, the school year is too short and something has got to give. The first thing to go should be fluff, and phys ed is fluff.*[36]

The State Education Department threatened legal action if the plan was implemented, but this may be the face of the future.

Our Failure to Provide Leadership

Exercise science is not a field noted for its nationally recognized leaders or authorities. We face the challenge of developing greater creativity in our practitioners—that is, their ability or talent to think and act innovatively. The growing private sector in wellness and fitness services demonstrates our field's failure to lead. Over the last several decades many of the leaders were nonprofessionals such as actress Jane Fonda, not leaders from American Alliance for Health, Physical Education, Recreation and Dance (AAHPERD), the American College of Sports Medicine (ACSM), or the disciplines.

The public has accepted professional models (for visual appeal) and ghost-writers (for information) as fitness leaders, so Beauty overshadows the Beast (professionals). We stood aside for outside leadership that emphasizes youth and appearance over knowledge and expertise. We largely ignored (as do the nonprofessional leaders) the needs of an aging population that does not want a young-people-only fitness center.

We need exercise scientists with strong skills in all of the communication sciences. We have not been very successful in communicating to the public the values of, or the need for, our field. One reason for this lack of success has been our narrowly defined education. In physical education, for example, the new leader needs to be very skill oriented (capable of demonstrating as well as teaching the skills used in any class) and, at the same time, broadly educated in the liberal arts and sciences, thus able to converse meaningfully with people in all academic fields. For too long, the physical educator has been relegated to the gym and has had the reputation of having few interests or abilities beyond the sports pages. That type of physical educator cannot survive in today's world, much less in the future.

Exercise scientists need more education in the liberal arts and interdisciplinary studies areas.[37] There are several reasons for suggesting this shift. One is supplied by James Conant, who was considered an opponent of physical education. He still expresses some compelling arguments for such a broadening of our educational background:

> Because the physical education teacher is likely to be a coach and because of the high visibility of the coaching staff, the road to administrative positions is open and attractive. . . . The future is likely to be like the past in this respect. Unless there is a change in the direction of this trend, I conclude that the physical education teacher should have an even wider general academic education than any other teacher [my emphasis]. . . . More likely than not, the [student] preparing to be a physical education teacher is, perhaps unconsciously, preparing to be an educational administrator. He [or she] needs to start early on a course of wide reading in the humanities and the social sciences [my emphasis].[38]

Many coaches eventually become administrators in the public schools. Conant's suggestions are meant to direct their training toward broader liberal arts studies that will make them more aware of the ideas and viewpoints of other disciplines. Although he touches on the justification for these wide studies, he misses one basic reason that should occur to most physical educators: a lack of ability to communicate.

A communications gap exists between exercise scientists and other educators simply because we cannot speak their language. People in our field sometimes seem out of touch with the liberal arts and with their required development of communication skills. Even if our field has become more academically respectable, we are unable to convince the greater academic community.

There is little value in our telling ourselves that our field is a respectable area of the educational process. We must sell it convincingly to those without ties to the field. We must broaden our horizons so that we will open new lines of communication to the many academic fields. Only when they begin to understand us (and we begin to understand them) will our field begin to achieve the respect that we believe it deserves.

Trends in Sport

This section briefly examines five trends that affect sport in the United States (**Table 15.6**). As in the other sections on trends, they are not given in order of importance. Each is important, and they are often interconnected.

The Drug Culture of Sport

Perhaps the most common view of sport today is that success at a high level requires drugs. The level of drug use found at the highest levels in some sports is scandalous. The Tour de France has come close to being destroyed by the extent of drug use not just by athletes, but by whole teams.[39]

In professional sports, such as baseball, records in areas such as home run hitting can no longer be taken seriously because of exposé of the high incidence of steroid use by the athletes who broke those records. Despite great concern about drug use, most professional sports have essentially toothless anti-drug rules.

Despite the growth of organizations such as World Anti-Doping Agency (WADA) to deal with drug usage in sports, the problem continues to grow, in

Table 15.6 Trends in Sport

Trend 1: The drug culture of sport

Trend 2: The professionalization of sport

Trend 3: The trivialization of sport

Trend 4: Violence in sport

Trend 5: Money drives the machine

part because it is still relatively easy to evade the uses with designer drugs that fly under the testing radar.

The Professionalization of Sport

We particularly need to make athletics more genuinely educational. One of our greatest failures is that we tend to lose sight of the purposes of physical education and education where school sport is concerned. We have made no significant effort to correct the gross ills of sports since the 1929 Carnegie Report (and even that had little noticeable effect on college practices). Many people outside the field question the value of school sports. If we do not work to demonstrate and practice the positive values, we may find sports disappearing from the trimmed budgets of the future.

The Trivialization of Sport

The growth of trashsports continues. *Trashsports* are so-called sports events with competitors who are personalities (usually minor ones) competing in designed sports events, usually at a low level of skill. The term was coined by a cartoon strip in the 1970s in response to sports programs such as *Network Battle of the Stars*. Other events use well-known athletes, chosen for their name recognition, rather than their skill in the event. Still others require athletic ability, but again use created sport-like activities, an adult version of children's competitive backyard games.

This trend causes a loss of the distinction between real sport and trashsport because television carries the trashsport in preference to real sport. Television has created and promoted these activities for two reasons. First, they are cheaper to produce than real sport because cheap talent is always available. They are another version of reality television. Second, they will be widely watched because even the least talented viewers believe (with some justification) that they themselves could compete on a fairly equal basis with the selected athletes.

Violence in Sport

Violence is increasingly a problem in sport in the United States. We are accustomed to hearing of riots at soccer matches in other nations, but we do not think of spectators as a problem here. Yet we are now seeing more acts of deliberate violence on the playing field, more disrespect and baiting of officials, more fights in the stands, and more victory riots after championship games. This has already become a serious problem in our society. We see it extending off the playing field and into personal relationships.[40]

It is a grave matter for our field, which claims to teach good sportsmanship and fair play. Is courtesy toward opponents dead? Has our society decided that it is acceptable to demonize our opponents, even in children's games? If this is true, what does it say about our society and its hopes for the future?

Money Drives the Machine

The focus of much sport today, even college sport, is money. The importance of a sport too often is based on the number of paid spectators, the number of viewers, and the money that changes hands, not on the quality of competition or the benefits to the competitors. Unfortunately, this model from professional sport travels downward to the lowest levels of age and skill. The result is our current emphasis on success over participation.

Private funding for school sports will continue to weaken the schools' control over their conduct and focus. That weakened focus is also an outcome of the decline in school budgets, which places control in the hands of the people who provide the money. The result may be the death of many school sports programs.

Again, Toward the Future

Carol Irwin and Frank Pettigrew interviewed the authors of two major books on the future of the field: Michael Ellis's *The Business of Physical Education* and John Massengale's *Trends Toward the Future in Physical Education*.[41] Based on those interviews, they made six recommendations for the profession of physical education, which apply well to the greater field of exercise science:

1. Have a better alliance between practitioners and researchers.
2. Market and promote your program.
3. Unify with health (a return to the holistic concern of the unified mind–body): Physical, intellectual, social, and emotional.[42]
4. Study the fragmentation (discipline versus profession) issue.
5. Revise teacher preparation programs (there is a trend to require additional certifications for employment).[43]
6. Have an open mind; think differently.

Looking toward the future, we might consider two points raised by Warren Fraleigh in discussing the curricular implications for our field.[44] The first is that, although a leisure society can provide greater opportunities for human fulfillment, it also can result in meaningless discretionary time that is simply wasted. We have rarely considered this side of the coin.

Furthermore, there is a larger question. Leisure time is not increasing except in comparison to the last century.[45] We actually have far less leisure time than those living in the past centuries when there were far more holidays. Daryl Siedentop suggests that the reputation of our field will improve only when leisure time is redefined to lose its work–leisure connection as nonwork that permits an individual to return to work refreshed and ready to do a better job. Instead, leisure should be defined in terms of its part in contributing to the good life; he believes that leisure's quality-of-life-enhancing potential should be stressed.[46]

Fraleigh's second point is the continuing trend of increasing attention to the needs and expressions of the human body. Although this trend has many positive benefits for better programs of physical education, it also can simply become "a simplistic, indulgent hedonism," a not-uncommon sight today.[47] Indeed, some of the more faddish physical activities of the recent past and present show that characteristic. It is noticeable in the health clubs that emphasize attractive facilities for socializing but hire only marginally prepared instructors.

Diversity is a mark of any large civilization. The strength of the American society has been, in large part, a result of the diversity of abilities and experiences brought into its culture by the many immigrants absorbed into its society. Being different should not be discouraged because from it often come new breakthroughs. A society that discourages diversity, preferring strict conformity instead, generally is less able to cope with change and has to improvise to meet the rapidly changing needs of a highly technological society.

In an overcrowded world, cooperation is essential to survival. One reason for the interest in the New Games concept is that it might be considered the athletics for the overcrowded society, with its emphasis on cooperation rather than competition. Competition is natural and will not disappear; however, survival in a mass society requires that people also learn the skills and value of cooperation.

Readiness for change is necessary in modern society. Change is inevitable; although some people will resist it, those who are more adept at survival will be prepared to accept it and learn to adapt. Educators face the difficult task of trying to develop this readiness for change or adaptability. They must prepare people not only for what is, but also for what will be, even though what is to come is unknown. Thus, teachers must prepare their students from a blind position—an ignorance of the future. But what is important is that students learn to adapt to and accept change; they must learn to work with new situations. This adaptability is critical to any individual's ability to cope with the modern world.

Throughout this text we have looked at our field as a broad field in the context of its historical past, its patterns of development, its function in today's society, and the most likely trends it will follow into the future. You now should have some idea of what our field is all about. I have tried to show the field as an important part of the total educational process, but without making exaggerated claims for it.

Our field is a worthy field. In its activities and experiences we can find elements of value to people of all ages and conditions. The greatest question that faces us today is not anything we have looked at directly in this text, rather it is a question concerning the future of our field: When you graduate and become a professional in the field, how will you change the field? What directions will the field take under your guidance and leadership?

Summary

This chapter discusses what the future holds for physical education, sport, and kinesiology. Predictions are highly unreliable. The chapter discusses trends in three areas: society, education, and physical education and sport. The following lists are not all-inclusive, nor are they ordered by importance, as all are important.

The trends in American society in broad terms are (1) the new multicultural society, (2) the decline of personal responsibility, (3) the growth of world change, and (4) constant change. In more specific terms, they are (1) the growing language gap, (2) growing economic inequality, (3) growth of the underclass population, (4) the new tribalism: growing ethnic conflict, (5) declining social conscience and cooperation, (6) family instability, (7) growth of the now generation, (8) growth of a world culture through the online world, (9) growth of a world techno-industrial economy, (10) changing leisure patterns, and (11) continuing ethical dilemmas.

The trends in American education are (1) disagreement about educational priorities, (2) education for a technological world, (3) the future curriculum: narrow or broad, (4) changing educational priorities, (5) declining student knowledge levels, (6) more accountability, (7) more testing, (8) changing school populations, (9) teacher education: specialist versus generalist, (10) whole-school involvement in teacher education, (11) higher teacher education standards, and (12) privatization of education.

The trends in exercise science are (1) new lifestyle needs, (2) holistic goals, (3) the discipline morass, (4) the field moving toward the real world, (5) expanding service focus, (6) service shift from public to private sector, (7) inequality of services, (8) the continuing decline of school service programs, and (9) the failure to provide leadership.

The trends in exercise science are (1) the drug culture of sport, (2) the professionalization of sport, (3) the trivialization of sport, (4) violence in sport, and (5) the increased focus of sport on money.

The greatest questions that face us today are: When you join our field, what will you do with it? What directions will the field take under your guidance and leadership?

Further Readings

Boyce, Barbara Ann. 2012. Redefining the EdD: Seeking a separate identity. *Quest* 64: 24–33.

Chodzko-Zajko, Wojtek, and Andiara Schwingel. 2009. Transnational strategies for the promotion of physical activity and active aging: The World Health Organization model of consensus building in international public health. *Quest* 61: 25–38.

Delbanco, Andrew. 2012. *College: What it was, is, and should be*. Princeton, NJ: Princeton Univ. Press.

Dunn, John M. 2009. The times are a changing: Implications for kinesiology. *Quest* 61: 268–277.

Ellis, Michael J. 1988. *The business of physical education: Future of the profession*. Champaign, IL: Human Kinetics.

Ennis, Catherine D. 2010. New directions in undergraduate and graduate education in kinesiology and physical education. *Quest* 62: 76–91.

Finkenberg, Mel. 2008. Future choices, future trends in technology in kinesiology and physical education. *Quest* 60: 434–442.

Gleick, James. 1999. *Faster*. New York: Pantheon.

Hochstetler, Douglas R. 2008. Handing each other along: Developing leadership in kinesiology. *Quest* 60: 331–334.

Ishee, Jimmy. 2009. The time is now and always has been: A mindset for the future. *Quest* 61: 259–267.

Ives, Jeffrey C., and Duane Knudson. 2007. Professional practice in exercise science: The need for greater disciplinary balance. *Sports Medicine* 37 (2): 103–115.

Keeling, Richard P., and Richard H. Hersh. 2011. *We're losing our minds: Rethinking American higher education*. New York: Palgrave Macmillan.

Kretchmar, Scott. 2007. What to do with meaning? A research conundrum for the 21st century. *Quest* 59: 373–383.

Sanders, Ross H., and John M. Dunn. 2010. The Bologna Accord: A model of cooperation and coordination. *Quest* 62: 92–105.

Spirduso, Waneen W. 2009. Staying afloat in an information-age sea change. *Quest* 61: 5–18.

Trudeau, François, and Roy J. Shephard. 2008. Is there a long-term health legacy of required physical education? *Sports Medicine* 38 (4): 265–270.

Ward, Phillip, and Paneyiotis Dontis, eds. 2001. *Physical education in the 21st century*. Lincoln: Department of Health and Human Performance, Univ. of Nebraska-Lincoln.

Zeigler, Earle F. 1994. Ten stances that have to be changed. In *Physical education and kinesiology in North America: Professional and scholarly foundations*. Champaign, IL: Stipes, 397–400.

Zlotkowski, Edward. 1997. Millennial expectations: Creating a new service agenda in higher education. *Quest* 49: 355–368.

Discussion Questions

1. Briefly discuss three trends in American society.

2. Briefly discuss three trends in American education.

3. What are the implications of privatization in American education?

4. What is a holistic approach to physical education? Why is it important?

5. What trends are appearing in American physical education and sport? What effect might those trends have on physical education and sport in the future?

6. Have physical educators provided national leadership in trying to meet our nation's needs? What are the implications of their success or failure?

7. What are the positive and negative effects of the discipline movement? Do you feel that it has helped or hindered our field's reputation? Defend your decision.

8. What is meant by the trivialization of sport? Give examples to illustrate the trend.

9. What are possible causes for the growing violence that we see in or that are connected to sport? Can you suggest solutions to end or lessen the problem?

10. Discuss Carol Irwin and Frank Pettigrew's six recommendations for the profession of physical education. Why are they useful, and what impact might they have on the field?

References

1. Phillips, Madge. 1979. The challenge of change for physical education in the 1980s: Sociological view. *Academy Papers* 13: 51.

2. Siedentop, Daryl. 1994. *Introduction to physical education, fitness, and sport.* 2nd ed. Mountain View, CA: Mayfield, 357–367.

3. Edginton, Christopher. 1990. Drivers of change: Opportunities in the 1990s. *JOPERD (Journal of Physical Education, Recreation and Dance)* (May–June): 11.

4. Hellison, Donald R. 1987. Dreaming the possible dream: The rise and triumph of physical education. In *Trends toward the future in physical education*, ed. John D. Massengale, Champaign, IL: Human Kinetics, 137.

5. Burt, John J. Three dreams: The future of HPERD at the cutting edge. In *Trends toward the future in physical education*, ed. John D. Massengale, 153–168.

6. Hoffman, Shirl J. Dreaming the impossible dream: The decline and fall of physical education. In *Trends toward the future in physical education*, ed. John D. Massengale, 135.

7. Zeigler, Earle F. 1989. Gearing up for the 1990s in North American sport and physical education. *Physical Educator* 46: 116–120.

8. Zeigler, Earle F. 1994. Physical education's 13 principal principles. *JOPERD (Journal of Physical Education, Recreation and Dance)* (September): 4–5; and Zeigler, Earle F. 1999. The profession must work "harder and smarter" to inform those officials who make decisions that affect the field. *Physical Educator* 56: 114–119.

9. Corbin, Charles B. 1993. Clues from dinosaurs, mules, and the bull snake: Our field in the 21st century. *Quest* 45: 546–556, 559.

10. Feingold, Ronald S. 1994. Making connections: An agenda for the future. *Quest* 46: 356–366.

11. Park, Roberta J. 1990. The past before us, transition toward the future. *Academy Papers* 24: 1–4.

12. Yen, Hope. 2010. This may be the year white babies are minority. *Raleigh (NC) News and Observer*, March 10.

13. Johnston, David Cay. 1999. Gap grows between rich and poor. *Raleigh (NC) News and Observer*, September 5.

14. Geyer, Georgie Anne. 1999. A scary look at America's possible future. *Raleigh (NC) News and Observer*, September 1.

15. Walinsky, Adam. 1995. The crisis of public order. *Atlantic Monthly*, July 39–41, 44, 46–49, 52–54.

16. Gleick, James. 1999. *Faster.* New York: Pantheon.

17. Freeman, William H. 1991. Mickey Mouse goes to Jurassic Park: The challenge of technology for leisure. Paper presented at the 106th Annual Convention of the American Alliance for Health, Physical Education, Recreation and Dance, San Francisco, CA.

18. McQueen, Anjetta. 1999. Technology stressing profs out. *Raleigh (NC) News and Observer*, September 1.

19. Gross, Richard E. 1978. Seven new cardinal principles. *Phi Delta Kappan* 60: 291–293.

20. Bloom, Benjamin S., ed. 1956. *Taxonomy of educational objectives: Handbook I: Cognitive domain.* New York: McKay; and Krathwohl, David R., Benjamin S. Bloom, and Bertram B. Masia, eds. 1964. *Taxonomy of educational objectives: Handbook II: Affective domain.* New York: McKay.

21. Bloom, *Taxonomy*, 7.

22. Lasch, Christopher. 1978. *The culture of narcissism.* New York: Norton.

23. Walberg, Herbert J., and Rebecca C. Greenberg. 1999. Educators should require evidence. *Phi Delta Kappa* 81 (October): 132–135.

24. Blankenship, Donna Gordon. 2010. New education standards put forth. *Raleigh (NC) News and Observer*, March 11.

25. Burniske, R. W. 1999. The teacher as skilled generalist. *Phi Delta Kappa* 81 (October): 121–122, 124, 126.

26. Ragon, Bruce M., and John P. Bennett. 1996. Something more to consider: Combining health education and physical education. *JOPERD (Journal of Physical Education, Recreation and Dance)* (January): 14–15.

27. Burt, Three dreams, 153–168.

28. Schoof, Renee. 2013. Bring playtime back to schools, experts say. McClatchy Newspapers, reprinted in *Raleigh (NC) News and Observer,* February 14, 8A; Renee Schoof. 2013. Experts want to revive recess. McClatchy Newspapers, reprinted in *Raleigh (NC) News and Observer,* February 17, 14A.

29. Zeigler, Gearing up for the 1990s. 116–120.

30. Irwin, Carol, and Frank Pettigrew. 1993. A look back to the future. *Physical Educator* 50: 173.

31. Rokosz, Frank. 1990. Quantifying the unquantifiable? *JOPERD (Journal of Physical Education, Recreation and Dance)* (August): 12.

32. King, Harry A. 1990. Practitioners and the scholar–theorists: An uncoordinated alliance. *JOPERD (Journal of Physical Education, Recreation and Dance)* (March): 34–35.

33. Irwin and Pettigrew, A look back to the future, 172–173.

34. Jones, C. Jessie, and Roberta E. Rikli. 1993. The gerontology movement—is it passing us by? *JOPERD (Journal of Physical Education, Recreation and Dance)* (January): 17–26.

35. Ellis, Michael J. 1988. *The business of physical education.* Champaign, IL: Human Kinetics.

36. Phys ed plan is exercise in reading. 1990. *Raleigh (NC) News and Observer,* October 14.

37. Whitson, David J., and Donald Macintosh. 1990. The scientization of physical education: Discourses of performance. *Quest* 42: 40–51; McKay, Jim, Jennifer M. Gore, and David Kirk. 1990. Beyond the limits of technocratic physical education. *Quest* 42: 52–76; and Zakrajsek, Dorothy, and William Pierce. 1993. Academic preparation and the academic consumer. *JOPERD (Journal of Physical Education, Recreation and Dance)* (May–June): 20–23, 31.

38. Conant, James B. 1963. *The education of American teachers.* New York: McGraw-Hill, 185–186.

39. Fraser, Adam. 2010. The drugs don't work. *Sports Pro* 19: 76–78, 80.

40. Nack, William, and Lester Munson. 1995. Sport's dirty secret. *Sports Illustrated*, August 31, 63–70, 73–74.

41. Irwin and Pettigrew, A look back to the future. 172–173.

42. Hellison, Donald. 1991. The whole person in physical education scholarship: Toward integration. *Quest* 43: 307–318.

43. Silvester, L. Jay. 1995. From education to certification. *JOPERD (Journal of Physical Education, Recreation and Dance)* (May–June): 4.

44. Fraleigh, Warren. 1979. A philosophic basis for curriculum content in physical education for the 1980s. *Academy Papers* 13: 20–26.

45. Haskell, William L. 1996. Physical activity, sport and health: Toward the next century. *Suppl., Research Quarterly for Exercise and Sport* 67 (3): 37–47.

46. Siedentop, Daryl. 1980. *Physical education: Introductory analysis*. 3rd ed. Dubuque, IA: Brown, 229–231.

47. Fraleigh, Philosophic basis, 20.

Index